D0070610

TOURO COLLEGE LIBRARY
Kings Hwy

WITHDRAWN

Series Editors:
Steven F. Warren, Ph.D.
Joe Reichle, Ph.D.

**Communication
and Language
Intervention
Series**

Volume 10

Promoting Social Communication

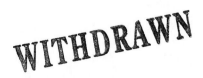

Also in the Communication
and Language Intervention Series:

TOURO COLLEGE LIBRARY
Kings Hwy

Communication
and Language
Intervention
Series

Volume 10

Promoting Social Communication

Children with Developmental Disabilities from Birth to Adolescence

edited by

Howard Goldstein, Ph.D., CCC-SLP

Professor and Chair
Department of Communication Disorders
Florida State University
Tallahassee, Florida

Louise A. Kaczmarek, Ph.D., CCC-SLP

Associate Professor
Department of Instruction and Learning
University of Pittsburgh
Pittsburgh, Pennsylvania

and

Kristina M. English, Ph.D., CCC-A

Assistant Professor
Department of Speech-Language Pathology
Duquesne University
Pittsburgh, Pennsylvania

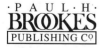

·P·A·U·L·H·
BROOKES
PUBLISHING CO

Baltimore • London • Toronto • Sydney

KH

·P A U L·H·
BROOKES
PUBLISHING C⁰

Paul H. Brookes Publishing Co.
Post Office Box 10624
Baltimore, Maryland 21285-0624

www.brookespublishing.com

Copyright © 2002 by Paul H. Brookes Publishing Co., Inc.
All rights reserved.

Typeset by A.W. Bennett, Inc., Hartland, Vermont.
Manufactured in the United States of America by
Thomson-Shore, Dexter, Michigan.

The cases described in this book are composites based on the authors' actual
experiences. Individuals' names have been changed, and identifying details
have been altered to protect confidentiality.

The two middle photographs on the cover are copyright © Digital Vision.
The bottom photograph on the cover is by Laura Shiver.

Library of Congress Cataloging-in-Publication Data

Promoting social communication: children with developmental disabilities
    from birth to adolescence / edited by Howard Goldstein, Louise A.
    Kaczmarek, and Kristina M. English.
        p.   cm.—(Communication and language intervention series ; v. 10)
        Included bibliographical references and index.
        ISBN 1-55766-521-4
        1. Developmentally disabled children—Language.   2. Communicative
disorders in children.   3. Communicative disorders in adolescence.
4. Social skills—Study and teaching.   5. Social interaction. I. Goldstein,
Howard, 1922– II. Kaczmarek, Louise A.   III. English, Kristina M., 1951–
IV. Communication and language intervention series ; 10.
HV891.P87   2002
618.92'85889—dc21

                                     200103539

British Library Cataloguing in Publication data are available from the British
Library.

10/25/04

Contents

Series Preface

The purpose of the *Communication and Language Intervention Series* is to provide meaningful foundations for the application of sound intervention designs to enhance the development of communication skills across the life span. We are endeavoring to achieve this purpose by providing readers with presentations of state-of-the-art theory, research, and practice.

In selecting topics, editors, and authors, we are not attempting to limit the contents of this series to viewpoints with which we agree or that we find most promising. We are assisted in our efforts to develop the series by an editorial advisory board consisting of prominent scholars representative of the range of issues and perspectives to be incorporated in the series.

We trust that the careful reader will find much that is provocative and controversial in this and other volumes. This will be necessary so to the extent that the work reported is truly on the so-called cutting edge, a mythical place where no sacred cows exist. The point is demonstrated time and again throughout this volume as the conventional wisdom is challenged (and occasionally confirmed) by the authors.

Readers of this and other volumes are encouraged to proceed with healthy skepticism. In order to achieve our purpose, we take on some difficult and controversial issues. Errors and misinterpretations inevitably are made. This is normal in the development of any field and should be welcomed as evidence that the field is moving toward and tackling difficult and weighty issues.

Well-conceived theory and research on development of both children with and children without disabilities are vitally important for researchers, educators, and clinicians committed to the development of optimal approaches to communication and language intervention. For this reason, each volume in this series includes chapters pertaining to both development and intervention.

The content of each volume reflects our view of the symbolic relationship between intervention and research: Demonstrations of what may work in intervention should lead to analysis of promising discoveries and insights from developmental work that may in turn fuel further refinement by intervention researchers.

An inherent goal of this series is to enhance the long-term development of the field by systematically furthering the dissemination of theoretically and empirically based scholarship and research. We prom-ise the reader an opportunity to participate in the development of this field through debates and discussions that occur throughout the pages of the *Communication and Language Intervention Series.*

Editorial Advisory Board

David Beukelman, Ph.D.
Department of Special Education
  and Communication Disorders
University of Nebraska–Lincoln
Lincoln, NE 68583

Diane Bricker, Ph.D.
College of Education
Center on Human Development
University of Oregon
Eugene, OR 97403

Philip Dale, Ph.D.
Department of Communication
  Science and Disorders
University of Missouri–Columbia
Columbia, MO 65211

Howard Goldstein, Ph.D.
Department of Communication
  Disorders
107 Regional Rehabilitation
  Center
Florida State University
Tallahassee, FL 32306

Laurence B. Leonard, Ph.D.
Department of Audiology and
  Speech Sciences
Purdue University
West Lafayette, IN 47907

Jon F. Miller, Ph.D.
Department of Communication
  Disorders
University of Wisconsin–Madison
Madison, WI 53706

Amy M. Wetherby, Ph.D.
Department of Communication
  Disorders
107 Regional Rehabilitation
  Center
Florida State University
Tallahassee, FL 32306

David E. Yoder, Ph.D.
Department of Medical Allied
  Health Professions
University of North Carolina at
  Chapel Hill
Chapel Hill, NC 27599

Editor emeritus
Richard L. Schiefelbusch, Ph.D.
Schiefelbusch Institute for Life Span Studies
University of Kansas
Lawrence, KS 66045

Contributors

The Editors

Howard Goldstein, Ph.D., CCC-SLP, Professor and Chair, Department of Communication Disorders, Florida State University, Tallahassee, FL 32306-1200

Dr. Goldstein is a professor in and the chair of the communication disorders department at Florida State University. His graduate training reflected an interdisciplinary perspective, melding communicative disorders, developmental psychology, and mental retardation research. He teaches courses in clinical methods, communication development, child language disorders, research strategies and tactics, and developmental disabilities. Dr. Goldstein has been involved in research and the education of children with developmental disabilities for the past 30 years. His work has focused on early intervention and the development of instructional approaches for teaching generalized language and social skills to children with severe disabilities. He also has worked with numerous school districts and health care agencies on a number of projects and research grants, including the development of in-service training initiatives, clinical research and development, and a distance education graduate training program. He is an American Speech-Language-Hearing Association fellow and a certified speech-language pathologist and has extensive expertise in training and supervising master's and doctoral students in communication sciences and disorders.

Louise A. Kaczmarek, Ph.D., CCC-SLP, Associate Professor, Department of Instruction and Learning and Department of Communication Science and Disorders, 4F21 Posvar Hall, University of Pittsburgh, Pittsburgh, PA 15260

Dr. Kaczmarek coordinates the early intervention and early childhood education programs at the University of Pittsburgh. Her research interests include classroom-based language intervention strategies, social skills, and family-centered practices in classroom-based programs. Dr. Kaczmarek also serves on the editorial boards of three journals: *Journal of Early Intervention, Topics in Early Childhood Special Education,* and *Education and Treatment of Children.*

Kristina M. English, Ph.D., CCC-A, Assistant Professor, Department of Speech-Language Pathology, 403 Fisher Hall, Duquesne University, Pittsburgh, PA 15282

Kristina M. English is a pediatric audiologist with a doctorate in education from San Diego State University and Claremont Graduate University. She currently is an assistant professor at the speech-language pathology department at Duquesne University. Dr. English is conducting research on friendship development among children with hearing impairments and also the development of counseling skills among professionals who serve these children and their families.

The Chapter Authors

Leonard Abbeduto, Ph.D., Professor and Chair of Educational Psychology, Waisman Center, University of Wisconsin–Madison, 1500 Highland Avenue, Madison, WI 53705

Dr. Abbeduto is an investigator at the Waisman Center and Professor and Chair of Educational Psychology at the University of Wisconsin–Madison. He is well know for his research on the language and communication problems of children, adolescents, and adults with mental retardation. His research has been funded for many years by National Institute of Child Health and Human Development. In 1996, Dr. Abbeduto received the Emil A. Steiger award for excellence in teaching from the University of Wisconsin–Madison. He is a fellow of the American Association on Mental Retardation.

William H. Brown, Ph.D., Associate Professor, Department of Educational Psychology, College of Education, University of South Carolina–Columbia, Columbia, SC 29208

Dr. Brown is an associate professor of early childhood special education in the Department of Educational Psychology and an Affiliated Faculty Member with the Institute for Families in Society at University of South Carolina–Columbia. He was a National Institute of Child Health and Human Development Trainee in Mental Retardation and received his doctorate in special education from Vanderbilt University in 1985. During his 26-year professional career, he has been a teacher, a parent trainer, a service coordinator, an executive director of a large university-affiliated early intervention program, a consultant to early childhood and early childhood special education programs, an advocate for enhanced services for young children and adults with disabilities, and President of the Nashville/Davidson County and Tennessee Association for Retarded Citizens. His current professional interests focus on early intervention, prevention, and family support services for infants, toddlers, preschoolers, and young children with and without disabilities as well as personnel preparation of early childhood and early childhood special educators.

Maureen A. Conroy, Ph.D., Associate Professor, University of Florida, Box 117050, Gainesville, FL 32611

Dr. Conroy is an associate professor in the Department of Special Education at the University of Florida. Her areas of interest include young children with communication and behavior problems.

Lisa Sharon Cushing, Ph.D., Research Associate, Vanderbilt University, Box 328 Peabody College, Nashville, TN 37203

Dr. Cushing is a research associate in the Department of Special Education at Vanderbilt University. She received her doctorate from the University of Oregon. Her interests include systems change, inclusive education, technical assistance strategies, and students with significant disabilities.

Christine Golden, M.A., Autism Specialist, Lawrence Public Schools, Prairie Park Elementary, 2711 Kensington, Lawrence, KS 66046

Ms. Golden is a third grade teacher with the Lawrence, Kansas, public schools and has accepted a position as Elementary Autism/SMH Consultant. Ms. Golden has a bachelor's degree in human development and family life and a master's degree in special education. She has more than 9 years experience as a teacher, staff trainer, and consultant for children with autism and developmental disabilities, their families, and general education classroom students.

Charles R. Greenwood, Ph.D., Senior Scientist, Juniper Gardens Children's Project, University of Kansas, 650 Minnesota Avenue, Second Floor, Kansas City, KS 66101

Dr. Greenwood is Senior Scientist and Director of the Juniper Gardens Children's Project. He has contributed extensively to the research on children's social and academic behavior in school and community settings.

Debra M. Kamps, Ph.D., Senior Scientist, Juniper Gardens Children's Project, University of Kansas, 650 Minnesota Avenue, Second Floor, Kansas City, KS 66101

Dr. Kamps is Senior Scientist at the Juniper Gardens Children's Project. She holds courtesy appointments in the Departments of Special Education and Human Development and Family Life at the University of Kansas. She has been a classroom teacher, consultant, researcher, and teacher trainer for more than 20 years across several disability areas including autism, developmental disabilities, and emotional and behavioral disorders.

Craig H. Kennedy, Ph.D., Associate Professor, Vanderbilt University, Box 328, Peabody College, Nashville, TN 37203

Dr. Kennedy is an associate professor in the Department of Special Education at Vanderbilt University. He received his doctorate from the University of California, Santa Barbara. His interests include social relationship development, problem behavior, and students with significant disabilities.

Tammy Kravits, M.A., Autism Consultant, Professional Behavior Management, Inc., 10401 Holmes Road, Suite 440, Kansas City, MO 64131

Ms. Kravits is a program consultant and staff trainer for Professional Behavior Management, Inc., in Kansas City. She is also currently a doctoral student in human development and family life at the University of Kansas. Ms. Kravits has 15 years experience in the field of applied behavior analysis working with families and children with autism, developmental disabilities, and behavioral disorders.

Shirley V. Leew, Ph.D., Speech-Language Pathologist, 202 26th Avenue NE, Calgary, Alberta, T2E 1Y9 Canada.

Dr. Leew is in private practice in Calgary, Canada, directing a social-pragmatic communication program for toddlers diagnosed with autism spectrum disorders. With Paul J. Yoder and Steven F. Warren, she is conducting prelinguistic intervention research.

Adriana Gonzalez Lopez, M.A., Assistant Director of Education, Melmark School, 2600 Wayland Road, Berwyn, PA 19312

Ms. Lopez is Assistant Director of Education at the Melmark School in Berwyn, Pennsylvania. Areas of interest include developmental disabilities, autism, and severe communication disorders. Ms. Lopez has 15 years experience in applied behavior analysis and teaching and consulting for students with disabilities and their families.

Lindee Morgan, M.S., CCC-SLP, Speech-Language Pathologist, Florida State University, 409 RRC, Tallahassee, FL 32306

Ms. Morgan is a doctoral candidate in speech-language pathology at Florida State University. Her research interests include literacy development and school-age language intervention.

Michelle Ross, M.A., Juniper Gardens Children's Project, University of Kansas, 650 Minnesota Avenue, Second Floor, Kansas City, KS 66101

Ms. Ross has a master's degree in developmental and child psychology and 5 years teaching and consulting experience with children with autism and their families. Areas of interest include autism, applied behavior analysis, and instructional programming for students with disabilities.

Katherine Short-Meyerson, Ph.D., Adjunct Faculty, Department of Educational Foundations, University of Wisconsin–Oshkosh, Oshkosh, WI 54901

Dr. Short-Meyerson earned her doctorate in educational psychology from the University of Wisconsin–Madison. She completed a post-doctoral fellowship at the Kennedy Center of Vanderbilt University. Her interests are language development, developmental disabilities, and research methods.

Cheryl A. Utley, Ph.D., Associate Research Professor, Juniper Gardens Children's Project, University of Kansas, 650 Minnesota Avenue, Second Floor, Kansas City, KS 66101

Dr. Utley received her doctorate degree in special education from the University of Wisconsin–Madison. Her research interests include the implementation of interventions to improve the academic and social behaviors of students with and without disabilities in multicultural and impoverished communities.

Dale Walker, Ph.D., Assistant Professor and Research Scientist, Juniper Gardens Children's Project, University of Kansas, 650 Minnesota Avenue, Second Floor, Kansas City, KS 66101

Dr. Walker is an assistant professor of human development and a research scientist and principal investigator with the Juniper Gardens Children's Project at the University of Kansas. Her research interests include early childhood intervention and education, language development, improving outcomes for children from poverty backgrounds, factors associated with risk and resilience, and observational assessment methodology.

Steven F. Warren, Ph.D., Professor of Human Development and Family Life, Director of the Kansas Mental Retardation and Developmental Disabilities Research Center, University of Kansas, 1052 Dole Human Development Center, Lawrence, Kansas 66045

Dr. Warren is Professor of Human Development and Family Life at the University of Kansas and Director of the Schiefelbusch Institute for Life

Span Studies' mental retardation center. He has conducted extensive research on communication and language development and intervention approaches over the past 25 years.

Paul J. Yoder, Ph.D., Research Professor, Vanderbilt University, Box 328, Peabody College, Nashville, TN 37203

Dr. Yoder has been studying adult–child interaction as it relates to children's communication and language development for more than 16 years.

Volume Preface

The purpose of this volume is to provide an overview of the literature on strategies for promoting social communication in individuals with developmental disabilities from early intervention through the school years. It is our hope that readers will derive greater awareness of the critically important role that social communication plays in the lives of children and adolescents with developmental disabilities and their families. By studying what is known about how interventionists might help to promote social communication from birth through adolescence, educators, clinicians, counselors, family members, and others will be better prepared to maximize the potential of individuals with developmental disabilities as they learn to navigate their social circumstances successfully.

We have assembled a group of world-class investigators who have contributed to this body of knowledge and asked them to summarize the current state of the art and science. In addition, as part of the second section of the book, we have asked many of them to solicit the help of interventionists with whom they have worked to help illustrate the application of scientific discoveries to educational practice.

The first section of the book presents the bases and models of developing social skills. This introductory section presents the basic foundations for understanding why and how one might want to improve the abilities of children and youth with developmental disabilities to interact with others in their social milieu. The first three chapters examine approaches to elucidating the development of social competence, frameworks for understanding the linguistic underpinnings of communication, and models for applying an interdisciplinary perspective to assessing social and communicative competence. It is important to gain insights into how a dynamic array of social and linguistic abilities interacts within social and cultural contexts to influence a variety of social, academic, and vocational outcomes.

The second section offers a chronological approach to promoting social communication from infancy through the school years. The chronology is divided into four age spans that correspond largely to different bodies of literature. Each of four review chapters seeks to analyze the empirical support for interventions designed to promote social and communicative interaction. Four companion chapters present illustrative case studies of social-communicative interventions. These chapters seek to clarify through case studies how the strategies discussed in the prior chapter might be applied. The final chapter provides a broader context by examining how social-communicative intervention efforts can affect general life achievements across the life span.

First and foremost, we hope that this volume will be helpful to people who are striving to maximize the potential of individuals with developmental disabilities. The book is written mainly for professionals and for students in education, speech-language pathology, psychology, and related fields. We also hope that this book will pique the interest of seasoned and budding researchers in contributing to this body of knowledge. The information summarized in this volume also may prove helpful for support groups, advocacy organizations, and policy makers who need to be aware of the potential outcomes for improving the lives of individuals with developmental disabilities through thoughtful and competent implementation of the various intervention approaches described.

We sincerely appreciate the efforts of the many investigators who have contributed to the large and diverse literature that served as a basis for this volume. We hope that the efforts of the authors who contributed to this volume have made this information more accessible to readers and that the insights embedded throughout this book will help to advance our understanding of developmental disabilities and the practices that promote the development of children and youth with special needs.

Acknowledgments

I am grateful for the guidance that has been provided over the years by my many colleagues and students. I offer a special thanks to John and Janice Baldwin who initially led me on the path to studying ways to teach social-communicative behavior to help improve everyday lives and our social order. My love and gratitude is insufficient to thank an understanding family, as Michelle, Alexa, and Evan tolerate my professional distractions far more than they should—H.G.

I would like to express my appreciation to Nicole Lewis and Moriah Brown, who worked ever so diligently and efficiently in searching for the articles and books I needed. In addition, Dr. Virginia Swisher and her doctoral writing seminars provided insightful feedback and further helped to facilitate my thinking on the assessment of social communication. Finally, I offer my love and thanks to Phil, Tom, and Jackie for their patience and understanding when this professional activity took precedence over our life as a family—L.A.K.

My appreciation is extended to both Howard and Louise, who have taught me more than they know. The opportunity to work with them has been a genuine honor. And as always, thanks and love to my wonderful family: Lewis, Jason, and Katie—K.M.E.

I

Bases and Models of Developing Social Skills

Howard Goldstein

A high quality of life for children with developmental disabilities and their families presupposes a lot of positive interactions within their social milieu. This book is based on this common-sense premise. Although most people expect to be accepted and active socially within their families, schools, communities, and unique cultural associations, for most of the 20th century, individuals with developmental disabilities were not accorded these same expectations. It was not uncommon for families of children with significant disabilities to be told that it might be best if their children were cared for in institutions; there, they would be kept safe and members of families and society would be shielded from unpleasant interactions.

Since the 1970s, society has made great strides in improving the lives of individuals with disabilities and their families. Children with disabilities are now included in the same classrooms as their peers without disabilities. They learn, eat, exercise, and play together within typical school environments. Children with disabilities can be seen within the broader community as well, taking part in camps, church functions, and recreational activities. They accompany their families to beaches, national monuments, and amusement parks. They attend sporting events and movies and frequent restaurants with family and friends.

Although each environment holds potential for interacting socially and building friendships, the potential may not always be realized. Although children with disabilities can be seen amidst the fabric of society, they may not always be woven into the fabric itself. It is our hope that a careful analysis of the threads that make up social competence and social-communicative functioning will further enhance the social outcomes of children with disabilities. This book summarizes the developments in fields that have helped us to define the essence of social behavior, to outline methods for assessing social behavior, and to develop procedures for enhancing social-communicative functioning.

The communicative interactions of individuals with developmental disabilities share common features with those of all humans. Some interactions are easy, pleasant, and rewarding; others are not. Indeed, impairments in social and communicative skills are not limited to individuals with developmental disabilities; however, they are the hallmark of some developmental disabilities (e.g., autism). This book focuses particularly on strategies for promoting social communication in those children whose disabilities inhibit typical patterns of social-communicative development. One should note, however, that many of these same strategies have broader applicability. Improved social functioning may be a valuable goal for all children and for our society as a whole.

Efforts within our educational system to include children with developmental disabilities in the least restrictive environments possible has spurred many positive changes in our public education system. Teachers, related services providers, administrators, and family members are better acquainted with strategies for individualizing instruction and minimizing the likelihood that children who are not progressing adequately will slip through the cracks. Coupled with a move toward higher academic expectations and objective standards, all children should have a greater opportunity to maximize their educational potential. These positive changes have not necessarily been directed toward improved social functioning, however. Research and its application to children with developmental disabilities has the potential to lead the way toward greater value being placed on social-communicative skill development, more objective assessments of social well-being, and more effective intervention procedures for teaching social-communicative skills and promoting relationship development.

In the first section of the book, we lay the foundation for more effective social-communicative interventions by examining models of social competence, the linguistic underpinnings of communication, and an interdisciplinary perspective on assessment. These chapters draw heavily from literature on early social and communication development and theories that may prove helpful in delineating the processes involved in social-communicative interaction and development. Chapter 1 explores social competence and its development in order to help us understand why and how one might want to improve the interaction abilities of children with developmental disabilities in their social milieu.

In addition, Goldstein and Morgan in this chapter review models that provide a framework for understanding how social interaction skills relate to other social outcomes, such as the development of relationships and friendships.

In Chapter 2, Abbeduto and Short-Meyerson view pragmatics—the social uses of language—from a process perspective in which participants in communication have a shared goal and collaborate to achieve that goal. The chapter considers the role of context in language performance, particularly the use of language scripts in recurring contexts. It puts forth the position that sequences of collaborative, context-dependent behaviors should be the focus of assessment and intervention rather than the isolated utterances that have traditionally been analyzed.

Chapter 3 provides an overview of the assessment of social communication that bridges the social and communicative competence literatures. In this chapter, Kaczmarek offers an interdisciplinary model of assessment that examines the effectiveness and appropriateness of social communication at three increasingly complex levels. Effectiveness or the measurement of function represents the convergence of social and communicative competence, whereas appropriateness or the measurement of form remains primarily distinct for social and communicative repertoires.

1

Social Interaction and Models of Friendship Development

Howard Goldstein and Lindee Morgan

What is the essence of social behavior that might be relevant to children with developmental disabilities? Because of the lack of a comprehensive theory of social behavior and its development, this question is not an easy one to answer. Based on the literature and perhaps an intuitive analysis, a number of goals for children with developmental disabilities can be proposed. At least five areas seem to be relevant, each building on the prior areas: 1) identifying social skills or behaviors that are possible objectives for intervention; 2) improving rates of social interaction; 3) enhancing social acceptance, by peers in particular; 4) encouraging children with developmental disabilities to develop relationships with people in their lives; and 5) enabling people with disabilities to develop mutual relationships or friendships that yield lasting and even intimate relationships. This conceptualization reflects an interventionist's perspective that is not readily apparent in the existing literature on social competence and social-communicative development. Indeed, as Newcomb and Bagwell (1995) pointed out in their review of 82 articles on children's friendships, investigators readily acknowledge an absence of a strong theoretical conceptualization to guide work in this area. Nevertheless, a number of frameworks have been proposed that may help people to begin to understand the complexities of social behavior and its development in children with disabilities.

DEVELOPMENTAL PERSPECTIVES

Most conceptualizations of social relationship development (e.g., Buhrmester, 1996; Furman, 1982) are based on Sullivan's (1953) theory of friendship development. Sullivan proposed that people have specific interpersonal needs at different stages in development and that different types of relationships best suit these needs at each stage. The social skills and competencies needed to be successful in social interactions are thought to develop within the context of these relationships (Buhrmester & Furman, 1986). Because these social skills and competencies are not specified, however, diverse approaches are evident in the literature (see Chapter 3). This diversity of approaches is not surprising because the primary focus of investigators tends to shift as they examine different populations, cultural groups, and age groups.

Sullivan (1953) asserted that people need social interaction and social input, such as tenderness, companionship, acceptance, and intimacy, to obtain happiness and psychological well-being. An underlying assumption is that when such interaction does not occur, people experience distress and maladjustment. Sullivan defined friendship as collaborative relationships. Friends are sensitive to the needs of one another and seek mutual satisfaction. Sullivan suggested that friendship relationships do not typically begin to emerge until the preadolescent period when the need for acceptance transforms. That is, the need for acceptance in the elementary school years is met by general peer group interaction, but this focus shifts to a need for interpersonal intimacy during adolescence and beyond.

Although one may question whether Sullivan's theoretical conceptualization has undergone direct empirical scrutiny, clearly his theory has helped direct investigators to observe and describe social behavior and relationships from a developmental perspective. Certainly those taking a behavioral perspective may wonder whether the theory of social needs has any real explanatory value or psychological reality. Sullivan's theory lacks specification of social behaviors and competencies that are expected to develop. Nevertheless, Sullivan's idea of scrutinizing the demands of social situations from a developmental perspective and acknowledging the changing value of companionship, peer acceptance, mutual satisfaction, and intimacy has great appeal for researchers. This concept is reflected in the developmental literature, in the chapters that follow, and in the milestones summarized next.

The first 3 years of social life typically are characterized by interactions with caregivers. Developmental approaches stress the development of parental bonds and attachment in infants. Warren and his colleagues (see Chapter 4) explain how a transactional model helps people to understand how social-communicative development is facilitated by the bidirectional, reciprocal influences of the child and the social environment. They provide a summary of social-communicative skills that typically are acquired during the first 2 years of life. In today's society, toddlers often are provided opportunities to interact with peers.

Toddlers' peer relationships mostly converge around playing together. At this stage, peer relationships cannot really be defined as friendships. Infants and toddlers rarely show mutual and stable preferences for specific peers (Furman, 1982). Discrimination between familiar and unfamiliar peers may be the major characteristic of the friendship literature devoted to this age group.

During the preschool years, however, peer interaction becomes more prominent, mostly in the context of mutual engagement in play activities. Gottman and his colleagues (Gottman, 1983; Gottman & Mettetal, 1986; Gottman & Parkhurst, 1980; Parker & Gottman, 1989) distinguish among the social requirements associated with different types of play. Parallel play places few demands on children to accommodate each other. By the time preschoolers begin to display nonstereotyped fantasy play, they are faced with many more social-communicative demands. Fantasy play requires social coordination as children continually negotiate play roles. Consequently, it has the potential for disagreement and conflict that take sophisticated social skills to resolve satisfactorily. By the end of the preschool period, there are heavy demands on children in terms of verbal skills, behavioral inhibition, and perspective taking. Preschoolers who are more familiar with one another display fantasy play more frequently (Matthews, 1978). Likewise, they are more likely to acknowledge one another as friends (Berndt & Perry, 1986; Furman & Buhrmester, 1992).

About 75% of preschoolers have been described as having friends (Hinde, Titmus, Easton, & Tamplin, 1985; Howes, 1983). Although preschool children may have friends, relationships at this stage can change from day to day. There is some evidence, however, for stability of friendships. In a study of friendship stability, Gershman and Hayes (1983) found that two thirds of preschool friendships remained stable over a 6-month period. Regardless of length, preschool friendships are thought to be important for social development (Furman, 1982). Gottman (1986) also pointed out the potential role of preschool friendships in affective development. He noted that fantasy play seems to provide a means for practicing roles and for resolving major fears. Corsaro (1985) noted three recurrent themes for preschool fantasy play: lost–found, danger–rescue, and death–rebirth. Consequently, fantasy play seems to provide an avenue for children to address their fears within the supportive context of peer interactions. Thus, early peer relationships, especially in the context of play, are not only a source of excitement and entertainment but also seem to play an important role in social, communicative, and affective development.

School-age children begin to develop deeper friendships around age 8 or 9 (Furman, 1982). These relationships are characterized by less egocentrism and a greater sensitivity to others. But as Sullivan (1953) pointed out, the major goal of this stage in development is acceptance by peers. Predictably, children are concerned about self-presentation and want to avoid rejection by their peers. Children begin to form peer groups that differ in status (Crockett, Losoff, & Petersen, 1984; Hartup, 1984). Most children highly value group membership, but it may contribute to insecurity as they also view membership as somewhat capricious. Peer group reactions often are gauged using sophisticated verbal behavior, namely negative evaluation gossip and teasing. Children can use these strategies to determine group attitudes and norms without risking personal exposure by engaging in the behaviors yet to be judged. Children with developmental disabilities are at social risk not only because peers may not deem their behavior acceptable but also because they lack the social and communicative sophistication required for expressing and responding to gossip and teasing effectively (Goldstein & Gallagher, 1992).

Adolescents acquire a desire for interpersonal intimacy. The major theme of this stage of development is self-exploration and self-definition (Gottman & Mettetal, 1986). Relationships at this stage begin to be characterized by self-disclosure, trust, commitment, respect, and similar value systems (Furman, 1982). Through discussions with friends, adolescents explore their identities, beliefs, and aspirations. Hence, talking is a primary problem-solving strategy. When coupled with a high level of emotional involvement, these interactions pave the way for romantic relationships, a special kind of friendship.

Buhrmester (1996) qualified this timeline by stating that needs emerge as children become occupied with new developmental issues and concerns. He suggests that these concerns dictate what children seek in relationships and why mutual and exclusive relationships develop. Friendship provides a context for tackling issues with which children are preoccupied. He suggests that an absence of friendships may have deleterious effects on social adjustment and the learning of life's lessons. Indeed, researchers have found that children who do not develop friendships due to peer relationship difficulties are at risk for social maladjustment in later life (see Dishion, Andrews, & Crosby, 1995; Parker & Asher, 1987).

Asher, Parker, and Walker (1996) differentiated between the concepts of peer acceptance and friendship. *Peer acceptance* refers to the extent to which children are liked and accepted by members of their peer group. In contrast, *friendship* is a dyadic construct that must include mutual liking between two individuals. Furman and Robbins (1985) suggested that some skills (e.g., intimacy) are better served in the context of friendship, whereas other skills (e.g., leadership) are likely to be acquired in peer group interactions. Therefore, the goals of social skills training programs should be to enhance peer interactions in general as well as to promote friendships.

These goals need to be examined with respect to children with developmental disabilities. Functional social-communicative objectives for a child with a disability may produce very different types of friendships from those of same-age peers due to delays in development. Indeed, Buhrmester (1996) suggested that the emergence of social behavior is influenced by multiple factors such as biological maturation, cognitive development, cultural expectations, and individuals' experiences. He suggested that these elements converge to define children's social needs and expectations at any given stage of development. Fulfilling these needs and expectations requires possession of certain knowledge, skills, and behaviors. The term *social competence* has come to refer to such knowledge, skills, and behaviors. Katz (1988), for example, used the term to refer to the initiation, development, and maintenance of relationships. Guralnick defined the construct as "the ability of young children to successfully and appropriately select and carry out their interpersonal goals" (1990, p. 4). The abilities to relate effectively to people and to be accepted by others are important outcomes of social competence (Quay, 1993).

Although social competence can be defined and described in myriad ways, the significance of social competence is unmistakable with respect to early development, particularly in children with disabilities (Farmer, Pearl, & Van Acker, 1996). Developmental changes motivate children to enter into new types of relationships. Within these new and more complex relationships, different social competencies are demanded. From this perspective, social competence plays a role in determining the quality of a child's friendships. This influence is bidirectional in that friendship also provides access to opportunities to improve one's social competence.

Friendship experiences might contribute to social competence in two ways (Buhrmester, 1996). First, friendship may provide exclusive opportunities to master certain social skills. For example, an adolescent without close friends may never be called on to discuss personal thoughts and feelings and, therefore, will not have the opportunity to practice and refine these skills. It also may limit the opportunities one has to learn observationally from a highly valued peer. Second, the feedback one receives through interactions with friends may play a role in shaping individual differences in social competence (Buhrmester, 1996). When friends react positively to a child's attempts at a new social skill, that skill is reinforced; however, when efforts evoke negative feedback from friends, use of a new skill is undermined. Hence, keeping in mind the complete hierarchy of goals proposed at the beginning of this chapter seems important. Conceptualizing these goals sequentially may do a disservice to children with disabilities because of the reciprocal influences of friendships and social skills. Many studies have documented lower frequencies of social interactions in young children with developmental disabilities than in typical children (see Odom & McEvoy, 1988). Clearly, this situation puts children with disabilities at risk for fewer peer relationships and fewer mutual friendships (Guralnick & Groom, 1988). Educators and researchers may need to target relationships and friendships as well as social skills and social interactions to maximize the benefits of intervention. The social competence that children bring to a situation affects their likelihood of succeeding in forming relationships. From this perspective, if children manage to make friends, they are more likely to learn more sophisticated social skills and, in turn, are more likely to continue to develop relationships and make friends.

The developmental perspective is most pervasive in the chapters in this book; however, the exploration of theories emanating from other perspectives promises to provide fresh insights into the nature of social competence and relationship development.

SOCIAL PSYCHOLOGICAL PERSPECTIVE

Theories of social interdependence developed in response to a proposal from Kurt Lewin (1946) that the essence of a group is the interdependence of its members. These early theories proposed that an intrinsic state of tension among group members motivates the movement toward the accomplishment of desired common goals. This tension motivates both cooperative and competitive behavior. We first examine these ideas with respect to the dyad (Kelley & Thibaut, 1978) followed by a discussion of interdependence within cooperative learning groups (Johnson & Johnson, 1998).

Interdependence theory (Kelley & Thibaut, 1978) has been used to explain behavior in dyadic interactions. How these dyadic interactions progress over time in turn determines whether relationships will be maintained or terminated. Essentially, patterns of behavior are determined by the consequences of interaction, which are based on a combination of the costs and rewards attributed to each participant in the dyad. Costs are those things that inhibit performance such as conflict, competition, and embarrassment. Rewards are the reinforcers that give pleasure and gratification. The accumulation of costs and rewards in an interaction determines the outcome of the situation. For satisfactory outcomes to be met, rewards must outweigh the costs incurred. Ultimately, the likelihood that the relationship will continue is based on mutually satisfactory outcomes.

Dyads tend to behave in ways that yield satisfactory outcomes for both participants. What is satisfactory, however, may differ per individual and situation. According to Kelley and Thibaut's (1978) interdependence theory, participants evaluate relationships based on two standards. The first standard is the *comparison level*, which is the minimum level of outcome deemed satisfactory for the maintenance of the relationship. This level is determined individually based on one's social experiences. The second standard is called the *alternatives comparison level*. This is the lowest level of outcomes a participant will accept in light of available alternative relationships given the present circumstances.

How can teachers support interactions between typical children and classmates with developmental disabilities in order to enhance the likelihood of a positive relationship developing? Because typical children are likely to have alternative opportunities to interact with other classmates, teachers should consider how to enhance peers' outcomes when interacting with classmates with disabilities. For example, teachers might increase the likelihood of relationship development by reducing costs and increasing rewards for typical peers. Perhaps this explains the success of peer support networks as described by Haring and Breen (1992). Peer networks may reduce costs and increase rewards by having teachers attach additional status and extra privileges to participants and by incorporating typical peer interaction with a common objective of improving the socialization of a child with disabilities.

The underlying premise of interdependence theory is consistent with social learning theory; both purport that social behavior will be extinguished unless it is reinforced at least intermittently. Social learning theory also recognizes the role that observational learning is likely to play in the initial learning of social behaviors (Bandura, 1977). Nonetheless, a condition of interdependence is access to rewards for each other's behavior with limited costs to each participant. What is critical then is to identify determinants of costs and rewards in child relationships. Kelley and Thibaut (1978) identified three factors that may serve as determinants of friendship: 1) ability, 2) proximity, and 3) similarity.

First, skills such as intelligence and taking another's perspective appear to promote dyad formation (Kelley & Thibaut, 1978). Children will be chosen as friends if they are able and willing to help others. Conversely, children are rejected if they fail to help others or if they induce anxiety or discomfort. In general, better-liked people are perceived to have more positive traits. Peers select friends who have desirable attributes, such as social skills and personality traits (Aboud & Mendelson,

1996). The value of certain abilities, however, may change with each relationship and situation. This is an issue to consider when planning intervention for children with developmental disabilities. In a study of preschool children's social initiations, Tremblay, Strain, Hendrickson, and Shores (1981) found that sharing, suggesting a play activity, affection, assistance, and rough-and-tumble play had a high probability of evoking a positive response from a peer. Children with disabilities who use these social interaction skills are more likely to be accepted by their peers (Strain, 1983). Abilities such as these may increase the peers' rewards and reduce costs in the situation.

Second, proximity affects whether individuals will come into contact and is usually related to similarity in backgrounds and values (Kelley & Thibaut, 1978). Simply put, individuals who are together more often are more likely to engage in interactions and develop relationships. Conversely, physical distance contributes to the costs of a relationship. This distinction comes into play in applications of the principle of least restrictive environments. Children who are included full time in general education classrooms may be more likely to develop relationships with typical peers than children who are placed in other environments or are mainstreamed for only portions of the day. Even children included in general education classrooms may experience different degrees of proximity to peers. The child with a disability who sits at a desk in the front of class next to the teacher may interact more with the teacher and less with peers when compared with a child with a disability who sits at a table amidst typical peers in the middle of the classroom.

Third, Kelley and Thibaut (1978) suggested that a dyad may begin to interact because of common characteristics. If individuals are similar, they anticipate good outcomes associated with interaction and therefore are more likely to initiate interaction. Rewards seem to be based on similarities between two people in that children often choose friends who are the same age, sex, and race (Aboud & Mendelson, 1996). Strain (1984) found that typical children tended to select other typical children or older, more cognitively mature children with disabilities as partners in interaction. Research has shown that even in schools of mixed demographic groupings, friends are still more similar to each other than to nonfriends (Goldman, 1981). Hartup (1996) hypothesized that children construct relationships that maximize interpersonal payoffs and that these choices are made on an experiential basis. With limited experience, physical characteristics are likely to play a larger role. Determining similarities in likes and dislikes or preferred and avoided activities takes time for individuals.

The identity of one's friends is a significant consideration in predicting outcomes. Access to friendship may be indicative of either a good developmental prognosis or a deviant one depending on the relationships in which one is involved. By virtue of having a disability, many children may be viewed as dissimilar from their peers. In planning intervention, consideration must be given to how to emphasize similarities that exist among children.

Johnson and Johnson (1998) applied interdependence theory to groups and advocated its application within the context of cooperative learning. They suggested that interdependence theory provides guidance as to how to best structure social skill interventions and, specifically, cooperative learning activities. Social interdependence exists when individuals share common goals and each individual's outcomes are affected by the actions of others (Johnson & Johnson, 1989). Positive interdependence creates "promotive interaction patterns" as individuals encourage and facilitate each other's efforts to reach the group's goals. In school environments, the group's goal is usually a learning task that needs to be completed. In cooperative learning groups, group members tend to promote each other's success by

- Giving and receiving help
- Exchanging resources and information
- Giving and receiving feedback on task work and teamwork behavior
- Challenging each other's reasoning and task strategies
- Encouraging one another to achieve
- Influencing and being influenced by other's behavior and reasoning
- Engaging in social and communicative skills needed for effective teamwork
- Evaluating how effectively the team is working and determining how teamwork can be improved

Johnson and Johnson (1989) reviewed a large body of literature that compares the impact of cooperative, competitive, and individualistic efforts on achievement and productivity. They suggested that three broad outcomes could be used to summarize the numerous dependent variables that have been investigated over the years: 1) effort to achieve, 2) positive relationships, and 3) psychological adjustment and social competence. First, cooperation, compared with competitive or individual efforts, tends to result in higher achievement, greater willingness to take on difficult tasks, better retention of what is learned, more creative thinking, improved generalization of learning to other situations, more positive attitudes toward tasks being completed, and more time on task (Johnson & Johnson, 1989).

Second, numerous studies have found that the development of positive interpersonal relationships is more likely to result from cooperative than competitive or individualistic learning efforts. Johnson and Johnson (1989) reviewed studies on relationships among white and minority students as well as students with and without disabilities. In both cases, working cooperatively created far more positive relationships among diverse and heterogeneous students than did learning in other situations. They also found greater acceptance in students' social judgments. They attributed this to factors such as more frequent, accurate, and open communication; better understanding of others' perspectives; and improved expectations for future interactions. The influence of positive relationships among group members can be powerful, as high morale, improved self-esteem, and increased motivation to achieve are likely to influence other outcomes such as absenteeism and school dropout.

The third set of outcomes involves influences on students' psychological adjustment and social competence. Cooperative groups depend on individuals' abilities to develop, maintain, and appropriately modify interdependent relationships with others to succeed in achieving goals. Thus, students must correctly perceive whether positive interdependence exists and whether they are meeting normative expectations for appropriate behavior within the situation. Psychological health can be promoted in cooperative efforts because 1) students realize that they are known, accepted, and liked by their peers; 2) they know that they contributed to their own, others', and the group's success; and 3) they can perceive themselves relative to others in a realistic manner that allows for multidimensional comparison based on complementary abilities. Individuals who are part of a cooperative effort also experience more opportunities to learn social skills from one another and to become more socially competent (Johnson & Johnson, 1989).

Johnson and Johnson (1998) suggested that friendships emerge out of a sense of mutual accomplishment and bonding from engaging in joint efforts. Positive interdependence exists when one perceives that one is linked with others in a way that one cannot succeed unless the group does and vice versa. To coordinate efforts to achieve mutual goals, students must get to know and trust each other, communicate accurately and unambiguously, accept and support each other, and resolve conflicts constructively (Johnson & Johnson, 1979, 1998). Clearly, placing children with developmental disabilities in a learning group and telling them to cooperate is not sufficient. To be successful, children with and without disabilities need to be taught the basic social-communicative skills that are needed to work together productively and to cope with breakdowns in interpersonal and group functioning. Allowing cooperative learning groups to function over a prolonged period may be advantageous. In addition, Putnam, Rynders, Johnson, and Johnson (1989) found that relationships became more positive when students with and without disabilities were taught social skills, were observed by the teacher, and were given individual feedback on the frequency of social skills use. The group development process and individual instruction should combine to enhance social skills, to promote higher achievement and productivity, and to facilitate positive relationships among group members.

Social interdependence theory has implications for many areas of human social endeavors, and it has been subjected to a good deal of empirical investigation in educational settings. Although cooperative learning groups have become widely accepted in education, refined protocols for its application are still lacking. In particular, techniques for facilitating effective learning groups and for adapting to the needs of diverse learners remain challenging to most teachers.

SOCIOLOGICAL PERSPECTIVE

Intergroup contact theory has been applied primarily to the reduction of prejudice among groups undergoing desegregation in schools, neighborhoods, and military units. It has not been specifically applied to the development of friendships and social competence among children. Yet, the principle of least restrictive environment is based at least in part on some of the same underlying assumptions as desegregation movements. When discussing interventions to increase the social interaction and inclusion of children with disabilities with typical peers, sociological and anthropological perspectives on intergroup dynamics may provide new insights.

Allport's (1954) contact theory held that positive effects of intergroup contact occur only in situations marked by four key conditions: equal group status within the situation; common goals; intergroup cooperation; and the support of authorities, laws, or customs. Equal group status within the situation helps to reduce bias and increase positive contact. Goldstein and Kaczmarek (1992) noted the problems with peer-mediated social interventions that allow children with disabilities to be placed in subservient roles. They sought to develop interventions in which typical peers were placed in the role of "buddy," as opposed to teacher, tutor, or babysitter. Institutional processes that maintain social boundaries and hierarchies can thwart equal group status. Practices such as tracking and specialized class placement may serve to limit social opportunities and stigmatize the student (Evans & Eder, 1993). These practices may perpetuate inequality when children with developmental disabilities attempt to enter the social networks of typical children.

Common goals among individuals help to decrease negative feelings by steering the focus toward the group effort. This concept can be examined with respect to the camaraderie that develops among members of a team. Sports teams furnish a prime example. For example, an interracial athletic team needs all of its members to achieve its goal of winning. The construct of intergroup cooperation is of course reminiscent of the cooperative learning groups described by Johnson and Johnson (1998).

Support of authorities tends to promote contact. Within the context of integrating children with disabilities, this concept can be illustrated throughout the administrative hierarchies of our educational systems. Superintendents and school board members communicate a set of norms to school principals and teachers. Teachers in turn model the behavior that they deem appropriate for interaction with groups of students. They can provide explicit instruction about disabilities, encourage contact among groups of children, offer suggestions for interaction, and answer questions. Pettigrew (1998) noted that Allport's (1954) original hypothesis not only influenced social policy but has been largely validated by experiments that explored the effects of the four key conditions posited.

Pettigrew (1998) also pointed out a number of problems with Allport's intergroup contact theory and subsequent attempts to extend the theory. Perhaps the most critical problem that he identified is that the theory says nothing about the processes by which contact among groups members changes attitudes and behavior. Whereas Allport (1954) predicted *when* positive contact effects will occur, Pettigrew (1998) suggested that four interrelated mediating processes help explain *how* and *why*. He proposed four interrelated processes that operate to mediate attitude change: learning about the out-group, changing behavior, generating affective ties, and in-group reappraisal. This chapter refers to children with disabilities as the out-group and typical peers as the in-group.

The process thought to be most important to changing attitudes and reducing prejudice toward out-groups is *learning about the out-group*. Through contact with children with developmental disabilities, typical peers may learn that the out-group shares many of the same values and interests as the in-group. They may learn that behavioral, physical, or cognitive differences do not necessarily interfere with positive interactions. When negative views of other groups are corrected, contact should reduce prejudice. Thus, typical children who are in contact with children with disabilities should learn about developmental disabilities, have less prejudice, and be more willing to interact with children with disabilities. Pettigrew (1998) pointed out that positive effects of contact situations are more common than this cognitive analysis would predict, most likely because other processes are involved, as well.

Changing one's behavior often is a precursor to attitude change. When put in new situations, people are required to conform to new expectations. Repeating such experiences leads to "feeling right," to further comfort, and in many cases even to advocacy. Children who interact with peers with developmental disabilities in learning and play activities will conform to classroom expectations, and if their behavior is reinforced, they will continue to repeat these experiences. When behavior changes, attitudes are sure to follow to resolve dissonance between old prejudices and new behavior.

It is common for children from both groups to experience anxiety during initial contact between groups. With continued contact, anxiety is reduced as long as negative experiences are avoided. Hence, positive emotions stemming from positive experiences can mediate intergroup contact effects. Empathy for a stigmatized out-group or an individual from an out-group also can improve attitudes toward the out-group (Batson et al., 1997; Reich & Purbhoo, 1975). In addition, positive emotions aroused by intergroup friendship can have an especially strong effect on changing attitudes (Pettigrew, 1998). In a study of preschoolers, LaFreniere and Charlesworth (1987) asked what drives cooperation. They found that devising a common task and goals did not ensure cooperation, but children who were friends were more successful at completing a group task. Facilitating successful cooperation initially seems important to foster more positive interactions, emotions, and relationships among individuals experiencing intergroup contact. These positive experiences in turn are likely to facilitate successful intergroup cooperative ventures.

Intergroup contact also results in in-group reappraisal. One can gain insights about one's own in-group norms and customs. This new perspective can reshape one's view of the world and lead to less provincial views of out-groups in general. Thus, more positive attitudes toward out-groups are likely to result from a reappraisal or questioning of the beliefs of one's own in-group, and one becomes more tolerant of the views, customs, and norms of out-groups. This process may help explain how opportunities for typical peers to engage in activities and interventions aimed at children with disabilities may reshape their view of such groups. For example, Haring and Breen (1992) reported that students who engaged in a peer support network intervention for students with disabilities reported more positive attitudes about disabilities following their participation.

Pettigrew's analysis (1998) also began to outline a longitudinal model or developmental progression that may help people understand how positive contact affects generalization across individuals, situations, and groups. Clearly, optimal intergroup contact requires time for cross-group friendships to develop. Friendship relationships imply the potential for extensive and repeated contact in a variety of social contexts. Allport (1954) recognized the potency of friendships when he suggested that intimate, meaningful contact was important. Pettigrew later speculated that intergroup friendship has potent effects because it invokes all four mediating processes.

In summary, Pettigrew (1998) provided a useful extension of Allport's (1954) original contact hypothesis. His review showed that considerable empirical support existed for Allport's general hypotheses in field and archival studies, national and international surveys, and laboratory experiments. This theoretical perspective helps to explain why contact alone is not likely to change behavior and attitudes toward students with developmental disabilities. Pettigrew's reformulated contact theory begins with a supportive societal and institutional context. Positive intergroup contact is associated with at least five situational factors: 1) equal group status within the situation, 2) common goals, 3) intergroup cooperation, 4) authority support, and 5) friendship potential. Under these conditions, early contacts are likely to overcome initial anxiety. Positive feelings about a member of the out-group are likely to result from positive experiences, but generalized effects are limited as the focus is on the individual and not on the out-group in general. Later, with established and repeated contact in optimal situations, prejudice is likely to be reduced, and this reduction is generalized across situations. Finally, if established contact evolves into a unified group, then maximum reduction in prejudice is expected. People begin to think of themselves in a larger group perspective that highlights similarities among all individuals and obscures the "we" and "they" boundaries. Effects may even generalize from the immediate out-group to other out-groups. This longitudinal model may prove helpful in understanding the many factors and long-term perspective that are needed in planning social interventions for children with developmental disabilities.

CONCLUSION

The three perspectives discussed—developmental, social psychological, and sociological—represent different approaches to designing interventions to improve social interaction and encourage friendship development in children with developmental disabilities. Although each perspective brings novel ideas into consideration, common themes can be identified among these theoretical perspectives.

Proximity is an important consideration within each theory. Interdependence theory (Kelley & Thibaut, 1978) defines proximity as a determinant of friendship. Contact theory posits that acquaintance and friendship development are positive effects of intergroup contact. This concept is given practical significance in Furman's observation (1982) that toddlers' friends are typically neighbors and classmates. The implication for children with developmental disabilities is obvious. Proximity to typical peers is a necessary but not sufficient condition for developing friendships. Likewise, similarity among peers increases the likelihood that children will interact. According to contact theory and interdependence theory, individuals are drawn to those who are like themselves in terms of age, gender, race, values, and interests. In terms of intervention, identifying similarities among individuals and pointing them out in a positive light may be beneficial as a starting point for interaction. This should help children learn that judgments of similarity need not be made on a superficial basis, such as physical characteristics.

Common goals or social needs play a role in each theory. The initiation of interactions and later peer relationships results from mutual social needs in Sullivan's (1953) developmental theory. According to interdependence theory and contact theory, positive group interactions are likely to result when group members share common goals. Cooperation may be a natural byproduct when one's outcomes are affected by the actions of other members. Successful cooperation in turn sets the stage for relationship development at a dyadic level or a reappraisal of the out-group in general. These observations point to the potential benefits of setting up situations in which children with developmental disabilities experience group interactions that require cooperative effort and support interdependence.

The relationship between social skills and friendship is considered from both the developmental and the social psychological perspective. Buhrmester (1996) discussed a bidirectional influence in that children with social skills are more likely to make friends, and having friends further supports the acquisition of social skills. Kelley and Thibaut (1978) referred to a person's ability to help others as a determinant of friendship. Obviously, children with greater levels of social competence are more likely to be accepted by peers and to be chosen as friends. Appropriate social skills provide a foundation for relationship and friendship development. What social skills should be taught to optimize the effects of intervention with children with developmental disabilities, however, continues to be difficult to ascertain. Furthermore, children need to discriminate when to use which social skills, and the variations and frequencies of demonstrations need to be considered. This discrimination is complicated by the need to adjust to the everchanging expectations of peers as children with developmental disabilities grow older. Thus, intervention agents need to be cognizant of these shifting demands and, when possible, plan ahead to equip children with the skills that will be needed in future social encounters.

Although dyads tend to behave in ways that yield positive outcomes for both participants (Kelley & Thibaut, 1978), one must guard against problems associated with dysfunctional or involuntary interactions. Coercive relationships can develop if individuals have unequal status and one peer is allowed to dominate another. Also, if peers are forced to interact with a child with a disability and not allowed to pursue more attractive alternatives, one should not expect positive interaction patterns to be sustained. Durable, positive relationships are based on a history of reinforcing interactions. The implications for this are twofold. First, teachers must set up contexts that increase the rewards and minimize the costs of interacting with children with disabilities. This can be done through activities that are novel, exciting, and produce a desired outcome. Second, teachers must recognize the need to teach children with disabilities social behaviors that peers value. Indeed, peers or networks of peers may be in the best position to help interventionists identify social behaviors that tend to reduce costs (e.g., embarrassment) and maximize rewards (e.g., acceptance by high status peers).

These theoretical perspectives highlight the need to scrutinize social competence and intervention efforts on behalf of children with developmental disabilities longitudinally. First, improving social interventions may begin with an examination of the objectives to be taught. Obviously, promoting both acceptance and friendship for children with developmental disabilities is important. Although it is important to train skills to optimize effectiveness in interactions such as conversational skills, prosocial behavior, and so forth, these alone may not be enough to foster friendships. Peers themselves will need to be the target of our intervention efforts. As can be seen in subsequent chapters, peers have served effectively as intervention agents, although the long-term benefits to typical peers and society in general have not been fully explored.

Second, we must acknowledge how the requirements of social competence change as children develop. The demands shift when one considers interactions within families, dyads, and peer groups. The need for relationships and friendships seems to be tied to one's social maturity and perhaps one's cognitive abilities. Research should begin to define with greater specificity the friendship needs emerging with each developmental stage and the developmental markers associated with these needs. This identification of developmental needs also requires an assessment of specific social competencies to be attained at each stage in development. Newcomb and Bagwell (1995) suggested that research should address features of friendship relations, such as temporal patterns in friendship development, age changes in friendship experiences, and the developmental significance of mutual or intimate friendship experiences.

One set of experiences worth examining further is cooperative learning groups and how to capitalize on this context for facilitating the development of social competence. The reciprocal nature of cooperation and social competence should not be overlooked. Allport (1954) and Johnson and Johnson (1998) pointed out that cooperation leads to more productivity and more positive outcomes than competitive situations do. LaFreniere and Charlesworth (1987) suggested that cooperation is more likely to happen if engaged individuals are friends. Thus, more effective cooperative learning experiences are likely to foster friendships, and friendships serve to produce more positive outcomes in cooperative interactions. Cooperative learning groups also may provide a context for testing contact theory using groups of typical children and children with developmental disabilities. Questions could be addressed regarding Pettigrew's (1998) processes that promote intergroup acceptance and the facilitation of relationships among group members.

Contact theory, in particular, offers some novel insights into efforts to integrate children with developmental disabilities into educational and community contexts. Much of the work from a developmental perspective has focused on interaction of individuals within dyads; group interactions are acknowledged in the context of affiliations and acceptance by cliques and one's peer group generally. Interdependence theory provides an analysis of interactive behavior largely at the level of the dyad as well, but the extension to cooperative learning groups provides a context for exploring how to set up interactions that can facilitate learning as well as the development of group interaction skills. Because typical peers are expected to identify skills and teach one another how to promote success within the group, the addition of children with disabilities to cooperative learning groups would seem a natural extension of this process. Contact theory focuses its attention on the inclusion of groups that are considered different and are subject to prejudice. This theory acknowledges the role of institutional or cultural norms and the influence of authority figures. Equal group status and the support of authority figures, rules, or laws are critical conditions that are required to promote inclusion and reduce prejudice.

Contact theory uniquely presents the concepts of equal status and support of authorities as well as the processes by which contact changes attitudes and behaviors. Status is an important issue with youth beginning in the middle elementary school years (Sullivan, 1953). Not all inclusive practices are implemented effectively. Children with developmental disabilities who are inadvertently placed at a lower status level are handicapped from the outset in the likelihood of being able to develop friendships and positive peer relationships. The support of authorities (e.g., teachers, school administrators, church leaders, parents) is critical to the success of interventions aimed at peer acceptance. Adult attitudes are directly modeled for children and provide a basis for determining what is acceptable in school and community contexts. If teachers treat children with developmental disabilities differently from their peers, the peers will do so, as well. A positive attitude of acceptance of differences must be adopted and practiced by adults for children to follow suit.

Although these theories seek to explain different aspects of social functioning, the ideas they present tend to support each other. An integration of these ideas may make for a more comprehensive theory of social behavior and social development. At the very least, they offer a broader perspective with which to explore strategies for evaluating social competence in children with developmental disabilities and designing interventions that will teach critical skills, promote social acceptance, provide opportunities for relationship development, and set the stage for the development of mutual or intimate relationships. Research and clinical endeavors need to move beyond counting rates of peer interaction and determining whether a child has friends. The theories presented should expand understanding of the complexity of the development of social-communicative skills, relationships, and friendships and the difficulty in developing effective interventions. We hope that this chapter and the chapters that follow will lead researchers and interventionists to consider a wide range of possibilities in tackling issues related to social interaction and the development of meaningful relationships for children with developmental disabilities.

REFERENCES

Aboud, F.E., & Mendelson, M.J. (1996). Determinants of friendship selection and quality: Developmental perspectives. In W.M. Bukowski, A.F. Newcomb, & W.W. Hartup (Eds.), *The company they keep: Friendship in childhood and adolescence* (pp. 87–112). New York: Cambridge University Press.

Allport, G.W. (1954). *The nature of prejudice.* Reading, MA: Addison-Wesley.

Asher, S.R., Parker, J.G., & Walker, D.L. (1996). Distinguishing friendship from acceptance: Implications for intervention and assessment. In W.M. Bukowski, A.F. Newcomb, & W.W. Hartup (Eds.), *The company they keep: Friendship in childhood and adolescence* (pp. 366–405). New York: Cambridge University Press.

Bandura, A. (1977). *Social learning theory.* Upper Saddle River, NJ: Prentice-Hall.

Batson, C.D., Polycarpou, M.P., Harmon-Jones, E., Imhoff, H.J., Mitchener, E.C., Bednar, L.L., Klein, T.R., & Highberger, L. (1997). Empathy and attitudes: Can feeling for a member of a stigmatized group improve feelings toward the group? *Journal of Personality and Social Psychology, 72,* 105–118.

Berndt, T.J., & Perry, T.B. (1986). Children's perceptions of friendships as supportive relationships. *Developmental Psychology, 22,* 640–648.

Buhrmester, D. (1996). Need fulfillment, interpersonal competence, and the developmental contexts of early adolescent friendship. In W.M. Bukowski, A.F. Newcomb, & W.W. Hartup (Eds.), *The company they keep: Friendship in childhood and adolescence* (pp. 158–185). New York: Cambridge University Press.

Buhrmester, D., & Furman, W. (1986). The changing functions of friends in childhood: A neo-Sullivanian perspective. In V.J. Derlega & B.A. Winstead (Eds.), *Friendship and social interaction* (pp. 41–62). New York: Springer-Verlag.

Corsaro, W.A. (1985). *Friendship and peer culture in the early years.* Stamford, CT: Ablex Publishing.

Crockett, L., Losoff, M., & Petersen, A.C. (1984). Perceptions of the peer group and friendship in early adolescence. *Journal of Early Adolescence, 4,* 155–181.

Dishion, T.J., Andrews, D.W., & Crosby, L. (1995). Anti-social boys and their friends in early adolescence: Relationship characteristics, quality, and interactional process. *Child Development, 66,* 139–151.

Evans, C., & Eder, D. (1993). "No exit": Processes of social isolation in the middle school. *Journal of Contemporary Ethnography, 22,* 139–170.

Farmer, T.W., Pearl, R., & Van Acker, R.M. (1996). Expanding the social skills deficit framework: A developmental synthesis perspective, classroom social networks, and implications for the social growth of students with disabilities. *Journal of Special Education, 30*(3), 232–256.

Furman, W. (1982). Children's friendships. In T. Field, G. Finley, A. Huston, H. Quay, & L. Troll (Eds.), *Review of human development* (pp. 327–342). New York: John Wiley & Sons.

Furman, W., & Buhrmester, D. (1992). Age and sex differences in perceptions of networks of personal relationships. *Child Development, 63,* 103–115.

Furman, W., & Robbins, P. (1985). What's the point? Issues in the selection of treatment objectives. In B.H. Schneider, K.H. Rubin, & J.E. Ledingham (Eds.), *Children's peer relations: Issues in assessment and intervention* (pp. 41–54). New York: Springer-Verlag.

Gershman, E.S., & Hayes, D.S. (1983). Differential stability of reciprocal friendships and unilateral relationships among preschool children. *Merrill-Palmer Quarterly, 29*(2), 169–177.

Goldman, J.A. (1981). The social interaction of preschool children in same-age versus mixed-age groupings. *Developmental Psychology, 21,* 644–650.

Goldstein, H., & Gallagher, T. (1992). Strategies for promoting the social-communicative competence of young children with specific language impairments. In S.L. Odom, S.R. McConnell, & M.A. McEvoy (Eds.), *Social competence of young children with disabilities: Nature, development, and intervention* (pp. 189–213). Baltimore: Paul H. Brookes Publishing Co.

Goldstein, H., & Kaczmarek, L. (1992). Promoting communicative interaction among children in integrated intervention settings. In S.F. Warren & J. Reichle (Series and Vol. Eds.), *Communication and language intervention series: Vol 1. Causes and effects in communication and language intervention* (pp. 81–111). Baltimore: Paul H. Brookes Publishing Co.

Gottman, J.M. (1983). How children become friends. *Monographs of the Society for Research in Child Development, 48*(3, Serial No. 201).

Gottman, J.M. (1986). The observation of social process. In J.M. Gottman & J.G. Parker (Eds.), *Conversation of friends: Speculation on affective development* (pp. 55–102). New York: Cambridge University Press.

Gottman, J.M., & Mettetal, G. (1986). Speculations about social and affective development: Friendships and acquaintanceship through adolescence. In J.M. Gottman & J.G. Parker (Eds.), *Conversation of friends: Speculation on affective development* (pp. 192–237). New York: Cambridge University Press.

Gottman, J.M., & Parkhurst, J.T. (1980). A developmental theory of friendship and acquaintanceship process. In W.A. Collins (Ed.), *Minnesota symposia on child development: Vol. 13. Development of cognition, affect, and social relations* (pp. 197–253). Mahwah, NJ: Lawrence Erlbaum Associates.

Guralnick, M.J. (1990). Social competence and early intervention. *Journal of Early Intervention, 14,* 3–14.

Guralnick, M.J., & Groom, J.M. (1988). Friendships of preschool children in mainstreamed playgroups. *Developmental Psychology, 24,* 495–604.

Haring, T.G., & Breen, C.G. (1992). A peer-mediated social network intervention to enhance to social integration of persons with moderate and severe disabilities. *Journal of Applied Behavior Analysis, 25,* 319–333.

Hartup, W.W. (1984). The peer context in middle childhood. In W.A. Collins (Ed.), *Development during middle childhood: The years from six to twelve* (pp. 240–282). Washington, DC: National Academy Press.

Hartup, W.W. (1996). The company they keep: Friendships and their developmental significance. *Child Development, 67,* 1–13.

Hinde, R.A., Titmus, G., Easton, D., & Tamplin, A. (1985). Incidence of "friendship" and behavior towards strong associates versus nonassociates in preschoolers. *Child Development, 56,* 234–245.

Howes, C. (1983). Patterns of friendship. *Child Development, 54,* 1041–1053.

Johnson, D.W., & Johnson, R.T. (1979). Conflict in the classroom: Controversy and learning. *Review of Educational Research, 49,* 51–70.

Johnson, D.W., & Johnson, R.T. (1989). *Cooperation and competition: Theory and research.* Edina, MN: Interaction Book Company.

Johnson, D.W., & Johnson, R.T. (1998). Cooperative learning and social interdependence theory. In R.S. Tindale, L. Heath, J. Edwards, E.J. Posavac, F.B. Bryant, Y. Suarez-Balcazar, E. Henderson-King, & J. Myers (Eds.), *Theory and research on small groups* (pp. 9–35). New York: Kluwer Academic/Plenum Publishers.

Katz, L. (1988). What should young children be learning? *American Educator, 23*(3), 44–45.

Kelley, H., & Thibaut, J. (1978). *Interpersonal relations: A theory of interdependence.* New York: John Wiley & Sons.

LaFreniere, P.J., & Charlesworth, W.R. (1987). Effects of friendship and dominance status on preschooler's resource utilization in a cooperative/competitive situation. *International Journal of Behavioral Development, 10,* 345–358.

Lewin, K. (1946). Behavior and development as a function of the total situation. In L. Carmichael (Ed.), *Manual of child psychology* (pp. 791–844). New York: John Wiley & Sons.

Matthews, W.S. (1978). Sex and familiarity effects upon the proportion of time young children spend in spontaneous fantasy play. *Journal of Genetic Psychology, 133,* 9–12.

Newcomb, A.F., & Bagwell, C.L. (1995). Children's friendship relations: A meta-analytic review. *Psychological Bulletin, 117,* 306–347.

Odom, S.L., & McEvoy, M.A. (1988). Integration of young children with handicaps and normally developing children. In S.L. Odom & M.B. Karnes (Eds.), *Early intervention for infants and children with handicaps: An empirical base* (pp. 241–267). Baltimore: Paul H. Brookes Publishing Co.

Parker, J.G., & Asher, S.R. (1987). Peer relations and later personal adjustment: Are low-accepted children at risk? *Psychological Bulletin, 102,* 357–389.

Parker, J.G., & Gottman, J. (1989). Social and emotional development in a relational context. In T. Berndt & G. Ladd (Eds.), *Peer relationships in child development* (pp. 95–131). New York: John Wiley & Sons.

Pettigrew, T.F. (1998). Intergroup contact theory. *Annual Review of Psychology, 49,* 65–85.

Putnam, J., Rynders, J., Johnson, R., & Johnson, D.W. (1989). Collaborative skill instruction for promoting positive interactions between mentally handicapped and nonhandicapped children. *Exceptional Children, 55,* 550–557.

Quay, L.C. (1993). Social competence in nonhandicapped, low interacting, and five handicapped groups of preschoolers. *Early Education and Development, 4,* 89–98.

Reich, C., & Purbhoo, M. (1975). The effect of cross-cultural contact. *Canadian Journal of Behavioural Sciences, 7,* 313–327.

Strain, P.S. (1983). Identification of social skill curriculum targets for severely handicapped children in mainstreamed preschools. *Applied Research in Mental Retardation, 4,* 369–382.

Strain, P.S. (1984). Social behavior patterns of nonhandicapped and handicapped-developmentally disabled friend pairs in mainstreamed preschools. *Analysis and Intervention in Developmental Disabilities, 4,* 15–28.

Sullivan, H.S. (1953). *The interpersonal theory of psychiatry.* New York: W.W. Norton.

Tremblay, A., Strain, P.S., Hendrickson, J.M., & Shores, R.E. (1981). Social interactions of normal preschool children: Using normative data for subject and target behavior selection. *Behavior Modification, 5,* 237–253.

2

Linguistic Influences on Social Interaction

Leonard Abbeduto and Katherine Short-Meyerson

Language is the foundation for most social interaction. People use language to acquire goods, services, and information and to make public their thoughts and feelings. They use language in informal encounters with friends and family and in more task-oriented or highly scripted encounters, such as those occurring in school and the workplace. They also use language in face-to-face encounters as well as in encounters with partners who are not visible to them, such as when they speak on the telephone. People use language to talk about events that are immediately perceptible and events that are abstract (e.g., hypothetical) or more distant in time and space. This chapter examines children's developing capacity to use language across these diverse types of social interactions. Questions about this capacity have traditionally been seen as being within the domain of pragmatics.

WHAT IS PRAGMATICS?

The term *pragmatics* is typically used to refer to the study of the ways in which speakers and listeners use language in social interaction (Levinson, 1983). In most conceptualizations of pragmatics (see McTear & Conti-Ramsden, 1992), a distinction is drawn between knowledge of the forms (i.e., phonology and morphosyntax) and content (i.e., semantics) of language, on the one hand, and knowledge of the ways in which those forms and contents can be used to achieve intended interpersonal goals (i.e., pragmatics), on the other. Consider, for example, the fact that speakers who are fluent in English have the ability to refer to the four-

L. Abbeduto's work on this chapter was supported by Grant Nos. R01 HD24356 and P30 HD03352 from the National Institute of Child Health and Human Development.

legged, barking family pet by its name (e.g., *Rover*) or by words such as *terrier, dog, canine, animal,* or *it.* This ability reflects knowledge of the forms and contents of language. In contrast, knowing when to use those words (e.g., knowing that *canine* is probably not a good choice when speaking to a toddler) reflects pragmatic knowledge.

Although there is consensus that pragmatics is the study of the social uses of language, there is considerable debate about its scope and methods (McTear & Conti-Ramsden, 1992). This debate has largely focused on three controversies:

- What is the relation between pragmatics and the other components of language (i.e., knowledge of form and content)?
- Is a competence-based or a performance-based account of pragmatics most useful?
- What is the proper unit of analysis in pragmatics?

Each of these controversies is discussed in the following sections. The discussion begins by considering the traditional, linguistically oriented approach to pragmatics and concludes by introducing an alternative model, one that takes a very different view of the three controversies compared with the traditional approach.

Relationship Between Pragmatics and Other Components of Language

Traditionally, pragmatics has been seen as separate from but related to the phonological, morphosyntactic, and semantic components of language (see Craig, 1995; McTear & Conti-Ramsden, 1992; Ninio & Snow, 1996). Just as there are thought to be syntactic categories (e.g., noun, verb) and rules for combining them into phrases and sentences (e.g., noun phrase → [determiner] + noun), so, too, are there pragmatic categories and rules. This concept is perhaps best illustrated by the work on speech acts (see Abbeduto & Benson, 1992, for a review). A speech act is the social function that an utterance is intended to perform in an interaction. Included among these functions are requests for information, requests for action, assertions, and commitments to a future course of action. Other categories of speech acts and finer distinctions within each category are possible, as well (see Ninio & Snow, 1996, for a coding scheme that includes dozens of speech act categories).

Although speech acts are performed through the utterance of a word, phrase, or sentence, a speech act is not isomorphic with any particular language form or content. A request for action, for example, can be expressed through any one of several linguistic expressions. "Sign this," "This needs to be signed," and "Could you sign this?," among other forms, could all be used to solicit a signature from an addressee. These forms differ in the directness with which they make the request for action and, consequently, are thought to vary in politeness, as well (Brown & Levinson, 1987). Therefore, rules governing the use of these forms would need to make reference to the social function of requesting an action and to the directness between that function and the various linguistic forms that could be used to encode it. Such rules would also need to refer to contextual factors associated with variations in politeness, such as the familiarity and social status of addressees, the emotional state of the speaker, the actions being performed at the time of the request, and the degree of effort anticipated for the addressee to comply with the request (Ninio & Snow, 1996; Nuccio & Abbeduto, 1993).

Just as any speech act can be performed by many different linguistic expressions, so, too, can any linguistic expression be mapped onto many different speech acts (Abbeduto & Benson, 1992). The sentence "That's mine," for instance, could be used to request the return of an object or to make a statement of fact. The *request* interpretation would be appropriate if the sentence was uttered by a child to a sibling who had grabbed a prized toy. In contrast, the *statement* interpretation would be appropriate if the sentence was uttered by a business tycoon while taking some business associates on a tour of properties recently amassed. In explaining how listeners arrive at different interpretations of the same utterance, the traditional view (e.g., Searle, 1975) assumes that any linguistic expression has associated with it a literal, or direct, interpretation that is context-independent and solely a function of the words that the expression contains and the morphological and semantic rules governing their combination. Further assumed is the idea that nonliteral, or indirect, speech act interpretations are then derived from the literal interpretation according to various context-sensitive rules or principles (e.g., Grice, 1975). For example, "That's mine" would be interpreted as a request rather than as a statement (i.e., its direct interpretation) if it were already mutually obvious to the speaker and listener that the referent belonged to the speaker. In this case, listeners purportedly assume that speakers adhere to the principle "Don't tell people what they already know" (Abbeduto, Furman, & Davies, 1989) and thus seek an interpretation other than the direct one (Abbeduto, Davies, & Furman, 1988; see Gibbs, 1983, for a contrasting view).

This traditional view of pragmatics has important implications for understanding the language problems of children and youth with developmental disabilities. It suggests that problems in linguistic performance may arise not just from deficits in the acquisition of linguistic forms and contents but also from a lack of pragmatic knowledge. Children may show impairments in requesting, for example, for reasons besides not being able to express this function linguistically. Rather, they may not understand or may not be motivated to express the function. Or, they may not know which forms to use in the service of the function. For example, a study by Nuccio and Abbeduto (1993) found that despite being able to produce polite forms (e.g., interrogatives, such as "Could you help me?") children and adolescents with mental retardation used impolite forms (e.g., imperatives, such as "Help me"; want/need statements, such as "I want help") for their requests more often than mental age–matched typically developing children. The traditional view also has expanded the focus of language intervention by reminding us to teach children with language impairments not only the linguistic forms and contents they lack but also how to use those forms and contents for social purposes (Abbeduto, 1984).

Despite these important contributions, the traditional linguistic view has been criticized for what is seen as a largely artificial distinction between language and its use in social interaction (Abbeduto, Evans, & Dolan, 2001). For example, there have been debates about which phenomena are pragmatic and which are semantic or morphosyntactic (see McTear & Conti-Ramsden, 1992; Ninio & Snow, 1996). More important, the traditional view assumes that pragmatic knowledge is somehow acquired, represented, and retrieved independently from knowledge of the other components of language. The fact is, however, that pragmatic categories and principles most likely motivate and shape the search for many linguistic forms and contents and vice versa (Craig, 1995).

There also is evidence that pragmatic knowledge is not stored or used independently of other linguistic knowledge. For example, direct, literal interpretations are not always considered before indirect, pragmatically derived interpretations; in fact, so-called direct interpretations may not even be considered at all in some contexts (Gibbs, 1983). The implication of this critique of the traditional view is that problems in language use and problems in language forms and contents are not so easily separated in either assessment or intervention.

Competence and Performance in Pragmatics

Although pragmatics is by definition the study of language use, it typically has been studied from the perspective of competence rather than from the perspective of performance. When addressing issues related to developmental disorders, this has led researchers to ask whether a child of a particular age or with a particular disorder has mastered various pragmatic categories and rules. For example, much research has focused on whether prelinguistic children have mastered basic categories of speech acts, such as requesting and declaring (see Ninio & Snow, 1996, for a review). In studies of later development, researchers have shifted their focus to rules. For example, Whitehurst and Sonnenschein (1985) studied the mastery of the difference rule (i.e., the rule that referential descriptions must encode the dimensions of difference between the intended referent and other potential referents). Other examples include rules governing the relationship between request politeness and addressee status (James, 1978), rules governing turn taking (Sacks, Schegloff, & Jefferson, 1974), and rules governing topic contributions (Brinton & Fujiki, 1989). From the competence perspective, pragmatic categories are similar in nature to linguistic categories, such as sentence and noun phrase, and pragmatic rules are similar to linguistic rules, such as a subject–verb agreement.

This competence-based approach to pragmatics is plagued by at least three problems. The first problem is that the approach assumes that the pragmatic categories and rules that govern communication are well-defined and deterministic in much the same way as linguistic categories and rules. In fact, pragmatic categories and rules seem to be descriptive of regularities in behavior that are less deterministic and more probabilistic. For example, many so-called pragmatic rules are violated with surprising frequency in daily conversation. Nevertheless, these violations are not seen as unnatural and certainly not as reflective of a communication disorder. Researchers often claim, for example, that the rules of turn taking dictate that no more than one person speaks at a time. In fact, as many as 5%–10% of speaker transitions violate this rule in the conversations of competent adults (Levinson, 1983). Moreover, most people have participated in conversations focused on emotion-laden topics (e.g., politics, religion) that contain even more violations of this one-speaker-at-a-time constraint. People typically view these conversations as heated or passionate rather than as poor exemplars of conversation or as reflections of a language-based disorder in the participants.

Indeed, the probabilistic nature of many pragmatic categories and rules leaves them with little explanatory power. For example, one "rule" of pragmatics is that speakers should make requests via forms that are indirect (e.g., "Would you be able to help me?") and that contain conventional politeness markers (e.g., "please") when speaking to someone with higher social standing than their own, but this does not allow researchers to predict precisely how people will express their requests in a given circumstance. Two speakers might adhere to the rule, but one might opt for "Could you help me, please?," whereas another might use "Would you please help me?" in the same situation. The same speaker might use different forms for the same request to the same addressee on different occasions while still adhering to the "rule." Thus, in contrast to the conventional definition of a linguistic rule, the pragmatic rules governing polite requesting seem poorly defined and less deterministic. In fact, it seems that the process of communication is essentially a probabilistic process in which people never know for sure if they and their partners have arrived at precisely the same representation of any symbolic behavior. Therefore, the precision and determinism implied by the concepts of pragmatic categories and pragmatic rules appear antithetical to the very nature of the communication process.

The second problem with the competence-based approach is that explaining communicative behavior in terms of categories and rules often diverts our attention away from some of the most interesting and perplexing issues in all of pragmatics. Consider the traditional account offered for the way in which a listener comprehends an indirect speech act. How might one recognize that "It sure is hot out" is a request to share the listener's lemonade? The traditional view assumes that listeners first compute a direct, literal reading of the sentence based on their knowledge of the form and content of English. Listeners then decide that this literal reading violates a rule of conversation that can be roughly paraphrased as "Don't tell people what they already know" (Abbeduto et al., 1989). Because listeners assume that speakers adhere to this rule, listeners conclude that the speaker of "It sure is hot" must have some other interpretation in mind. Listeners then use the context of the utterance to arrive at the indirect interpretation. In fact, there is considerable evidence that listeners, including young children and individuals with developmental disabilities (Abbeduto et al., 1988; Abbeduto, Nuccio, Al-Mabuk, Rotto, & Maas, 1992), use context in the process of speech act comprehension. But there is also a considerable amount of psychological activity that is ignored or trivialized using this traditional account. For example, it fails to consider how listeners identify the relevant context and integrate it in real time with information derived from the speaker's utterance.

The third problem with the competence-based approach is that explaining regularities in language use by reference to well-defined, deterministic categories and rules obscures the fact that many of these regularities owe their origins to constraints on human behavior and social interaction, rather than to some independently acquired pragmatic knowledge (Prideaux, 1991). Perhaps the most obvious example of this is the rule that speakers typically take turns at talking. Speakers most likely adhere to this rule not to ensure that the resulting discourse is well-formed relative to some discourse standard but rather because of the difficulty of talking and listening at the same time given limited attentional resources (Craig, 1995). Calling a regularity in language use a pragmatic rule is at best misleading and at worst diverts attention from important questions about the origins of these regularities or the absence of such regularities in the behavior of children and youth with developmental disabilities.

The fact that pragmatics may involve regularities that are not describable in terms of traditional rules and categories raises important issues for those concerned with assessment and intervention in children and youth who have disabilities. If not categories and rules, what should be assessed and taught? The next section considers this issue further. Worth noting here, however, is that assessment and intervention must consider all of the linguistic and nonlinguistic sources of information that speakers and listeners use during communication as well as the ways in which their use of that information is constrained by the cognitive, linguistic, and social resources available to them (Abbeduto et al., 2001).

Unit of Analysis

In the traditional view, the unit of analysis is the *utterance*,[1] and each utterance of interest is analyzed to determine whether it displays properties that make for well-formed, coherent, or otherwise *acceptable* discourse. Here are three examples of this approach:

- In the area of referential communication, interest has focused mainly on whether speakers include in each utterance all the information necessary for listeners to identify the intended referent (Whitehurst & Sonnenschein, 1985).
- In the study of speech acts, considerable effort has been devoted to determining whether each utterance of interest expresses an identifiable speech act and the relative rates of different speech acts (Ninio & Snow, 1996).
- In the area of topic skills, researchers have studied whether (and to what degree) each utterance of interest is on- or off-topic (Brinton & Fujiki, 1989).

---

[1]Although the definition of an utterance is frequently vague, it typically corresponds to a linguistic unit of varying size but is no larger than a sentence.

This traditional view can be thought of as a product approach. It is based on the assumption that a linguistic interaction is simply a collection of utterances and that the utterances can be evaluated using criteria that are independent of the participants, their objectives, and the process of generating the utterances (Clark, 1996).

Clark (1996) proposed an alternative, collaborative, process-oriented model of linguistic interaction that emphasizes multiple units of analysis, performance over competence, and regularities over rules. In Clark's model, the participants have a shared goal and collaborate to achieve that goal. The goal may be as narrow as wanting to make a purchase in a store or as general as wanting to reminisce about the past. Achieving the goal often requires addressing various subgoals along the way (e.g., gaining the store clerk's attention before one can make a purchase). When collaborating, each participant engages in behaviors that represent a step toward the goal, and this requires that each participant's behavior is contingent on the behavior and needs of the other participant. Examples of the types of goal-directed, contingent behaviors in which participants engage include

- Checking on background assumptions held by the other participants (e.g., "Did you ever bake cookies before?" as a prelude to an episode of baking)
- Soliciting and providing feedback concerning the ways in which each other's utterances have been interpreted (e.g., "Do you know the one I mean?" or "Which cookie cutter?")
- Initiating and completing exchanges that bring the talk closer toward achievement of the goal (e.g., asking or answering a question)
- Evaluating the knowledge that is shared and tailoring one's utterances and interpretations accordingly (e.g., using the pronoun *it* only after its referent has been introduced)

The collaborative model leads us away from an exclusive concern with utterances and their static, context-independent properties and toward the collaborative behaviors and the discourse goals that motivate them. Focusing on goal-directed collaboration, however, necessitates a consideration of units of analysis other than the utterance. This can be seen by considering the collaborative view of reference making, speech acts, and topic organization.

In the collaborative view, establishing a speaker's intended referents is more complicated than in the traditional view. Establishing referents is typically accomplished over a number of successive speaker and listener utterances (Wilkes-Gibbs & Clark, 1992). The speaker first evaluates the knowledge shared with the listener and thereby identifies the types of utterances that are likely to be effective vehicles for reference making. The speaker also may engage in more overt preparatory behaviors, such as gaining the listener's attention or directing attention to a particular entity or location, before producing the referential utterance. Once the utterance has been produced, the listener must provide evidence of understanding the speaker's intent (e.g., by acknowledging it or by requesting clarification). The speaker may need to make revisions in the original utterance or provide additional information that will evoke further feedback from the listener, and so on. Moreover, speakers and listeners use the physical, linguistic, and social context in which each utterance is embedded as a source of information for establishing the intended referents (Ackerman, Szymanski, & Silver, 1990). In studying reference making, therefore, the unit of analysis is the referential sequence of collaborative behaviors (e.g., attempts to solicit or provide feedback on comprehension) and context-use behaviors (e.g., "filling in" missing information with context).

The collaborative view of speech acts also focuses on sequences of utterances rather than on isolated utterances. When making requests, for example, speakers often precede their requests with utterances designed to establish whether the ultimate request is likely to be successful (Levinson, 1983; Schegloff, 1990). For example, before uttering the request "Could I have a piece of chocolate?" a speaker might check on the availability of the desired object with "Is there any chocolate left?" These preparatory utterances, or pre-requests, often are sufficient to solicit compliance from the listener without the speaker even making the request (e.g., "Is there any chocolate left?" is quite transparent as to the nature of the forthcoming request, which may enable the addressee to preempt the request with a response such as "Would you like some?"). In other instances, these pre-requests may lead to extended sequences in which the listener may attempt to block the speaker's issuing of the request (e.g., the addressee might respond to "Is there any chocolate left?" with something such as "What chocolate?" or "You're not hungry already, are you?"). In all such sequences, listeners use their shared knowledge and the context to interpret utterances (Abbeduto & Benson, 1992). In the case of speech acts, therefore, the collaborative view leads to an examination of sequences of utterances (or speech acts), the use of context for expressing and interpreting utterances, and collaborative behaviors (including various listener responses that anticipate or block subsequent speech acts).

In the area of topic skills, there is considerable evidence that the link between utterances has less to do with a topic than with the goal that motivates the discourse in the first place. Achieving one's goals often requires addressing a number of subgoals, and these subgoals and the utterances produced to accomplish them may not be linked in any obvious semantic way (Schegloff, 1990). Consider, for example, the following pair of utterances, each of which is uttered by a different speaker.

Speaker 1:   How's that beautiful house of yours?
Speaker 2:   Did you know that Mary and I separated?

In this sequence, the second speaker's utterance is not a semantically contingent response to the first speaker's question let alone on the topic of "that beautiful house." Nevertheless, the utterance is appropriate for the goal of the conversation (i.e., to catch up) and as a prelude to further discussion about the topic (e.g., perhaps the second speaker no longer lives in the house in question). Thus, utterances that are off-topic compared to the previous utterance may well be seen as appropriate by the conversational participants and may help to move the interaction toward the goal. In the collaborative view, then, utterances should be evaluated not for their adherence to the topic of a prior utterance but rather for their utility in achieving the goal that motivates the interaction.

In summary, we promote the study of collaborative, context-dependent pragmatic behaviors and their sequential organization. In our view, the focus of pragmatic assessment and intervention for children and youth with disabilities should not be on well-defined, deterministic pragmatic categories, rules, or products. Rather, assessment and intervention should focus on the process of communication and behaviors such as checking on background assumptions, tracking and evaluating shared knowledge, soliciting and providing feedback concerning comprehension, and initiating and completing exchanges that accomplish tasks that bring the participants closer to their goal.

PRAGMATIC DEVELOPMENT: CONTEXT AND COLLABORATION

This section elaborates on the collaborative process model of communication and illustrates the ways in which it can inform researchers about the communicative performance of immature language users. The section begins by considering the importance of context in the process of communication and how context influences children's comprehension and expression of language and the ways in which context is represented. The section then reviews what is known about the development of some key collaborative behaviors.

Contextual Influences on Communication

The idea that the context of a linguistic interaction influences the behavior of the participants in important ways has long been recognized (e.g., Sperber & Wilson, 1986). In the collaborative process model, participants must produce utterances that are appropriate for the goal of the exchange and for the point in the interaction at which they occur (i.e., they must be contingent). Participants must interpret the utterances they hear relative to the goal and the information that has been shared to that point in the exchange (Clark, 1996). In short, the decisions that language users make must be contextually sensitive (Abbeduto & Rosenberg, 1992).

Considerable research on typically developing children has shown that even during the toddler and preschool years, many decisions about language use are contextually constrained. Research has revealed that preschoolers tailor their utterances according to the age of their listeners. For example, they produce shorter, syntactically simpler utterances when speaking to a younger child than when speaking to a peer or an adult (Shatz & Gelman, 1973). They also are more likely to use politeness markers (e.g., "please") and syntactically indirect forms (e.g., "May I?") to make requests for objects or actions when addressing adults than when addressing peers or younger children (e.g., Camras, Pristo, & Brown, 1985). These adjustments are not based solely on simple associations between particular language forms and the physical markers of age. Instead, these adjustments are motivated by assumptions about differences in the ability and authority of adults and children (Abbeduto, 1984; Sonnenschein, 1986).

Preschoolers also formulate their utterances in ways that are sensitive to the *history* they share with their listener. For example, they provide more detail and make less use of pronouns when retelling an event for listeners who have no previous knowledge of the event than for listeners who witnessed the event with them (Menig-Peterson, 1975). They also provide less information to listeners whom they know well than to less familiar listeners (Sonnenschein, 1986). They are more polite when making a request of an unfamiliar listener than of a familiar one (Ervin-Tripp, Guo, & Lampert, 1990).

Comprehension, as well as expression, shows signs of being contextually constrained during the preschool years. For example, 3-year-olds can use a speaker's previous utterances (Shatz, 1978) as context for deciding among alternative interpretations of the sentences they hear. Preschoolers can even use the relative spatial positions of the speaker and listener as context, as demonstrated by the finding that they interpret a sentence such as "Would you like to play on the bike?" as a request for the addressee to do the action named if the speaker and addressee are facing each other but not if the addressee is instead facing the object named (Reeder & Wakefield, 1987). In fact, even 2-year-olds sometimes use context to make decisions about the intended meaning of a sentence (Shatz & McCloskey, 1984).

Despite the sensitivity of typically developing preschoolers to context, there is much they need to learn. Their use of context is often limited to information that is explicitly stated or otherwise immediately perceptible. They are less likely to use information that must be inferred from socially constructed categories. In a study by Ackerman and colleagues (1990), for example, even kindergarten children were poor compared with older children and adults at interpreting ambiguous referential expressions, such as "Go get that gift we bought," in accordance with the age or gender of the recipient of the object referred to by the speaker. Moreover, preschoolers and even older children sometimes engage in only a cursory analysis of the context, as when they assume that other people share all the contextual information that they themselves possess (Ackerman et al., 1990). In other instances, however, preschoolers may be overly sensitive to context and thereby fail to conduct the requisite linguistic analyses of the utterances they hear, as when they interpret a garbled or incomplete utterance as a request simply because the speaker and addressee are facing each other, something that older children and adults are reluctant to do (e.g., Reeder & Wakefield, 1987). In short, the task of learning to use context begins early and develops gradually over the course of the preschool years and beyond (Abbeduto, Short-Meyerson, Benson, Dolish, & Weissman, 1998).

The development of context use has important implications for understanding and treating the language problems of children and youth with disabilities. Inappropriate or immature uses of language in social interaction may reflect 1) a failure to process relevant contextual information or 2) a failure to recognize its implications for language expression and comprehension. There is considerable evidence that people with mental retardation are delayed (relative to chronological age expectations) in all aspects of context use examined to date (e.g., Abbeduto, 1984; Abbeduto, Davies, & Furman, 1988; Abbeduto, Davies, Solesby, & Furman, 1991; Abbeduto et al., 1998; Bliss, 1985; Nuccio & Abbeduto, 1993; Oetting & Rice, 1991). Therefore, targeting context use in assessment and intervention for this population is important. Unfortunately, with the exception of a few highly specialized language processing tasks (e.g., comprehension of idioms; Ezell & Goldstein, 1991), procedures for including context use in assessment or intervention have yet to be developed (Rosenberg & Abbeduto, 1993).

Problems in context use could also lead to a failure to demonstrate mastery of particular lexical items or syntactic forms during an assessment or to generalize a trained item or form beyond the training setting. This situation can occur if the individual with developmental disabilities fails to recognize the assessment or intervention situation as a relevant context for using communication skills that are in his or her repertoire. In the case of assessment, this means that a language form of interest must be evoked or prompted in a variety of contexts that are representative of its typical occurrence. In the case of intervention, this fact means that a language form should be taught along with discriminations of the contexts that are appropriate and inappropriate for its use (Rosenberg & Abbeduto, 1993). Determining whether contextual factors are eliciting problem behaviors that inhibit or preclude appropriate language behaviors on the part of the individual with developmental disabilities may also be necessary (Horner, 1994).

Scripts as Generalized Contexts for Language Use

At first glance, the diverse situations in which people use language make explaining the apparent ease with which people use context difficult, but the diversity may be more apparent than real. Many of the contexts in which people use language are quite routine and predictable. Consider, for example, the many similarities across different occasions of eating dinner at a restaurant. Patrons typically wait to be seated. A member of the wait staff greets them and shows them to a table. Someone else brings a menu, returns to take their order, and so on. Even a more *natural* conversation with a friend typically unfolds in a fairly predictable manner. Greetings are followed by "catching up" talk (i.e., a sharing of news about families or mutual friends), future meetings or events are planned, and then the conversation comes to a close with various linguistic expressions of departure. Such examples are not intended to dismiss the impressive psychological work that occurs during any social interaction. Instead, the point is that the contexts of language use do not vary infinitely. There are important regularities across contexts. Language users can exploit these regularities to make the task of language expression and comprehension manageable, provided that they are able to detect the regularities. In fact, considerable evidence reveals that language users of all ages do so, and these representations of the routine aspects of events have been referred to as scripts (Schank & Abelson, 1977).

A *script* is a schema for a familiar, repeatedly experienced event in which people interact with each other or act on objects to achieve some goal (Goodman, Duchan, & Sonnenmeier, 1994; Mandler, 1984). Like other forms of schematic representation, scripts are hierarchically organized and general in form (Goodman et al., 1994; Nelson, 1986).

Scripts are organized temporally and causally, which distinguishes them from other forms of schematic representation (Eiser, Eiser, & Lang, 1989; Ross & Berg, 1990; Slackman, Hudson, & Fivush, 1986). Scripts tie together the various elements of the event (Hudson, Fivush, & Kuebli, 1992; Nelson & Gruendel, 1981, 1986; Ross & Berg, 1990). Because of this wholeness, they involve expectations that direct aspects of cognitive processing, such as inference making, comprehension, and prediction of upcoming activities or behaviors (Abelson, 1981; Bianco & Tiberghien, 1991). This allows one to induce, and reason about, new information (Goodman et al., 1994).

Although young children organize their knowledge of events into scripts similar to adults (Duchan, 1991; Fivush & Slackman, 1986; French, 1986; Nelson & Gruendel, 1981, 1986), their scripts are typically skeletal in form compared with those of adults (Hudson et al., 1992). As children develop, their scripts become more elaborate (McCartney & Nelson, 1981; Nelson, 1986; Nelson & Gruendel, 1986). The fact that children's scripts are incomplete may influence their use of language in social interaction in two ways. First, incomplete scripts provide an impoverished context within which to make decisions about language use and, thus, limit one's ability to engage in effective collaboration. Second, incomplete scripts guarantee that the child will encounter *new* information when participating in an event. Because new information requires effortful processing, fewer cognitive resources will be available for planning talk and processing the talk of others. Thus, collaboration will be adversely affected by incomplete script knowledge.

In fact, there is considerable evidence that the completeness of children's scripts can influence their participation in social interaction in fairly dramatic ways (Chapman et al., 1992). Nelson and colleagues (Nelson & Greundel, 1979; Nelson & Seidman, 1984) examined preschoolers' spontaneous social play and found that interactions based on routine events were longer, more structurally complex, and included more participant agreement as to goals than did interactions not focused on routine events. Independent assessments of preschool and young school-age children's script knowledge also have been found to predict their linguistic performance when enacting those events with other children during play. Furman and Walden (1990) found that dyads of 3- to 5-year-olds who were enacting routine events took more speaking turns and were more likely to respond appropriately to their partner's obligating turns (e.g., questions) when both members of the dyad were highly familiar with the script for the event than when neither member was familiar with the script. In another study of enactments of routine events during dyadic play, Short-Meyerson (1997; Short-Meyerson & Abbeduto, 1997) found that topic maintenance and comprehension (as reflected by noncomprehension signaling) were better when both members of the dyad had substantial knowledge of the script for the event than when only one member of the dyad had such knowledge. Thus, many linguistic dimensions of social interaction are constrained by script completeness.

This research on scripts has two implications for understanding and treating the language and communication problems of children and youth with developmental disabilities. First, it raises the possibility that at least some of the communication problems experienced by children and youth with developmental disabilities are due to problems in acquiring and using effective scripts for the events in their lives. For example, these individuals might have cognitive limitations that require more exposure to routine events before they are able to construct a complete script compared with their typically developing peers. Moreover, unique life experiences (e.g., placement in special classes) may limit their exposure to important social events and may even result in development of atypical scripts. Second, a particularly vexing problem for language intervention is the often noted failure of children and youth with developmental disabilities to generalize trained language skills beyond the therapeutic setting (Rosenberg & Abbeduto, 1993). The research on scripts implies that this failure to generalize may reflect, in part, deficits in script knowledge. Particularly relevant in this regard would be deficits stemming from a lack of knowledge of how to integrate new language skills into the routine event. Generalization of new language skills might also be limited if the individual with developmental disabilities must devote too many cognitive resources to processing other, nonlinguistic, aspects of ongoing events.

In light of these implications, assessment and intervention for children and youth with developmental disabilities should target script knowledge. Procedures for assessing script knowledge have been outlined by Duchan (1991) and Westby (1980, 1988). Techniques for improving children's scripts have been developed by a number of investigators (Goldstein & Cisar, 1992; Goldstein, Wickstrom, Hoyson, Jamieson, & Odom, 1988; Robertson & Weismer, 1997).

Collaborative Behaviors

In the collaborative process approach to communication, the participants are seen as engaging in at least two types of language behaviors that ensure that they arrive at "a meeting of the minds" (i.e., establish shared knowledge). First, the participants try to make explicit the relevant background knowledge that they share with each other at the outset. Before launching into a story about a fellow student, for example, the speaker might try to determine whether the audience knows the student (e.g., "Do you know Bill from Mrs. Jones' class?"). These background-checking behaviors allow the speaker to shape the story in ways suited to the audience and may even eliminate the need for the story altogether. Second, participants engage in a process that Clark (1996) referred to as grounding. In grounding, the listener provides the speaker with feedback about the way in which his or her utterances have been interpreted. In many cases, grounding is achieved by explicit linguistic signals. For example, a listener, may respond to "Joe did it again" with "Did what?" if unclear about the speaker's intent or with "Oh no!" if confident about the interpretation. In some cases, however, grounding may be achieved nonlinguistically (e.g., through an "approving" nod of the head). Failure to engage in such background-checking or grounding behaviors will all but ensure that the participants will fail to understand each other.

Typically developing toddlers and preschoolers have been found to engage in several behaviors designed to check on shared background knowledge and to ground their utterances. Short-Meyerson and Abbeduto (1997) found that when 4- to 5-year-olds enact familiar events (e.g., baking cookies), they solicit information about their partner's script for the event (e.g., "Ever bake cookies before?") and provide information about the extensiveness of their own scripts (e.g., "I know how to mix the dough"). They also use these behaviors in contextually appropriate ways; for example, they are more likely to provide and solicit script-based information when they or their partner has an incomplete script for the event than when they both have complete scripts (Short-Meyerson & Abbeduto, 1997). In addition, children as young as 2 years of age signal noncomprehension of their partner's messages (Revelle, Wellman, & Karabenick, 1985; Shatz & O'Reilly, 1990) and respond to such signals from others (Anslemi, Tomasello, & Acunzo, 1986; Brinton, Fujiki, Winkler, & Loeb, 1986) at least under some circumstances.

Despite the early emergence of behaviors for establishing shared knowledge, these behaviors are used in rather limited ways by preschoolers. Short-Meyerson (1997) found that younger dyads of preschoolers were less likely than older ones to solicit and provide information about their script knowledge at appropriate points during script-based play. In addition, preschoolers are more likely to respond to some types of noncomprehension signals from their partners (e.g., a nonspecific request for repetition, such as "What?") than to other types (e.g., a request for specification, such as "Which cookie?"), and not all of their responses supply the information sought (Gallagher, 1981). Even school-age children do not signal noncomprehension of all types of incomprehensible messages (Abbeduto, Short-Meyerson, Benson, &

Dolish, 1997; Lempers & Elrod, 1983; Revelle et al., 1985). In fact, the ability to engage in effective collaboration continues to develop well into adolescence (Anderson, Clark, & Mullin, 1994; Ricard, 1993).

The fact that behaviors for establishing shared knowledge play a critical role in linguistic interaction has important implications for assessing and treating the language problems of children and youth with developmental disabilities. In particular, language problems displayed in social interaction by these individuals may reflect not a lack of the requisite linguistic tools but rather a failure to recognize how such tools can be used to facilitate collaboration or even that there is a need for collaboration. Although there has been only limited research on collaborative behaviors in people with developmental disabilities, the evidence to date suggests that they have delays (relative to chronological age expectations) in at least grounding (Abbeduto et al., 1991; Abbeduto et al., 1997, 1998; Ezell & Goldstein, 1991; Fujiki & Brinton, 1993). Procedures for assessing and treating delays in linguistic collaboration, however, are limited. An exception is an attempt by Ezell and Goldstein (1991) to teach children with developmental disabilities to monitor their comprehension and to ask for clarification when processing idiomatic expressions.

CONSTRAINTS ON CONTEXT USE AND COLLABORATION

In the collaborative process model, there is not a one-to-one correspondence between particular language forms and particular components or elements of collaboration. Instead, collaboration is seen as a process that requires flexible, goal-directed use of language forms. Collaboration is motivated and shaped by a variety of linguistic, cognitive, and social skills (see Abbeduto, 1991; Abbeduto & Hesketh, 1997). The implication for assessment and intervention is that understanding and treating the causes of communication problems in children and youth with developmental disabilities requires attention to far more than just language. Next, we consider the connections between language use in social interaction and the various capabilities on which it draws; namely, speech and language production and comprehension skills, cognitive skills, and interpersonal abilities are considered.

Speech and Language

There is no doubt that successful participation in social interaction requires knowledge of the forms and contents of language as well as the ability to have access to that knowledge as needed during speaking and listening. After all, language is the principal tool by which people communicate with each other (Abbeduto & Hesketh, 1997; Clark, 1996). Children and youth with developmental disabilities typically have not acquired the speech and language tools expected for their ages (Rosenberg & Abbeduto, 1993). Because they have fewer tools, their participation in the collaborative process will be limited, as well. For example, if one has not acquired the morphological form for marking the past tense of verbs, talking about past events is decidedly more difficult than when that form has been mastered. Speech and language problems, however, may influence communication and its development in more indirect ways, as well.

Individuals with serious impairments in the processes involved in speaking, for example, may adopt approaches to interaction to circumvent those impairments—patterns that may be less than optimal for their long-term developmental progress. Rice (1993) reported that children with specific language impairments who produced speech of low intelligibility often produced short responses to the initiations of their partners. They also were more likely to direct their initiations to adults rather than to peers. Short or minimal responses may reflect an attempt to *speak no more than necessary* either because of physical difficulties or because spoken communication leads to negative reactions from others (e.g., looks of confusion, teasing). Initiations to adults may be more likely to be successful because adults are more skilled in constructing the meaning of low intelligibility messages than are other children. Whatever the motivation, however, this approach to interaction is likely to decrease the already tenuous standing of these individuals among their typical peers (Rice, 1993).

Abbeduto and his colleagues (1998) found that among children and adolescents with mental retardation, individuals with poorer expressive language skills (measured in terms of lexical diversity, mean length of utterance, and intelligibility) were more likely to guess at the intended referent of ambiguous messages rather than signal noncomprehension. Also important, even the participants with the most limited expressive skills could be assumed to have mastered the linguistic forms needed to signal noncomprehension (e.g., "Which one?"). Abbeduto and colleagues argued that their participants were using a nonverbal response strategy similar to the one observed by Rice (1993). They suggested that although this strategy may have at first reflected an attempt to participate in communication despite limited linguistic and articulatory skills, it persisted even after the requisite skills had been acquired.

Communication is affected not only by the ability of the individual with a developmental disability to express language forms and contents but also by the ways in which he or she approaches the task of understanding language. This is suggested by the results of a recent study involving children and adolescents with mental retardation. In this study, Abbeduto and his colleagues (1997) found that scores on the Test for Reception of Grammar (TROG) (Bishop, 1982) predicted (i.e., were correlated with) the use of noncomprehension signals in response to nominally ambiguous referential expressions. In the TROG, the participant is required to select the one picture from four that matches the meaning of a word, phrase, or sentence spoken by the examiner. In interpreting the correlation observed in this study, one should note that all of the participants had the receptive skills needed to construct a syntactic-semantic representation of the problematic referential expressions, as demonstrated by their ability to respond correctly to linguistically identical but unambiguous versions of the referential expressions. Abbeduto, Short-Meyerson, et al. (1997) suggested that the correlation reflected the fact that both tasks—noncomprehension signaling and the TROG—require an analysis of the match between a spoken message and a set of potential referents. Individuals who are impulsive or unsystematic in their analysis of the message–potential referent match tend to do poorly on both tasks, whereas those who are more systematic in their analysis tend to do well.

It is important to note that individuals with limited language skills may be able to overcome these limitations and communicate effectively in a variety of contexts (Rosenberg & Abbeduto, 1993). Abbeduto, Davies, and Furman (1988) and Abbeduto, Davies, et al. (1991) offered examples of individuals with mental retardation displaying communication in advance of their linguistic skills. Such asynchronies may be possible because communication involves the use of nonlinguistic tools (e.g., eye gaze, gesture) as well as linguistic tools (Clark, 1996). Nonverbal compensatory strategies, such as those described previously, may be effective in some instances, as well. In addition, many everyday communicative tasks often can be completed quite effectively when using only simple language. Consequently, impairments in more complex domains of syntax and the like may have a limited impact on performance (Abbeduto & Rosenberg, 1992). Finally, because communication draws on many domains of expertise beyond the purely linguistic, the impact of impairments in the linguistic domain may be offset by strengths elsewhere in the psychological systems that support communication (e.g., cognition).

Cognition

The collaborative process model presupposes that cognitive skills (e.g., memory) are intimately involved in each and every instance of communication. In this model, communication is conceptualized as a real-time, probabilistic process of collaboration that requires the flexible use of language in ways that are sensitive to the dynamic network of shared knowledge and context that evolves during interaction. This process inevitably will be constrained by the knowledge of the world that the participants can bring to bear on the interaction and on the integrity and efficiency of the information processing systems available to them. The cognitive impairments that define mental retardation ensure that individuals with mental retardation will experience problems in communication relative to chronological age expectations (Abbeduto & Hesketh, 1997). In fact, communicative performance has been found to conform more closely to mental age (measured by nonverbal means) than to chronological age expectations in dozens of studies involving numerous aspects of linguistic communication with individuals of varying ages and severity of intellectual impairments (Abbeduto & Rosenberg, 1992).

In assessing and treating the communication problems of people with developmental disabilities, therefore, recognizing three ways in which their cognitive impairments may contribute to these problems is especially important. First, people with developmental disabilities will have more limited knowledge about the world compared with their typically developing peers. Thus, they will be making decisions about language within a less rich and informative context. For example, individuals with mental retardation are slower to construct social categories such as *male, female, adult,* and *child* over the course of development. This limits their ability to exploit these categories when making inferences about a speaker's intended referents (Abbeduto et al., 1991; Abbeduto et al., 1998). They also know less about objects and how they can act on those objects. This limits their ability to exploit this knowledge when deciding among alternative speech acts for the sentences they hear (Abbeduto et al., 1988). They also have difficulty benefiting from repeated exposure to recurring events and stimuli (Merrill, Goodwyn, & Gooding, 1996). Thus, they will have less detailed scripts for events that may be the topics of conversation. Treating the communication problems of individuals with developmental disabilities, therefore, will require attention to their knowledge base, particularly their understanding of recurring events in their daily lives.

Second, children and youth with developmental disabilities are likely to have fewer cognitive resources available to them and be less skilled in recruiting and directing those resources effectively (Merrill et al., 1996). Although such limitations are likely to have pervasive influences on communication, their effects will be greatest at those points in the interaction, or in those contexts, associated with the greatest cognitive demands. For example, Evans and her colleagues (Craig &

Evans, 1993; Evans, 1996) have shown that transitions between speaking turns are particularly cognitively demanding and that children with specific language impairment and limited expressive language capabilities are more likely to make grammatical errors in utterances at those transitions than in utterances that are *turn internal*. Evans also found such errors to be more frequent when the social demands were greatest (e.g., when the child was oriented toward rather than away from the partner). The implication for assessment is that the use of language should be sampled across a range of conditions varying in processing demands. Capacity limitations could be targeted in intervention by teaching individuals to make more effective use of the resources they have available. Alternatively, these limitations could be circumvented by using various prosthetics, or supports, such as verbal or visual reminders of the range of acceptable responses or interpretations for a particular discourse context (Whitehurst & Sonnenschein, 1985).

Third, there is considerable variability among individuals with developmental disabilities in the severity of their cognitive impairments (Rosenberg & Abbeduto, 1993). Moreover, research has documented that there also is variability in the profile of impairments across cognitive processes and that this variability is related to etiology. For example, individuals with Down syndrome typically display more severe impairments in auditory short-term memory than in visual short-term memory (Marcell & Weeks, 1988; Wang & Bellugi, 1994). Individuals with fragile X syndrome have greater difficulty in processing sequential information than in processing simultaneous information (Abbeduto & Hagerman, 1997; Dykens, Hodapp, & Leckman, 1994; Hagerman, 1999). Such variations in profiles of cognitive impairments will likely lead to different communicative impairments, as well. Assessment and intervention for children and youth with developmental disabilities will need to take account of these and other cognitive sources of variability in communication (Abbeduto & Hesketh, 1997).

Interpersonal Cognition

The process of communication involves two or more people arriving at a *meeting of the minds*. This notion is embodied in Clark's (1996) collaborative process model. Each participant in a linguistic interaction collaborates by making and interpreting contributions to conversations according to the knowledge that he or she shares and the goal of the interaction. Some of this shared knowledge is stated explicitly during the course of the interaction, but much of it must be inferred. For example, in deciding how much detail to provide when giving location directions, a speaker considers whether the listener is a "native" to the locale and, thus, familiar with important landmarks (Clark, 1996). Similarly, a preschooler who engages in child-directed language (i.e., the simplified register used for speaking to young children) when interacting with an unfamiliar toddler (Shatz & Gelman, 1973) may be making inferences about the informational needs and capabilities of younger children. In short, communication depends on the ability to understand and evaluate other people's beliefs, desires, and intentions, or what has been referred to as a *theory of mind* (Frith, 1996).

Since the 1990s, there has been considerable research on typically developing children's acquisition of a theory of mind (e.g., Baron-Cohen, Tager-Flusberg, & Cohen, 1994). This research has shown that although infants evidence surprisingly sophisticated understanding of intentionality and other processes subsumed by a theory of mind, achieving a mature theory of mind is a gradual and protracted process that continues into the school years and beyond. This raises the possibility that individuals with developmental disabilities may be slow to acquire a theory of mind and that the delay, in turn, will negatively affect their communication. In fact, a number of investigators have sought to determine to what extent the communication and social problems that define autism are a manifestation of delays in acquiring a theory of mind (Frith, 1996).

Evidence is beginning to accumulate that other developmental disabilities in addition to autism are associated with impairments in theory of mind. Children and adolescents with mental retardation of non-specific etiology have been found to do more poorly on false belief and other theory of mind tasks than expected for their chronological ages (e.g., Garner, Callias, & Turk, 1999; Tager-Flusberg & Sullivan, 1994a, 1994b) and in some instances even for their mental ages (Benson, Abbeduto, Short, Nuccio, & Maas, 1993). There also is evidence of differences in the extensiveness of theory of the mind impairments across different mental retardation syndromes (Abbeduto et al., in press). Correlations between theory of mind impairments and some aspects of communication, such as requesting confirmation of a referent choice (e.g., "You mean the blue one?"), have been observed for individuals with mental retardation, as well (Abbeduto et al., 1998). Such findings suggest that language assessment and intervention for children and youth with developmental disabilities must pay attention to the ways in which impairments in interpersonal cognition constrain communication.

CONCLUSION

Communication is a process of collaboration. It entails the flexible and goal-directed use of language in a way that is sensitive to, and builds on, the shared knowledge of the participants. This view implies that assessment and intervention should

- Recognize the intimate connection between language use and language form and content
- Focus on units and regularities that are not necessarily concordant with traditional linguistic categories (e.g., sentence or even utterance) or pragmatic rules (e.g., one speaker at a time)
- Focus on behaviors that allow individuals to establish shared knowledge, such as background checking and grounding
- Consider the role of context in language performance, with particular attention to recurring, or scripted, contexts of language use
- Attend not only to the linguistic tools available to individuals, but also to the ways in which they adapt to linguistic limitations and to the strategies they bring to the task of language understanding
- Consider how the communicative process is shaped by knowledge of the world, information processing capacity limitations, and interpersonal knowledge

Adherence to these and other implications of the collaborative view will require some dramatic changes in assessment and intervention practices. These changes, however, will lead to meaningful improvements in real-life social settings for children and youth with developmental disabilities.

REFERENCES

Abbeduto, L. (1984). Situational influences on mentally retarded and nonretarded children's production of directives. *Applied Psycholinguistics, 5,* 147–166.

Abbeduto, L. (1991). The development of verbal communication in persons with mild to moderate mental retardation. In N. Bray (Ed.), *International review of research in mental retardation* (pp. 91–115). San Diego: Academic Press.

Abbeduto, L., & Benson, G. (1992). Speech act development in nondisabled children and individuals with mental retardation. In R. Chapman (Ed.), *Processes in language acquisition and disorders* (pp. 257–278). St. Louis: Mosby.

Abbeduto, L., Davies, B., & Furman, L. (1988). The development of speech act comprehension in mentally retarded individuals and nonretarded children. *Child Development, 59,* 1460–1472.

Abbeduto, L., Davies, B., Solesby, S., & Furman, L. (1991). Identifying the referents of spoken messages: The use of context and clarification requests by children with and without mental retardation. *American Journal on Mental Retardation, 95,* 551–562.

Abbeduto, L., Evans, J., & Dolan, T. (2001). Theoretical perspectives on language and communication problems in mental retardation and developmental disabilities. *Mental Retardation and Developmental Disabilities Research Reviews, 1,* 45–55.

Abbeduto, L.. Furman, L., & Davies, B. (1989). Relation between the receptive language and mental age of persons with mental retardation. *American Journal on Mental Retardation, 93,* 535–543.

Abbeduto, L., & Hagerman, R. (1997). Language and communication in fragile X syndrome. *Mental Retardation and Developmental Disabilities Research Reviews, 3,* 313–322.

Abbeduto, L., & Hesketh, L.J. (1997). Pragmatic development in individuals with mental retardation: Learning to use language in social interactions. *Mental Retardation and Developmental Disabilities Research Reviews, 3,* 323–333.

Abbeduto, L., Nuccio, J., Al-Mabuk, R., Rotto, P., & Maas, F. (1992). Interpreting and responding to spoken language: Children's recognition and use of a speaker's goal. *Journal of Child Language, 19,* 677–693.

Abbeduto, L., Pavetto, M., Kesin, E., Weissman, M.D., Karodottir, S., O'Brien, A., & Cawthon, S. (in press). The language and cognitive profile of Down syndrome: Evidence from a comparison with fragile X syndrome. *Down Syndrome Research and Practice.*

Abbeduto, L., & Rosenberg, S. (1992). Linguistic communication in persons with mental retardation. In S.F. Warren & J. Reichle (Series & Vol. Eds.), *Communication and language intervention series: Vol. 1. Causes and effects in communication and language intervention* (pp. 331–359). Baltimore: Paul H. Brookes Publishing Co.

Abbeduto, L., Short-Meyerson, K., Benson, G., & Dolish, J. (1997). Signaling of noncomprehension by children and adolescents with mental retardation: Effects of problem type and speaker identity. *Journal of Speech, Language, and Hearing Research, 40,* 20–32.

Abbeduto, L., Short-Meyerson, K., Benson, G., Dolish, J., & Weissman, M. (1998). Understanding referential expressions: Use of common ground by children and adolescents with mental retardation. *Journal of Speech, Language, and Hearing Research, 41,* 348–362.

Abelson, R.P. (1981). Psychological status of the script concept. *American Psychologist, 36,* 715–729.

Ackerman, B.P., Szymanski, J., & Silver, D. (1990). Children's use of the common ground in interpreting ambiguous referential utterances. *Developmental Psychology, 26,* 234–245.

Anderson, A.H., Clark, A., & Mullin, J. (1994). Interactive communication between children: Learning how to make language work in dialogue. *Journal of Child Language, 21,* 439–464.

Anslemi, D., Tomasello, M., & Acunzo, M. (1986). Young children's responses to neutral and specific contingent queries. *Journal of Child Language, 13,* 135–144.

Baron-Cohen, S., Tager-Flusberg, H., & Cohen, D.J. (Eds.). (1994). *Understanding other minds: Perspectives from autism.* Oxford, England: Oxford University Press.

Benson, G., Abbeduto, L., Short, K., Nuccio, J.B., & Maas, F. (1993). Development of a theory of mind in persons with mental retardation. *American Journal on Mental Retardation, 98,* 427–433.

Bianco, M., & Tiberghien, G. (1991). Influence of script structure on reference resolution and concept recognition in 8- and 11-year-old children. *Cahiers de Psychologie Cognitive, 11,* 481–518.

Bishop, D. (1982). *Test for Reception of Grammar (TROG).* Unpublished test.

Bliss, L.S. (1985). The development of persuasive strategies by mentally retarded children. *Applied Research in Mental Retardation, 6,* 437–447.

Brinton, B., & Fujiki, M. (1989). *Conversational management with language-impaired children: Pragmatic assessment and intervention.* Gaithersburg, MD: Aspen Publishers.

Brinton, B., Fujiki, M., Winkler, E., & Loeb, D.F. (1986). Responses to requests for clarification in linguistically normal and language-impaired children. *Journal of Speech and Hearing Disorders, 51,* 370–378.

Brown, P., & Levinson, S.C. (1987). *Politeness: Some universals in language usage.* Cambridge, England: Cambridge University Press.

Camras, L.A., Pristo, T.M., & Brown, M.J.K. (1985). Directive choice by children and adults: Affect, situation, and linguistic politeness. *Merrill-Palmer Quarterly, 31,* 19–31.

Chapman, R.S., Streim, N.W., Crais, E.R., Salmon, D., Strand, E.A., & Negri, N.A. (1992). Child talk: Assumptions of a developmental process model for early language learning. In R.S. Chapman (Ed.), *Processes in language acquisition and disorders* (pp. 3–19). St. Louis: Mosby.

Clark, H.H. (1996). *Using language.* New York: Cambridge University Press.

Craig, H.K. (1995). Pragmatic impairments. In P. Fletcher & B. MacWhinney (Eds.), *The handbook of child language* (pp. 623–640). Oxford, England: Blackwell.

Craig, H.K., & Evans, J.L. (1993). Pragmatics and SLI: Within-group variations in discourse behaviors. *Journal of Speech and Hearing Research, 36,* 777–789.

Duchan, J. (1991). Everyday events: Their role in language assessment and intervention. In T. Gallagher (Ed.), *Pragmatics of language: Clinical practice issues* (pp. 43–98). San Diego: Singular Publishing Group.

Dykens, E.M., Hodapp, R.M., & Leckman, J.F. (1994). *Behavior and development in fragile X syndrome.* Thousand Oaks, CA: Sage Publications.

Eiser, C., Eiser, J.R., & Lang, J. (1989). Scripts in children's reports of medical events. *European Journal of Psychology of Education, 4,* 377–384.

Ervin-Tripp, S., Guo, J., & Lampert, M. (1990). Politeness and persuasion in children's control acts. *Journal of Pragmatics, 14,* 307–331.

Evans, J.L. (1996). SLI subgroups: Interaction between discourse constraints and morphosyntactic deficits. *Journal of Speech and Hearing Research, 39,* 655–660.

Ezell, H.K., & Goldstein, H. (1991). Observational learning of comprehension monitoring skills in children who exhibit mental retardation. *Journal of Speech and Hearing Research, 34,* 141–154.

Fivush, R., & Slackman, E. (1986). The acquisition and development of scripts. In K. Nelson (Ed.), *Event knowledge: Structure and function in development.* Mahwah, NJ: Lawrence Erlbaum Associates.

French, L.A. (1986). The language of events. In K. Nelson (Ed.), *Event knowledge: Structure and function in development* (pp. 119–136). Mahwah, NJ: Lawrence Erlbaum Associates.

Frith, U. (1996). Social communication and its disorder in autism and Asperger syndrome. *Journal of Psychopharmacology, 10,* 48–53.

Fujiki, M., & Brinton, B. (1993). Comprehension monitoring skills of adults with mental retardation. *Research in Developmental Disabilities, 14,* 409–421.

Furman, L.N., & Walden, T.A. (1990). Effects of script knowledge on preschool children's communicative interactions. *Developmental Psychology, 26,* 227–233.

Gallagher, T.M. (1981). Contingent query sequences within adult-child discourse. *Journal of Child Language, 8,* 51–62.

Garner, C., Callias, M., & Turk, J. (1999). Executive function and theory of mind performance of boys with fragile-X syndrome. *Journal of Intellectual Disability Research, 43,* 466–474.

Gibbs, R.W., Jr. (1983). Do people always process the literal meanings of indirect requests? *Journal of Experimental Psychology: Learning, Memory, and Cognition, 9,* 524–533.

Goldstein, H., & Cisar, C.L. (1992). Promoting interaction during sociodramatic play: Teaching scripts to typical preschoolers and classmates with disabilities. *Journal of Applied Behavior Analysis, 25,* 265–280.

Goldstein, H., Wickstrom, S., Hoyson, M., Jamieson, B., & Odom, S. (1988). Effects of sociodramatic script training on social and communicative interaction. *Education and Treatment of Children, 11,* 97–117.

Goodman, G.S., Duchan, J.F., & Sonnenmeier, R.M. (1994). Children's development of scriptal knowledge. In J.F. Duchan, L.E. Hewitt, & R.M. Sonnenmeier (Eds.), *Pragmatics: From theory to practice.* Upper Saddle River, NJ: Prentice-Hall.

Grice, H.P. (1975). Logic and conversation. In P. Cole & J.L. Morgan (Eds.), *Syntax and semantics: Speech acts* (pp. 41–58). San Diego: Academic Press.

Hagerman, R.J. (1999). Clinical and molecular aspects of fragile X syndrome. In H. Tager-Flusberg (Ed.), *Neurodevelopmental disorders* (pp. 27–42). Cambridge, MA: The MIT Press.

Horner, R.H. (1994). Functional assessment: Contributions and future directions. *Journal of Applied Behavior Analysis, 27,* 401–404.

Hudson, J.S., Fivush, R., & Kuebli, J. (1992). Scripts and episodes: The development of event memory. *Applied Cognitive Psychology, 6,* 483–505.

James, S.L. (1978). Effect of listener age and situation on the politeness of children's directives. *Journal of Psycholinguistic Research, 7,* 307–317.

Lempers, J.D., & Elrod, M.M. (1983). Children's appraisal of different sources of referential communicative inadequacies. *Child Development, 54,* 509–515.

Levinson, S.C. (1983). *Pragmatics.* Cambridge, England: Cambridge University Press.

Mandler, J.M. (1984). Scripts and scenes. In J.M. Mandler (Ed.), *Stories, scripts, and scenes: Aspects of schema theory.* Mahwah, NJ: Lawrence Erlbaum Associates.

Marcell, M.M., & Weeks, S.L. (1988). Short-term memory difficulties and Down's syndrome. *Journal of Mental Deficiency Research, 32,* 153–162.

McCartney, K.A., & Nelson, K. (1981). Children's use of scripts in story recall. *Discourse Processes, 4,* 59–70.

McTear, M.F., & Conti-Ramsden, G. (1992) *Pragmatic disability in children.* London: Whurr Publishers.

Menig-Peterson, C.L. (1975). The modification of communicative behavior in preschool-aged children as a function of the listener's perspective. *Child Development, 46,* 1015–1018.

Merrill, E., Goodwyn, E.H., & Gooding, H.L. (1996). Mental retardation and the acquisition of automatic processing. *American Journal on Mental Retardation, 101,* 49–62.

Nelson, K. (1986). *Event knowledge: Structure and function in development.* Mahwah, NJ: Lawrence Erlbaum Associates.

Nelson, K., & Gruendel, J.M. (1979). At morning it's lunchtime: A scriptal view of children's dialogues. *Discourse Processes, 2,* 73–94.

Nelson, K., & Gruendel, J. (1981). Generalized event representations: Basic building blocks of cognitive development. In M.E. Lamb & A.L. Brown (Eds.), *Advances in developmental psychology* (Vol. 1). Mahwah, NJ: Lawrence Erlbaum Associates.

Nelson, K., & Gruendel, J. (1986). Children's scripts. In K. Nelson (Ed.), *Event knowledge: Structure and function in development* (pp. 21–46). Mahwah, NJ: Lawrence Erlbaum Associates.

Nelson, K., & Seidman, S. (1984). Playing with scripts. In I. Bretherton (Ed.), *Symbolic play: The development of social understanding.* San Diego: Academic Press.

Ninio, A., & Snow, C.E. (1996). *Pragmatic development.* Boulder, CO: Westview Press.

Nuccio, J., & Abbeduto, L. (1993). Dynamic contextual variables and the directives of persons with mental retardation. *American Journal on Mental Retardation, 97,* 547–558.

Oetting, J.B., & Rice, M.L. (1991). Influence of the social context on pragmatic skills of adults with mental retardation. *American Journal on Mental Retardation, 95,* 435–443.

Prideaux, G.D. (1991). Syntactic form and textual rhetoric: The cognitive basis for certain pragmatic principles. *Journal of Pragmatics, 16,* 113–129.

Reeder, K., & Wakefield, J. (1987). The development of young children's speech act comprehension: How much language is necessary? *Applied Psycholinguistics, 8,* 1–18.

Revelle, G.L., Wellman, H.M., & Karabenick, J.D. (1985). Comprehension monitoring in preschool children. *Child Development, 56,* 654–663.

Ricard, R.J. (1993). Conversational coordination: Collaboration for effective communication. *Applied Psycholinguistics, 14,* 387–412.

Rice, M.L. (1993). "Don't talk to him; he's weird": A social consequences account of language and social interactions. In S.F. Warren & J. Reichle (Series Eds.) & A.P. Kaiser & D.B. Gray (Vol. Eds.), *Communication and language intervention series: Vol. 2. Enhancing children's communication: Research foundations for intervention* (pp. 139–158). Baltimore: Paul H. Brookes Publishing Co.

Robertson, S.B., & Weismer, S.E. (1997). The influence of peer models on the play scripts of children with specific language impairment. *Journal of Speech, Language, and Hearing Research, 40,* 49–61.

Rosenberg, S., & Abbeduto, L. (1993). *Language and communication in mental retardation: Development, processes, and intervention.* Mahwah, NJ: Lawrence Erlbaum Associates.

Ross, B.L., & Berg C.A. (1990). Individual differences in script reports: Implications for language assessment. *Topics in Language Disorders, 10,* 30–44.

Sacks, H., Schegloff, E., & Jefferson, G. (1974). A simplest systematics for the organization of turn-taking in conversation. *Language, 50,* 696–735.

Schank, R.C., & Abelson, R.P. (1977). *Scripts, plans, goals, and understanding.* Mahwah, NJ: Lawrence Erlbaum Associates.

Schegloff, E.A. (1990). On the organization of sequences as a source of "coherence" in talk-in-interaction. In B. Dorval (Ed.), *Conversational organization and its development* (pp. 51–77). Stamford, CT: Ablex Publishing.

Searle, J.R. (1975). Indirect speech acts. In P. Cole & J.L. Morgan (Eds), *Syntax and semantics* (Vol. 3, pp. 59–82). New York: Academic Press.

Shatz, M. (1978). On the development of communicative understandings: An early strategy for interpreting and responding to messages. *Cognitive Psychology, 10,* 271–301.

Shatz, M., & Gelman, R. (1973). The development of communication skills: Modifications in the speech of young children as a function of listener. *Monographs of the Society for Research in Child Development, 38* (No. 152).

Shatz, M., & McCloskey, L. (1984). Answering appropriately: A developmental perspective on conversational knowledge. In S. Kuczaj (Ed.), *Discourse development: Progress in cognitive development research* (pp. 20–36). New York: Springer-Verlag.

Shatz, M., & O'Reilly, A.W. (1990). Conversational or communicative skill? A reassessment of two-year-olds' behavior in miscommunication episodes. *Journal of Child Language, 17,* 131–146.

Short-Meyerson, K.J. (1997). *Preschoolers' establishment of mutual knowledge during script-based play.* Unpublished doctoral dissertation, University of Wisconsin–Madison.

Short-Meyerson, K., & Abbeduto, L. (1997). Preschoolers' communication during scripted interaction. *Journal of Child Language, 24,* 469–493.

Slackman, E.A., Hudson, J.A., & Fivush, R. (1986). Actions, actors, links and goals: The structure of children's event representations. In K. Nelson (Ed.), *Event knowledge: Structure and function in development.* Mahwah, NJ: Lawrence Erlbaum Associates.

Sonnenschein, S. (1986). Development of referential communication: Deciding that a message is uninformative. *Developmental Psychology, 22,* 164–168.

Sperber, D., & Wilson, D. (1986). *Relevance: Communication and cognition.* Cambridge, MA: Harvard University Press.

Tager-Flusberg, H., & Sullivan, K. (1994a). Predicting and explaining behavior: A comparison of autistic, mentally retarded and normal children. *Journal of Child Psychology and Psychiatry, 35,* 1059–1075.

Tager-Flusberg, H., & Sullivan, K. (1994b). A second look at second-order belief attribution in autism. *Journal of Autism and Developmental Disorders, 24,* 577–586.

Wang, W.P., & Bellugi, U. (1994). Evidence from two genetic syndromes for a dissociation between verbal and visual-spatial short-term memory. *Journal of Clinical and Experimental Neuropsychology, 16,* 317–322.

Westby, C.E. (1980). Assessment of cognitive and language abilities through play. *Language, Speech, and Hearing Services in Schools, 11,* 154–168.

Westby, C.E. (1988). Children's play: Reflections of social competence. *Seminars in Speech and Language, 9,* 1–14.

Whitehurst, G.J., & Sonnenschein, S. (1985). The development of communication: A functional analysis. In G.J. Whitehurst (Ed.), *Annals of child development* (pp. 1–48). Stamford, CT: JAI Press.

Wilkes-Gibbs, D., & Clark, H.H. (1992). Coordinating beliefs in conversation. *Journal of Memory and Language, 31,* 183–194.

3

Assessment of Social-Communicative Competence

An Interdisciplinary Model

Louise A. Kaczmarek

Although social and communicative competence have been studied separately, there has been growing acknowledgement of their interrelatedness. Language is considered a primary mediator of social interaction and an inherent aspect of social development (Gallagher, 1991; Goldstein & Kaczmarek, 1992). In fact, Prutting (1982) urged speech-language pathologists to view pragmatics as social competence, and Thompson (1996) asserted that communicative competence is a combination of social and linguistic competence. Some researchers have suggested that social and communicative competence represent different views of the same phenomenon with differences being more theoretical than real (Odom, McConnell, & McEvoy, 1992; Windsor, 1995). Others (Fujiki & Brinton, 1994; Prizant & Wetherby, 1990) have put forth the transactional model (Sameroff, 1987) as a framework for understanding the relationship between the two.

These theoretical positions have emerged from research on children's social and language development. The development of communication, which eventually leads to the development of language, begins at birth within the context of social interaction with caregivers (Bruner, 1975; Prizant & Wetherby, 1990; Snow, 1984). As they grow older, children continue to improve their communication skills within the context of social interactions. At the same time, children's abilities to communicate assist them in becoming more socially competent. This relationship between social and language development can be seen in the correlation between behavior and language disorders. Children diagnosed with behavior and emotional disorders have a higher incidence of language disorders (Mack & Warr-Leeper, 1992; Miniutti, 1991), and children with communication disorders have a higher incidence of behavior and emotional disorders (Baker & Cantwell, 1982; Baltaxe & Simmons, 1988).

The purpose of this chapter is to provide an overview of the assessment of social communication that is grounded theoretically in the interrelated conceptualizations of social and communicative competence. The chapter summarizes the convergent conceptualizations, delineates an assessment model based on these conceptualizations, and outlines specific strategies for assessing social communication. Although specific instruments for measuring social communication are mentioned, the chapter is not intended to be an exhaustive review of available instruments.

COMMONALITIES AMONG THEORIES AND MODELS

In Chapters 1 and 2, theories and models of social and communicative competence are reviewed. From these discussions, it should be apparent that conceptualizations of both social and communicative competence share two features. First, they relate to an individual's ability to accomplish specified functions, tasks, or goals that emerge from the physical and social context. Second, these conceptualizations purport that individuals possess a repertoire of forms or strategies that are matched to the specific cultural, social, and linguistic requirements of the context. The assessment model presented in this chapter is based on the position that social and communicative competence converge in their evaluation of function but, despite some common considerations, diverge in their evaluation of form. Function is evaluated in terms of effectiveness, which is the child's impact on the environment. Form is evaluated in terms of appropriateness, which is the extent to which behaviors fit the expected values, conventions, and criteria of the context. These relationships are depicted in Figure 3.1.

Function and Goals

Models of social and communicative competence appear to intersect in their consideration of function. Social competence is viewed in relation to social tasks (McFall, 1982), situations (Dodge, McClaskey, & Feldman, 1985), or problems (Rubin & Krasnor, 1986). When confronted with a social problem, children set social goals (Rubin & Krasnor, 1986). In the communicative competence literature, the terms *functions* (Halliday, 1975), *intents* (Miller, 1981) and *conversational acts* (Dore, 1978) appear to be similar to social goals. In at least some of the research con-

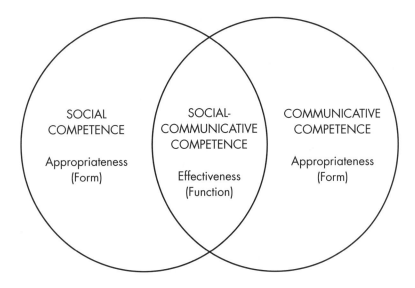

Figure 3.1.   The convergence of social-communicative competence.

ducted in the two fields, there is little difference among the social tasks and functions addressed. For example, Rubin's analysis of the social goals of children (e.g., Rubin & Krasnor, 1986; Rubin & Rose-Krasnor, 1992) and several taxonomies of communicative functions (Dore, 1975; Halliday, 1975) overlap considerably. Guralnick's (1992) model of social competence even referred to these same basic goals as social-communicative skills. Similarly, Clark (1996; Clark & Bly, 1995) extended the concept of communicative functions in his model of pragmatics by proposing that these basic functions operate in adjacency pairs (Schegloff & Sacks, 1973) within discourse (e.g., question–answer, request–promise, greeting–greeting) as "local projects."

Models of social and communicative competence often include more complex goals or tasks that are achieved through the sequencing of multiple steps of these basic functions. For example, Dodge and colleagues' analysis of social tasks (Dodge et al., 1985) appears implicitly to consider higher-level functions (e.g., group entry, peer provocations). On the same note, Guralnick's model (1992) explicitly acknowledges social tasks that are achieved by integrating and sequencing social-communicative skills as a higher level of social competence. Another example is Clark's model of pragmatics (Clark, 1996; Clark & Bly, 1995) that refers to "global projects" that are accomplished through the use of a series of "local projects."

The social competence literature suggests that as children get older, the sophistication of their social tasks or goals changes (Crick & Dodge,

1994; Rubin & Krasnor, 1986). Rubin and Rose-Krasnor, for example, suggested that "goals appear to become more numerous, more complex, more other oriented, and more likely to involve social comparison as children grow older" (1992, p. 297). Children display goals early in their development that appear to be focused at the social-communicative level of Guralnick's hierarchical model. As children get older, the goals increasingly emphasize the second social task level. To illustrate, toddlers are likely to seek proximity and attention from adults, whereas elementary school children are likely to seek attention and information from peers and to initiate friendships (Rubin & Krasnor, 1986). Adolescents organize themselves into mixed-gender peer groups to attend movies, sporting events, and concerts or to simply hang out and are concerned with enhancing their status among peers (Parker, Rubin, Price, & DeRosier, 1995).

Some children with disabilities lack certain social and communicative functions (e.g., Craig & Washington, 1993; Wetherby & Prutting, 1984). Other children may demonstrate a social or communicative function, but their relative rates in comparison to other functions or to the rates of peers and adults may be seriously out of balance (e.g., Adams & Bishop, 1989; Bishop, Hartley, & Weir, 1994; Rubin & Borwick, 1984; Rubin, Bream, & Rose-Krasnor, 1991).

Form and Strategies

There are a multitude of ways in which any given function, task, or goal can be accomplished. In the social competence literature, tasks and goals are completed by using *strategies,* whereas *forms* is the preferred term in the communication literature. Any linguistic form can be analyzed from a variety of perspectives (e.g., phonology, semantics, syntax). The choice of forms or strategies to achieve a particular function or goal varies within and across individuals. Both social and communication scientists agree that a variety of factors influence an individual's selection of form (e.g., Baltaxe, 1977; Crick & Dodge, 1994; Kaczmarek, 1990; Rubin & Krasnor, 1986). These include the immediate context, the perceived and known characteristics of social and communicative partners, existing knowledge, and culture. Information processing proponents view the ability to match an appropriate form to context to be a result of specific cognitive processes (e.g., Crick & Dodge, 1994; Rubin & Krasnor, 1986), whereas the behavioral position views the match in terms of the extent to which stimulus and response generalization are achieved (e.g., Kaczmarek, 1990; O'Neill & Reichle, 1993).

Perspective taking also influences form. As children get older, the strategies they use reflect an increasing ability to place their perspective in the context of others'. Selman (1980) offered a developmental model of perspective taking in the resolution of social conflict. Similarly, the use of language in social contexts requires perspective taking (see Chapter 2 for a more complete discussion). As children develop, their ability to take the perspective of others is exhibited in their acquisition of linguistic collaboration, including establishing shared background knowledge, grounding (Clark, 1996), and initiating and completing exchanges that allow them to achieve a shared goal.

Children with deficient social or communicative competence frequently display forms that do not match the contextual requirements and are considered inappropriate for achieving a given goal. For example, they may use challenging behaviors (Durand & Crimmins, 1988; Taylor & Carr, 1992), echolalia (Prizant & Duchan, 1981; Prizant & Rydell, 1984), aggressive behaviors (Rubin et al., 1991; Rubin, Moller, & Emptage, 1987), or less advanced forms (Folger & Chapman, 1978; Gallagher & Craig, 1984) to achieve specific functions. Less competent children often have a restricted set of forms for accomplishing specific functions (e.g., Craig, 1995; Rubin et al., 1987; Rubin et al., 1991). Thus, they are not as flexible in adjusting their social or communicative forms to fit the context.

Although there are some commonalities in the consideration of form, social and communicative competence models maintain separate emphases. Social competence is concerned with relationships between children and those with whom they interact. Some of the most central interests in evaluating social appropriateness concern children's positive and negative behaviors and examining the thinking processes involved in social situations. Communicative competence models, however, evaluate appropriateness from the perspective of the linguistic, paralinguistic, and nonverbal aspects of utterances and the relationships between utterances in connected discourse (e.g., Baltaxe, 1977; Bishop & Adams, 1989).

AN INTERDISCIPLINARY ASSESSMENT MODEL

Obtaining a comprehensive understanding of a child's social competence requires multiple measures that draw on the perspectives of the significant social agents in the child's environment (Gresham, 1986; Odom et al., 1992). The social communication assessment model presented in this chapter represents just such a conceptual framework within which multiple measures can be organized. The model consists of a 3 × 3 matrix (see Figure 3.2). The left side of the matrix represents three levels of social-communicative performance that are similar to the indicators of social competence described by Odom, McConnell, et al. (1992). The top of the matrix consists of three aspects of social-communicative competence: the separate conceptualizations of social and communicative appropriateness and the convergent conceptualization of social-communicative effectiveness.

Levels of Social Communication

Within the assessment model, there are three levels. The first two levels are derived from the commonalities between Guralnick's (1992) model of social competence and Clark's model (1996; Clark & Bly, 1995) of pragmatics. The terminology for the first two levels is based on Guralnick's model.

Social-Communicative Skills Level

At the first level are social-communicative skills, which according to Guralnick (1992) emerge as a result of the integration of basic language, cognitive, affective, and motor development. These skills are considered isolated, static behaviors, such as the basic social and communicative functions proposed by Dore (1975), Halliday (1975), and Rubin and Krasnor (1986). Assessment of these social-communicative skills, such as object requests or greetings, is typically considered to be at the molecular level (McFall, 1982; Prutting & Kirchner, 1983).

Social-Communicative Task Performance Level

The middle level represents higher level functions that require the integration and sequencing of the basic functions, what Clark (1996; Clark & Bly, 1995) called "global projects" and those in the social competence literature refer to as "social tasks" (Dodge, Pettit, McClaskey, & Brown, 1986; Goldfried & D'Zurilla, 1969). At this level, multiple social-communicative skills are integrated, organized, and sequenced to produce strategies used in the completion of more complex social tasks within the ongoing, changing social context. The emergent strategies also are influenced by the companion's characteristics and their shared knowledge. For example, a child who wishes to join a group of children in block play might approach the group, stand and watch the group in play for a few seconds, pick up a car and play in parallel to the group, and respond by saying, "Me, too. Let's buy some food for a picnic," when a child with another car says, "I'm going to the store." Contrast this example to one in which a child approaches the group and grabs the toy from another child saying, "I wanna play, too."

| | Appropriateness | | Effectiveness |
	Social	Communicative	Social-communicative
	• Partner characteristics • Physical environment • Cultural considerations		
Social-communicative skills	• Coding positive/negative behaviors • Social interaction rating scales	• Direct observation of linguistic, paralinguistic, and nonverbal characteristics of utterances • Pragmatics rating scales	• General characteristics of interaction • Social assertiveness and responsiveness • Social and communicative functions • Impact on social partners • Analysis of challenging behaviors
Social-communicative task performance	• Social cognition	• Discourse skills	• Length of interactions • Accomplishment of social tasks • Ecological inventories
Overall social-communicative performance	• Global social measures	• Global communication measures	• Peer acceptance • Friendships • Social networks

Figure 3.2. Social communication assessment model showing how different dimensions of social-communicative competence (top) interact with three levels of performance (left) to yield various assessment targets.

Overall Social-Communicative Performance

In the areas of social and communicative appropriateness, overall social-communicative performance focuses respectively on global measures of social and communicative competence. Under social-communicative effectiveness, outcomes such as peer acceptance, friendship, and membership in social networks are considered. Assessment at this level might reveal, for example, that a child is not particularly popular with most of his classmates but that he nevertheless has a best friend and plays with three or four other children in his class.

Aspects of Social-Communicative Competence

The aspects of social-communicative competence to consider include social appropriateness, communicative appropriateness, and social-communicative effectiveness.

Social Appropriateness

Social appropriateness refers to judgments by others that a child's social behaviors and thinking processes assist in establishing and maintaining effective interactions and relationships with others and assist in achieving interpersonal goals. At the social-communicative skill level, judgments focus on the social acceptability of individual behaviors (i.e., positive and negative quality) used in interacting with others. Judgments at the social-communicative task level focus on the child's social problem-solving skills and the achievement of social tasks. Social appropriateness is judged in relation to the contexts, situations, or tasks in which social behaviors are displayed (Goldfried & D'Zurilla, 1969). Decisions about appropriateness also must take into account such factors as cultural expectations, the physical environment, and the characteristics of the interacting partner(s). For example, a certain amount of rough-and-tumble play is tolerated on the playground or even promoted in a friendly game of football as long as the ages and body sizes of the children are similar. Such play would not be considered acceptable, however, in the classroom or the school cafeteria.

Communicative Appropriateness

Communicative appropriateness refers to judgments by others that the child's utterances and discourse skills suit communicative intents and permit the child to help others achieve their communicative intents. At the social-communicative skill level, communicative appropriateness is judged by examining the linguistic, paralinguistic, and nonverbal elements of utterances. At this level, assessors want to know if a child's utterances effectively communicate what the child wants to say. At the social-communicative task level, the elements of discourse (i.e., conversation) are examined. Like social appropriateness, communicative appropriateness takes into account the physical, social, and cultural context of the communication as well as the characteristics of communicative partners. For example, the use of direct commands as a method of requesting is acceptable for young children who are learning to talk; however, direct commands generally would not be considered polite if used by older children to address adults even though they might be tolerated among peers and considered appropriate when addressing very young children.

Social-Communicative Effectiveness

Effectiveness is the measurement of function and refers to judgments from the child's perspective that his or her social-communicative skills and performance of social-communicative tasks are successful. Success may be measured in terms of the extent to which a child is socially accepted by peers, has friends, and belongs to social networks. Although a professional or parent may make the judgment of effectiveness at the social-communicative skill or social task levels, it must be measured from the child's perspective. For example, when a child obtains a toy from another by hitting, the child's behavior is viewed as effective because the action resulted in getting the toy, even though the form used to obtain the toy probably would be considered by others, including the peer, as inappropriate.

ASSESSING SOCIAL-COMMUNICATIVE SKILLS

Social-communicative skills can be assessed with the use of direct observation in natural environments and analogue and role-play situations as well as by gathering information from others.

Direct Observation in Natural Environments

Observation is the most direct method of assessing the appropriateness and effectiveness of children's social-communicative skills. Direct observation may be used to assist in the identification of children for intervention, to gather information for programming planning, and to monitor the effects of intervention. Situations in which children and youth may be observed vary in the degree of structure from unconstrained natural environments, to analogue environments in which some variables are managed, to tightly controlled role-play situations.

Social and communicative interaction data usually are collected using a direct observation coding system. In such systems, observers may record behaviors as they occur or the interactions may be videotaped for later coding. Videotaping has the obvious advantage of being a permanent record of what occurred; however, it should be acknowledged that videotaping is an edited version of events. More subtle nuances of social behaviors may be difficult to observe on videotape, and camera angles may obscure important behaviors.

Because of the difficulty of coding every behavioral event that occurs, behaviors are usually sampled. Sampling methods include whole interval, partial interval, and momentary time sampling (Odom & Ogawa, 1992; Repp, Barton, & Brulle, 1987). It is important that behavioral sampling methods reflect the actual behavioral frequencies. The partial interval coding system (i.e., dividing the observation time into equal time intervals, usually 5–10 seconds, and recording a behavior if it occurs during the interval) is the most frequently used sampling method (Odom & Ogawa, 1992). Repp and colleagues (1987) reviewed studies of various methods, concluding that intervals of up to 10 seconds are accurate, with 5 seconds being more accurate than 10. In addition, they found that inserting a 5-second recording period between each observational interval did not compromise accuracy.

Computer-assisted methods of data collection are readily available (Brown, Odom, & Holcombe, 1996) and not only contribute to the ease of data collection but also reduce the amount of time necessary to analyze data. Nevertheless, practitioners who are unlikely to have the hardware and software available should not be discouraged from developing or implementing paper-and-pencil recording techniques. For example, English, Shafer, Goldstein, and Kaczmarek (1997) offered a simple paper-and-pencil format for collecting basic social-communicative interaction data.

Collecting observational data in a variety of situations and with a variety of partners increases the accuracy and comprehensiveness of the assessment of a child's social-communicative skills. Data should be viewed within each environment rather than collapsed across environments, which may obscure a child's situation-specific profile (Foster, Inderbitzen, & Nangle, 1993). The field unfortunately has not provided much guidance as to how much observational data represents adequate sampling (Foster et al., 1993), although the purpose of collecting data will influence this decision. For example, more comprehensive sampling is appropriate if the purpose is to determine whether a child requires intervention. Yet, monitoring intervention progress usually requires relatively short recording periods on a periodic schedule.

The validity of direct observation may be affected by a number of factors. For example, the presence of observers may affect the social behaviors children display (Brody, Stoneman, & Wheatley, 1984). Observer effects typically are overcome when observers or video cameras are present on a regular basis. Similarly, the more contrived the situation in which data are collected, the less likely the behaviors displayed correspond to the child's repertoire in the natural environment. Pettit, McClaskey, Brown, and Dodge (1987) found that children's behaviors in analogue environments did not correlate well with their behaviors in the natural environment. This lack of correspondence also was found when children's performances in the natural environment were compared with their behaviors in role-play situations (Kazdin, Matson, & Esveldt-Dawson, 1984; Van Hasselt, Hersen, & Bellack, 1981). The issues of validity are further compounded by the age and developmental sophistication of the children being observed. Bierman and Montminy (1993) described how the validity of direct observation is affected from preschool through adolescence. They indicated that social-communicative interactions of preschool children are relatively short and discrete and can be readily observed in preschool environments. As children enter the grade school years, however, significant peer interactions occur increasingly in more private contexts. Peer interactions are less likely in classroom environments because they are more highly structured, and observational codes are less likely to capture the nuances of critical social events. In adolescence, children's social behaviors have become so sophisticated that no set of skills adequately captures the multiple domains of adolescent peer interactions. Although role-play tests have been used with this age group (Freedman, Rosenthal, Donahoe, Schlundt, & McFall, 1978), more indirect methods of assessment such as reflective reasoning tasks (e.g., Rubin & Krasnor, 1986) and peer ratings may be more appropriate (Pope & Bierman, 1991). Environments and situations in which direct observations may take place are described next from least to most contrived.

Observation in Natural Environments

Children typically are observed in relatively unstructured environments, such as free play in classrooms for preschoolers, playgrounds for elementary school students, and the cafeteria for middle and high school students. Children also may be observed at home (e.g., playtime, dinnertime) and in community environments (e.g., playgrounds, recreation programs).

Observations in natural environments offer the best face validity of the direct observation methods (Vaughn & Haager, 1994); however, some direct observation measures correlate better than others with social outcome measures. Frequency of interaction, for example, was found to correlate poorly with peer acceptance (Asher, Markell, & Hymel, 1981), whereas the quality of children's behaviors as determined by positive and negative ratings (see LaGreca & Stark, 1986, for a review) was more predictive of peer social acceptance.

Coding or videotaping children's behaviors in natural environments can often be challenging because it may not always be possible to get close enough to capture the most detailed level of interaction without special microphones. Consequently, it is usually easier to collect general data such as initiations and responses than to collect information at more specific levels such as social or communicative functions (Foster et al., 1993). If recording equipment can be used successfully in a natural environment, the interactions among children can be transcribed to serve as language samples that can be coded to assist in determining the communicative appropriateness of a child's interaction skills. Direct observation in natural environments can be very time consuming and expensive (Voeller, 1994). In addition, it may not be ideal for some social skills that occur relatively infrequently (Foster et al., 1993; Vaughn & Haager, 1994).

Observation in Analogue Situations

Analogue situations are simulations of situations that occur in the natural environment. They are usually set up to resemble a social task but can be set up to evoke specific social-communicative skills. Analogue situations have been used to assess the social skills of children of all ages on such tasks as peer group entry (e.g., Dodge et al., 1986; Putallaz & Gottman, 1981) and responses to provocation (e.g., Dodge, 1986; Dodge et al., 1986). Some analogue situations are designed to use peer confederates who are coached or scripted to simulate specific situations (e.g., Dodge et al., 1986). Putallaz (1983), for example, used child actors who executed a script to create a peer entry situation as well as the need for help, conflict management, and resumption of dyadic play. Specific social-communicative skills within simulated tasks can then be analyzed, usually with a code similar to those used in observation in the natural environment.

Analogue situations also have been used successfully to sample parent–child interactions. A parent is asked to play with the child in typical fashion (Martinez, 1987; Yoder, Davies, & Bishop, 1994) or to teach the child how to do something such as operate a busy box. The interactions may take place in a laboratory, clinic, classroom, or the family's home. The interactions are usually videotaped or audiotaped.

Language samples (see Miller, 1981) are traditionally collected in what might be considered analogue environments. A child typically interacts with a speech-language pathologist who focuses on eliciting a representative sample of the child's productive language. The clinician assembles a set of materials (e.g., toys, books), some familiar and some unfamiliar, that serve as props in the interaction. The clinician uses a variety of interaction strategies that facilitate the child's productive language, such as following the child's lead, minimal questions or demands, self-talk (i.e., describing one's own actions while playing with toys), and parallel play with minimal talking. Sometimes the clinician also may set up situations that are known to elicit certain communicative functions, such as enclosing an interesting object in a transparent but difficult-to-open container for prompting requests for assistance (see Wetherby & Prutting, 1984). The session is recorded on audiotape or videotape. The child's language is transcribed with relevant notes about nonverbal actions and communications. The transcript is then analyzed by examining pragmatics and any other aspect of language that appear to be interfering with a child's functional communication. Language samples also may be collected from the natural environment, but unless recording equipment is relatively sophisticated (e.g., FM microphones), the results may be disappointing.

Like language samples, play-based assessment (e.g., Linder, 1993) and functional analyses of challenging behaviors (Carr et al., 1994; Iwata, Vollmer, & Zarcone, 1990) also occur in analogue environments in which interaction takes place with the evaluator. Linder's format for play-based assessment also incorporates opportunities for parent–child and peer interaction.

Observations in analogue environments are less time-consuming and less expensive than naturalistic observations. They provide the evaluator with greater control over the characteristics of the social context. When analogue situations are set up apart from the noisy hustle and bustle of the classroom, coding and recording children's interactions are usually easier. Similar to direct observation in natural environments, children's behaviors in analogue environments are well correlated with social acceptance measures (see Gresham, 1986); however, there is no guarantee that behaviors displayed in analogue environments relate to those displayed in natural environments (Pettit et al., 1987). The external validity of the behaviors is likely to be related to the degree of control exercised over a child's behavior in an analogue environment. Situations in which examiners implement nonintrusive techniques such as following the child's lead and parallel play are more likely to reflect natural environment behaviors than tightly controlled situations designed to structure a child's behavior through questions and other direct elicitation techniques. Children's performances in analogue situations can be confirmed with parents and other adults who are familiar with their behavior in other environments in order to gain a better understanding of the external validity of children's behaviors.

Role-Play Situations

In role-play situations, an examiner describes an interpersonal vignette usually addressing some issue relevant to the age of the child. The child is then prompted to respond with one or two sentences to the situation as if it were occurring in real life. A variety of vignettes usually are presented, such as giving and receiving compliments, standing up for oneself, and denying an unreasonable request. The entire procedure is videotaped and the child's responses are rated for their appropriateness and skillfulness. Examples of some of these measures are the Behavioral Test of Interpersonal Competence for Children–Revised (BTICC–R, Hughes et al., 1989), the Social Skills Test for Children (Williamson, Moody, Granberry, Lethermon, & Blouin, 1983), and the Adolescent Problems Inventory (Freedman et al., 1978). This technique is seldom used with younger children and is often designed to correspond with the specific skills addressed in an intervention (Foster et al., 1993). The specific tools and the technique itself may have limited utility with children and youth with significant disabilities, especially in the cognitive and language domains.

Obtaining Information About Social-Communicative Skills from Others

Gathering information about the appropriateness and effectiveness of social-communicative skills from family members, teachers, and, as appropriate, peers is an essential aspect of assessment practice that serves two purposes. First, it is an important source of information when direct observation is not possible because of a child's age, lack of access to critical environments (e.g., home, community), or the fear that observer effects will skew the data collected. Second, it supplements direct observation data by providing a more comprehensive picture of a child's skills and by validating the direct observation results.

Teachers in preschool and elementary classrooms have multiple opportunities to observe children's social interactions and thus are an important source of information about children's social-communicative skills. Although teachers have been shown to be both reliable and valid reporters of children's positive and negative social behaviors (e.g., Achenbach & Edelbrock, 1978), few measures have been developed to focus specifically on social-communicative skills. Most rating scales measure overall social competence (e.g., Social Skills Rating System; Gresham & Elliott, 1990), although they usually include some items focusing on social-communicative skills. These instruments generally consist of a broad range of positive and negative social behaviors, including school-specific behaviors. Teachers typically rate the frequency of these behaviors. Teacher ratings of children's behaviors have less validity as children grow older, as many critical, age-appropriate social skills are displayed outside of classroom environments and the view of teachers (Bierman & Montminy, 1993).

Family members, especially parents, have a unique perspective on the social and communicative skills of children, especially in environments that teachers and others have few opportunities to see. Many of the social skills rating tools include forms that have been developed specifically for parents. These tools are similar to those of teachers, but many are adapted to include behaviors displayed at home rather than school. There are also a number of parent report instruments in the area of language (see Dale, 1996). Although many include questions related to pragmatics, few offer an in-depth focus on pragmatics.

As children grow older, peers have more opportunities to observe the critical social-communicative skills of other children (Hymel & Rubin, 1985; Pope & Bierman, 1991) as well as greater social cognitive awareness to be able to rate the behaviors of others accurately. Most peer ratings tools, however, are focused on peers' perceptions of children's behaviors and social status rather than on ratings of specific skills (Foster et al., 1993). In the absence of specific instruments, peers, teachers, and family members can be interviewed to obtain assessment information or can be asked to complete practitioner-generated questionnaires about children's social-communicative skills.

Factors to Consider When Rating the Appropriateness of Social-Communicative Skills

The assessment model advocates that professionals make judgments about the social and communicative appropriateness of children's social-communicative behaviors. When making such judgments, it is critical that professionals understand that decisions about appropriateness are often value judgments. The criteria for appropriateness are not always well defined, and although many judgments might be straightforward (e.g., unprovoked aggression, incorrect object name) other decisions are more complex and equivocal (e.g., aggression as self-defense, lack of eye contact with adults) and may need to take into account a child's culture or subculture. Bishop and Adams (1989) showed that when rating the inappropriateness of child utterances, there were high correlations among the independent ratings of three professionals. In addition, Leinonen and Smith (1994) demonstrated that independent raters without expertise in child language disorders were not necessarily in agreement about the appropriateness of the pragmatic abilities of children with language disorders. This study also showed that the raters viewed some of the behaviors of the therapists as inappropriate, suggesting that adult interaction styles were not as "natural" as assumed by professionals and may have contributed to the problematic discourse. In another study, Prutting and Kirchner (1987) suggested that pragmatic parameters be marked inappropriate only if they are shown to have a negative impact on interaction and not simply because they are different. To assist professionals in making sound judgments about appropriateness, there appear to be at least three factors common to both social and communicative perspectives that should be considered— namely, partner characteristics, the physical environment, and the child's culture.

When judging the appropriateness of a social-communicative skill, it is essential to consider the characteristics of the partner with whom a child is interacting. Behavior varies depending on social and communicative partners. Employees act and talk to their bosses differently from their colleagues. Adult language to children varies depending on the ages of the children. In short, people adjust their behavior in accordance with such perceived or known partner characteristics as demographics (e.g., age, gender, race, occupation, social status), personal factors (e.g., familiarity, mood, personality), and unique personal history. Behavior that is acceptable with one's best friend may be totally inappropriate with one's parent. Behavior toward a parent who had a good day at work may be totally inappropriate after the parent has experienced a distressing incident.

Research shows that at least some of these stylistic variations in interaction skills are apparent as early as the preschool years. For example, children have been shown to adjust their communicative styles and communicative functions to partners of different ages. Preschoolers grammatically simplified their utterances (Sachs & Devin, 1976; Shatz & Gelman, 1973) and used more imperatives (Corsaro, 1979b, Sachs & Devin, 1976) and attention-getters (Sachs & Devin, 1976; Shatz

& Gelman, 1973) when talking to younger children than adults and peers. Children asked more internal-state questions of infants and more external-world questions of mothers and peers (Sachs & Devin, 1976). They were more likely to seek attention, address nonspecific initiations, and ask permission for self-action of teachers than peers; peers were more likely to be the recipients of requests for action, termination, and object goals than teachers (Krasnor, 1982). In addition to displaying more directives and exchanging less information, typical children who interacted with classmates who had mild developmental delays also asked for more message clarifications than they did of children without disabilities (Guralnick & Paul-Brown, 1989). Preschoolers with mild disabilities displayed similar patterns to typical children when they expressed more directives, asked fewer questions, and gave less information to children who were younger (Guralnick & Paul-Brown, 1986).

Being able to conceptualize and utilize all relevant partner characteristics in an interaction is a developmental phenomenon. As children grow older, they show greater flexibility, differentiation, and variation in their selection of social strategies in accordance with the age, gender, and other characteristics of their social partners (Berg, 1989; Levin & Rubin, 1983; Piche, Rubin, & Michlin, 1978; Rubin & Krasnor, 1983). Similarly, older children were shown to have more skill at considering partner characteristics when inferring other people's feelings than younger children (Gnepp, 1989a, 1989b).

The physical environment is another essential consideration in judging the appropriateness of a social-communicative skill. People interact and communicate differently depending on the physical environment. The impersonal and inanimate features of the environment influence children's selection of social goals and strategies (Rubin & Rose-Krasnor, 1992). Acceptable behavior in classrooms is different from that in playgrounds, ballparks, libraries, and churches. Each environment has its range of socially acceptable behaviors.

Although partner characteristics and the physical environment are essential considerations in making judgments about appropriateness, they are superceded in importance by culture. What is considered appropriate behavior toward varying partners and in different environments is largely determined by culture. Culture refers to the common social norms, beliefs, attitudes, and values that govern the roles, behaviors, communication patterns, and affective styles of those who identify with the culture (Betancourt & Lopez, 1993). Culture not only encompasses those who belong to specific ethnic, racial, and language groups but can also include subcultural groups within a larger culture or groups that cross ethnic and geographic boundaries, such as those with common religious beliefs (McCollum & McBride, 1997). Culture plays a significant role in shaping children's social and communicative behaviors (Clancy, 1986; Harkness & Super, 1995; Walker, Messinger, Fogel, & Karns, 1992). Children begin to learn the behaviors specific to a culture from birth through the parenting practices and behaviors of caregivers (e.g., Martinez, 1987; Ochs & Schieffelin, 1984). Parent–child interaction styles specific to the culture shape a child's social-communicative competence. Japanese mothers tend to use more upper body physical movements, whereas American mothers tend to hold and touch their infants more continuously (Fogel, Toda, & Kawai, 1988). American mothers respond more often to infant vocalizations than Japanese mothers (Fogel et al., 1988). Mexican American mothers typically interact nonverbally with their young infants (Garcia Coll, 1990). Because of these cultural variations in parenting styles, children will display a variety of social-communicative styles. High-context cultures are more attuned to nonverbal behaviors and messages, the environmental context, and relationships than low-context cultures, which rely more on information conveyed through words (Hecht, Andersen, & Ribeau, 1989; Lynch, 1998). Asian, Native American, Latino, and African American cultural groups are examples of high-context cultures. Anglo-European, German, and Scandinavian groups are examples of low-context cultures.

The paralinguistic and nonverbal behaviors that accompany speech, such as intonation, eye contact, touch, social distance, posture, facial expressions, and bodily gestures, are culturally specific behaviors (Lynch, 1998; Pennycook, 1985). Children in different cultures may display similar behaviors, but the meaning attributed to them may vary with cultural beliefs and values (Rubin, 1998). The meaning of eye contact, for example, differs among cultures. For Anglo-European Americans, direct eye contact is a sign of trustworthiness and sincerity (Asante & Davis, 1989). For Latino groups, however, sustained eye contact conveys disrespect, and for Asian groups eye contact between strangers is considered shameful (Lynch, 1998). Similarly, cultural standards vary for what is considered comfortable and acceptable distance between social partners. Anglo-European Americans maintain distances of about an arm's length, whereas Latinos, southern Europeans, Middle Easterners, and African Americans prefer closer proximity and Asians greater proximity (Lynch, 1998).

These culturally determined nonverbal and paralinguistic behaviors relate to the standards of politeness for particular cultural groups. Politeness is a "system that regulates what is said and how it is said in all sorts of interactions" (Ninio & Snow, 1999, p. 364). The system of politeness tells people how to treat other members of their cultural group in ways that maintain the group's beliefs, norms, and values. When judgments are made about the appropriateness of social-communicative behaviors, assessors at least partially consider politeness and must be careful not to impose the rules of their cultural group on children who belong to other groups.

Due to the diversity of the population of the United States of America, taking into account the cultural background of the children and families served is imperative when making judgments about the appropriateness of social and communicative behaviors. The beliefs and norms of a child's culture must provide the lens through which the appropriateness of social-communicative skills is judged. Children must not be penalized because their cultural heritage has shaped them in ways that differ from the dominant culture. Practitioners and researchers should become aware of their own cultural identities and how culture affects their beliefs and practices (Lynch, 1998). They need an understanding of the cultural practices, values, and beliefs of the children with whom they work. By engaging families in conversations about their values and beliefs; working closely with families as partners; and studying the practices, values, and beliefs of other cultures, practitioners and researchers can begin to establish cross-cultural competence (Lynch, 1998).

Social Appropriateness of Social-Communicative Skills

Children whose social behaviors are appropriate are considered more socially competent than those who display inappropriate (e.g., aggressive, aversive) behaviors. Appropriate behaviors strengthen a child's interactions and relationships with others and result in such outcomes as social acceptance, friendships, and membership in social networks. Yet, inappropriate behaviors inhibit social interactions, relationships, and positive outcomes and may ultimately lead to significant negative consequences that may be sustained into adulthood (see Asher & Parker, 1989).

Observational Coding of Positive and Negative Skills

The most common method of rating the appropriateness of a child's social-communicative skills is through direct observation in natural and analogue environments. Many direct observational coding systems make judgments about the positive and negative qualities of social behaviors (see Odom & Ogawa, 1992). Many codes explicitly define negative behaviors and consider all other behaviors that do not fit the negative definition(s) as positive (e.g., Brown et al., 1996; Goldstein, Kaczmarek, Pennington, & Shafer, 1992). These codes typically include one or more negative categories. Other social behavior codes explicitly rate every behavior as either positive or negative (e.g., Brady, 1997; Davis, Brady, Hamilton, McEvoy, & Williams, 1994). Practitioners may easily observe a child's social behaviors in naturalistic or analogue environments and keep a tally of positive and negative behaviors, noting the specific types of negative behaviors displayed; however, in selecting or developing a more comprehensive coding system, practitioners may find it easier to consider a code in which negative categories are included among the list of other categories. Such codes require only one decision (i.e., behavioral category) when a behavior is displayed rather than two (i.e., behavioral category plus negative or positive valence). Once the data have been collected, the types and frequencies of specific negative and positive behaviors can be tallied.

Rating Social Interactions

Rating scales offer an alternative to direct observation that may be less expensive and time-consuming (Beckman & Lieber, 1994; Bishop, 1998), more sensitive to the nuances of intervention and the significance of social behavior in context (Jacobson, Tianen, Willie, & Aytch, 1986), and more representative of typical behavior if completed by someone who knows a child well (Bishop, 1998). Unfortunately, there are few such scales focusing solely on basic social interaction skills. Two rating scales that are devoted to the social interaction skills of young children are the Ghuman-Folstein Screen for Social Interaction (Ghuman, Freund, Reiss, Serwint, & Folstein, 1998) and the Social Strategy Rating Scale (Beckman & Lieber, 1994). The Ghuman-Folstein Screen is a parent/caregiver questionnaire designed to measure basic reciprocal social interactions of children ages 6 months to 5 years across a variety of social situations (e.g., peers, caregivers, play, meals) that are typically not accessible to direct observation. Behaviors are rated along a four-point frequency continuum. The Social Strategy Rating Scale evaluates the ability of young children with disabilities to engage in key social strategies with adults and peers across a variety of social situations. Strategies are rated on a five-point frequency continuum and a three-point appropriateness scale. Both tools offer initial psychometric data.

Communicative Appropriateness of Social-Communicative Skills

Pragmatics is the study of language use in social contexts. As stated in Chapter 2, there are two theoretical approaches to the study of pragmatics—formalism and functionalism (Craig, 1995; Prutting, 1982). Our analysis of communicative appropriateness is constructed from the perspective of functionalism, which views pragmatics as the framework from which to study the other components of language (Prutting, 1982). Thus, in an assessment of children's communicative appropriateness, one must first determine how and the extent to which the more formal aspects of a child's utterances (e.g., syntax, phonology) deviate from developmental and/or cultural expectations and then decide how and the extent to which they interfere with the child's ability to function. In other words, an examination of the formal aspects of utterances must ultimately answer the question of how well the formal characteristics of children's utterances serve their communicative intents within specific contexts (i.e., the role of initiator) and assist them in collaborating with others in achieving their communicative goals (i.e., the role of responder).

Direct Observation of Pragmatics

Examination of the communicative appropriateness of social-communicative skills focuses on the linguistic, paralinguistic, and nonverbal elements of utterances. Discourse skills, which are another important aspect of pragmatics, are examined at the social task performance level because they deal with the sequencing of utterances within conversations. Analyses of the formal linguistic elements refer to the phonological, morphological, semantic, and syntactic characteristics of utterances. Particular consideration is given to the specificity and accuracy of word choice (Prutting & Kirchner, 1983, 1987). The paralinguistic elements of utterances include intonation, stress patterns, vocal intensity, voice quality, fluency, and intelligibility (Prutting & Kirchner, 1983, 1987). Nonverbal aspects of utterances refer to the nonverbal behaviors that accompany utterances such as physical proximity, body movements and posture, physical contact with communicative partners, facial expressions, and eye contact. Nonverbal elements also include gestures and other nonverbal behaviors that in and of themselves have communicative intent (e.g., handing an object to another, waving) and do not necessarily have to be accompanied by speech. Inclusion of communicative gestures independent of speech permits the analysis of the communicative expressions of children who are in the prelinguistic stages of language development or whose primary mode of expressive communication is nonverbal.

Language samples provide the basis for analyzing the formal linguistic elements of utterances from data collected in naturalistic environments rather than from standardized tests. Computer programs such as the CHILDES system (MacWhinney, 1999) and Systematic Analysis of Language Transcripts (SALT; Miller, 1996) are available to aid in these analyses, as well as those of pragmatics. Prutting and Kirchner (1983, 1987) provided a Pragmatic Protocol for children ages 5 years or older from which the verbal, nonverbal, and paralinguistic elements of pragmatics can be examined. In their format for molar analysis, clinicians judge various aspects of pragmatics as appropriate or inappropriate. They recommend observing a child for 15 minutes of unstructured, spontaneous conversation with a communicative partner before completing the protocol. The validity of the judgments might be enhanced if a team makes these decisions, rather than individuals. The Pragmatics Protocol format also may serve as the framework for more detailed molecular analysis (Prutting & Kirchner, 1983).

Rating Pragmatic Behaviors

Bishop (1998) developed a 70-item rating scale to measure children's communication behaviors that are not easily assessed using conventional methods. The tool consists of nine subscales: 1) speech output—intelligibility and fluency, 2) syntax, 3) inappropriate initiation, 4) coherence, 5) stereotyped conversation, 6) use of conversational context, 7) conversational rapport, 8) social relationships, and 9) interests. Items are rated on a three-point scale from "definitely applies," to "applies somewhat," to "does not apply." Most items are descriptions of inappropriate behaviors, although most subscales include several appropriate items. Subscales 3 through 7 represent a pragmatics composite scale. All subscales except for coherence, social relationships, and interests fit into the assessment model at the level of communicative appropriateness of social-communicative skills. A number of the psychometric properties of the tool have been evaluated.

The Early Social-Communicative Scales (Seibert, Hogan, & Mundy, 1982) provide a cognitive developmental framework for the assessment of social-communicative skills in the first 2 years of life. The scales may be administered as a parent questionnaire or formal test. They utilize five organizational levels similar to those of Piaget's sensorimotor period and eight developmental dimensions based on three primary pragmatic functions (i.e., social interaction, joint attention, behavioral regulation).

Effectiveness of Social-Communicative Skills

The effectiveness of social-communicative skills is measured by determining the extent to which a child's individual social-communicative skills accomplish the child's apparent function. To fully understand the social impact of a child's social-communicative skills, one must examine the following: 1) the general characteristics of the child's interactions, 2) the level of assertiveness and responsiveness, 3) the social and communicative functions displayed, 4) the impact of the child's social-communicative skills on others, and 5) the social-communicative effectiveness of challenging behaviors.

General Characteristics of a Child's Interactions

The general information that is collected about a child's social-communicative repertoire should address the following questions:

1. With whom (i.e., adults versus peers) does the child interact?
2. What modes of interaction (i.e., vocal/verbal versus nonverbal/ gestural) does a child use and to what extent?
3. Are there some environments in which a child interacts more or better?

With younger children, these data are best collected through direct observation with additional information gathered from other sources. With older children, the information may need to be collected from families, teachers, and peers.

Social Assertiveness and Responsiveness

A child's level of social assertiveness tells us how often the child seeks social contact and the level of social responsiveness tells us how often the child reciprocates social contact. Two assessment questions are pertinent to these two aspects of social-communicative skills: How socially assertive and responsive is the child? How does a child's level of assertiveness and responsiveness compare with that of other children interacting in the environment?

The identification of initiations and responses is one of the most commonly used metrics in the assessment of both social (e.g., LaGreca & Stark, 1986; Odom & Ogawa, 1992) and communicative competence (e.g., Rice, Sell, & Hadley, 1991; Roberts, Prizant, & McWilliam, 1995). Although specific definitions may vary somewhat, initiations and responses represent the most basic index of a child's social-communicative skills. In the communicative competence literature, initiations and responses are considered aspects of turn taking (Prutting & Kirchner, 1983; Roberts et al., 1995).

An initiation is a behavior whose goal is engagement with another person. Some definitions of initiation are topographical (e.g., Brown, Ragland, & Fox, 1988; McConnell, Sisson, Cort, & Strain, 1991), whereas others are temporal (e.g., Strain, 1984; Guralnick, Connor, Hammond,

Gottman, & Kinnish, 1995). Topographical definitions focus simply on the function of the behavior, such as any behavior directed toward a peer (Brady, 1997); any behavior directed toward a peer that attempts to evoke a social response (Kamps et al., 1992; McEvoy et al., 1988); any behavior "directed to a peer that could occasion a response" (Davis et al., 1994; p. 622); or touching another, handing an object to another, or using another's name (Chandler, Fowler, & Lubeck, 1992). Temporal definitions, however, add a time dimension. They usually refer to social behaviors that occur after a specified number of seconds of no interaction; emphasis is placed on starting an interaction after a period of no interaction.

A response is a behavior by another person that follows an initiation. In other words, a response reciprocates an initiation. Responding to an initiation is assisting in the fulfillment of a function asserted by another. Like initiations, definitions of response can be temporal (e.g., Brady, 1997; Hecimovic, Fox, Shores, & Strain, 1985) or topographical (e.g., Brown et al., 1988; Chandler et al., 1992). They also can combine both features (e.g., Guralnick & Weinhouse, 1984; Kamps et al., 1992; Kohler et al., 1995). Temporal definitions emphasize that the responding behavior must occur within a certain number of seconds of the initiation. Topographical definitions usually require that the content of the response be related to the content of the initiation.

When assessing children at this level, evaluators should be concerned with the extent to which the child initiates interactions and responds to the initiations of others. Initiations and responses are coded typically during naturalistic or analogue environments and are summarized as frequencies, rates, or percentages of utterances. Initiations provide information about a child's social assertiveness, and responses provide a measure of a child's responsiveness. Fey (1986) used the parameters of assertiveness and responsiveness to describe four types of social-conversational patterns. This paradigm might be broadened to refer generally to all social interactions: 1) active interactors (high levels of assertiveness and responsiveness), 2) responsive interactors (low assertiveness, high responsiveness), 3) assertive interactors (high assertiveness, low responsiveness), and 4) noninteractors (low assertiveness and responsiveness).

Comparison of a child's level of initiations and responses to that of peers or adults within a given analogue or naturalistic environment sheds light on the child's role within that environment. For example, by calculating each child's initiations as a proportion of the total number initiations by all children, comparisons can be made to determine whether a child dominates or is dominated by the initiations of others or whether the child shares equally in initiating interaction. Children who make about as many initiations as they receive demonstrate one defining feature of reciprocal interaction (Greenwood, Walker, Todd, & Hops, 1981).

Social and Communicative Functions

In addressing the functional aspects of a child's social-communicative skills, assessors should be interested in learning which social and communicative functions the child displays. This information is determined by applying various social and communicative taxonomies to data collected through direct observation. The information also can be obtained by asking caregivers, teachers, and peers (in the case of older students) to recall the types of social-communicative functions a child displays.

Taxonomies represent more detailed analyses of the functions of social-communicative skills than initiations and responses. By assessing a child's social-communicative skills using a taxonomy, evaluators can determine the specific functions that a child displays and those that might be targeted as instructional objectives. Taxonomies are derived typically from descriptive research of children's social (e.g., Dodge et al., 1985; Krasnor & Rubin, 1983) and communicative (e.g., Bates, 1976; Dore, 1975; Halliday, 1975) interactions. Some taxonomies such as those developed by Strain (1983; Kohler & Strain, 1997) and Goldstein (Goldstein et al., 1992) emphasize those behaviors that have been found through descriptive research to have greater than chance probabilities of eliciting positive responses from peers (e.g., Ferrell, 1990; Tremblay, Strain, Hendrickson, & Shores, 1981).

Some social skill taxonomies use initiations and responses as the first level of analysis with specific functions as a secondary analytical level (e.g., Kohler & Strain, 1997; McConnell et al., 1991). For example, Kohler and Strain (1997) identified seven types of child initiations and five types of responses (see Table 3.1). Other social skill taxonomies utilize specific functions as the primary level of analysis with the supplementary coding of each skill as an initiation or response (Guralnick, Connor, Hammond et al., 1995; Strain, 1984). For example, Guralnick and Groom (1985) offered a very extensive taxonomy of social behaviors, many of which may be coded as initiations if they begin an interaction (see Table 3.1). Coding schemes based on information processing models differentiate between goals and the strategies used to achieve those goals (Brown et al., 1996; Rubin & Krasnor, 1986). Strategies that represent individual behaviors would be considered at the social-communicative skill level, whereas goals fit in at the social task perfor-

Table 3.1. Coding system taxonomies at the social-communicative skill level

Kohler and Strain (1997)	Guralnick and Groom (1985)[a]	Brown et al. (1996)	Goldstein et al. (1992)
Social initiations	Gains the attention of peer[b,c]	Affiliatives/affection	Request for information
Play organizer	Uses peer as a resource[b,c]	Calling	Request for action
Share	Leads peers in activities—positive and neutral[c]	Comments	Request for clarification
Assistance	Leads peers in activities—negative[c]	Complimentary statement	Request for attention
Compliment	Imitates peer	Gestural communication	Comments
Affection	Expresses affection to peer[b]	Needs statements	Other assertives
Negative	Expresses hostility to peer[b]	Object aggression	General responses
General comment	Competes for equipment[b]	Personal aggression	Imitative responses
Immediate responses	Competes with peer for adult's attention[c]	Physical assistance	Responses to requests for information
Yes	Shows pride in product or attribute to peer	Play noises	Unintelligible utterances
No	Follows peer's activity without specific directions to do so[b]	Questions	Nonverbal requests for action
Ignores	Follows lead of peer in response to verbal or nonverbal directions[b]	Requests/command	Nonverbal general responses
General	Refuses to follow or ignores peer's directions or requests	Role assignment	Nonverbal imitative responses
Negative		Share/trade	Nonverbal social behaviors
Social concurrents		Suggestions	Vocal nonsocial behaviors
Same as initiations			Nonverbal negative behavior
Continued play			
Associative play			

[a]Many categories may also be coded as initiations.
[b]Includes further subcategories.
[c]Judged as successful or unsuccessful.

mance level of our analysis. The Brown and colleagues (1996) coding system includes examples of social-communicative strategies in Table 3.1 and social goals in Table 3.2.

Numerous taxonomies of communicative intents, many of which were derived by analyzing the prelinguistic behaviors and utterances of children of different ages, are available in the pragmatics literature (Miller, 1981). Because initiations and responses are considered a separate aspect of pragmatics called "turn taking" (Prutting & Kirchner, 1983), taxonomies of communicative intents generally are not as immediately linked to initiations and responses in the same way as those taxonomies emerging from the social competence literature. Categories of communicative intent tend to include such categories as requests, responses to requests, statements, and acknowledgements. Requests and statements are intents that typically correspond to specific sentence types. Requests are conveyed with questions and imperative sentences, and statements are conveyed with declarative sentences. Responses to requests and acknowledgements reciprocate requests and statements, respectively. Taxonomies for young children are quite simple (Bates, 1976; Dore, 1975; Halliday, 1975), whereas those for older children can be quite elaborate (Dore, 1978; Halliday, 1975; Tough, 1977).

Fey (1986) offered an intermediate alternative organized into four main categories (assertive conversational acts, responsive conversational acts, imitations, and other) with a total of 15 categories at its most fine-grained level. Fey's taxonomy was modified to include nonverbal behaviors as well when it was adapted for use with preschoolers with disabilities (see Table 3.1; Goldstein et al., 1992). Goldstein and colleagues further simplified the coding scheme in subsequent studies (English, Goldstein, Shafer, & Kaczmarek, 1997; Goldstein, English, Shafer, & Kaczmarek, 1997).

Impact on Social Partners

Three levels of increasingly specific analyses can be used to describe the impact of a child's social-communicative skills on social partners. The first level focuses on an analysis of the effectiveness of a child's initiations and responses. It addresses the questions, "To what extent are a child's initiations responded to by others, and to what extent does a child respond to the initiations of others?" The second level focuses on the questions, "To what extent do others respond to a child's specific social-communicative functions, and to what functions of others does the child respond." The third level examines the questions, "To what extent does the child succeed in achieving the specific purposes/intent of social-communicative attempts, and to what extent does the child

Table 3.2. Social task coding schemes

Social goals (Brown et al., 1996)	Peer group entry behaviors (Dodge et al., 1986)	Conflict resolution (Guralnick et al., 1998)	
Aggression	Behavior content codes	Initiator/companion interaction strategies	Provide clarification
Assistance	Strong demand	No apparent consequence	Initiates information
Attention	Request for information	Unrelated or digression	Insult
Comfort-support	Weak demand	Insist—positive	
Information-seeking	Request for agreement	Mitigate or minimize threat	Initial directive type
Information-providing	Sociable	Provide instruction	Mitigated directive
Object-related	Agree or comply	Unmitigated directive—companion	Unmitigated directive (10 types)
Other action	Give information	Mitigated directive—companion	
Pretend play	Greeting	Refuse with reason	Primary purpose of episode
Self-action	Get attention	Provide reason for noncompliance	Seek object
Stop-action	Kibitz	Postpone	Direct action in play
Cannot see or hear	Statements about self	Counter-compromise	Provide instruction
	Disagree, with rule cited	Conditional	Other
	Disagree, with reason cited	Accept proposal	
	Disagree, with no rule or reason cited	Reject proposal	Episode resolution
	Contentious/disruptive	Compliance or concurrence with directive	Full and complete compliance
	Incoherent behavior	Request reason for prior directive	Modified compliance
	Change of orientation	Request reason for noncompliance	Switch topic
		Information-seeking request	Self-solution
	Physical orientation markers	Concurrence-seeking request	
	Hover	Request clarification	
	Approach the group	Provide reason for prior directive	
	Nonverbal synchrony with the group's activity	Informative response	
	Proximal but not engaged in the group's activity	Concurrence with concurrence-seeking request	
	Disengage from group		

participate in assisting others to achieve their specific social-communicative purposes?" In keeping with the empirical foundation of the concept of effectiveness (Krasnor, 1982), the three questions are best answered by data collected through direct observation in naturalistic or analogue environments. The data to answer all three questions are usually expressed as a percentage or proportion (e.g., the number of successful initiations divided by the total number of initiations; the number of responses a child makes to others' initiations divided by the total number of initiations others make to him or her).

Responding to high proportions of initiations by others and receiving responses to a high proportion of one's own initiations are critical aspects of reciprocal social interaction (Greenwood et al., 1981), an indication of social competence. Children who do not respond readily to the social bids of others require support to assist them in responding. Children who initiate but who do not succeed in soliciting responses from others may require further analyses in the areas of social and communicative appropriateness to determine how their initiations might be changed to make them more effective. Kaczmarek, Evans, and Stever (1995) found, for example, that children who did not make eye contact when they initiated were less likely to receive responses from their communicative partners than those who did make eye contact.

The measurement of responses to social-communicative functions provides a more elaborate view of a child's social-communicative effectiveness than the more basic initiation-response level and highlights both functions that are effective as well as those whose effectiveness might be targeted for intervention. From a pragmatics perspective, this level of analysis assesses the intended illocutionary effect (Searle, 1969) because it examines the extent to which a communicative act gets a response without determining compliance. For example, a success at this level would be credited if the target child requested a toy from another child and the other child responded, "No, maybe later." The child's communicative act received a response, but the purpose of the target child's communication was not fulfilled.

At the most detailed analysis of effectiveness, the focus is on receiving responses and responding in ways that achieve the specific intents of the social-communicative skills. From the pragmatics perspective, it deals with the intended perlocutionary effect (Searle, 1969) because the response must specifically fulfill the intended purpose. So, in the example above, a success at this level would only be credited if the target child obtained the toy following his request.

Some observation systems have function-specific criteria for success (e.g., Guralnick, Connor, Hammond, et al., 1995; Roberts et al., 1995). Others have standard criteria applicable across functions (e.g.,

Brown et al., 1996; Rubin & Krasnor, 1986). Some coding schemes for measuring communicative effectiveness (e.g., Guralnick & Paul-Brown, 1986; Roberts et al., 1995) offer a detailed taxonomy for coding responses to some communicative functions (e.g., requests) that differentiates per-locutionary effects from the illocutionary effects.

Social-Communicative Effectiveness of Challenging Behaviors

Some children display challenging behaviors, such as having tantrums, crying, screaming, throwing things, biting, kicking, and hitting. Such be-haviors are clearly inappropriate and socially unacceptable. In a general sense, they tend to discourage the social bids of other children. At first glance, these behaviors may not be considered very socially effective; however, studies have shown that many challenging behaviors, despite their negative nature, do function socially and communicatively to gain the attention of others (Durand, Crimmins, Caulfield, & Taylor, 1989; Taylor & Carr, 1992), stop demands imposed by others (Carr & Newsom, 1985; Carr, Taylor, & Robinson, 1991), and acquire objects or activities from others (Day, Rea, Schussler, Larsen, & Johnson, 1988; Durand & Crimmins, 1988). In short, for many children these behav-iors are very effective social-communicative skills.

Functional assessment is a set of procedures that can be used to determine whether a child's challenging behaviors function socially and communicatively and to assist in the development of an intervention program to replace the challenging behaviors with functional, appro-priate alternatives. The key to determining the functions of challenging behaviors is the identification of the antecedent and consequent stim-uli that control them. The relationships between challenging behaviors and environmental stimuli can be complex because one challenging behavior (e.g., hitting) can function in many different ways (e.g., to escape demands, to obtain objects, to gain attention) and different challenging behaviors (e.g., hitting, screaming, running away) can have the same function (e.g., escape demands). Gathering information from others, direct observation in the natural environment, and systematic manipulations in analogue environments are three complementary strategies that assist in identifying the social-communicative functions of challenging behaviors (Carr et al., 1994; O'Neill, Horner, Albin, Storey, & Sprague, 1990). Data gathered from others and from direct observa-tions form the basis for generating hypotheses about the functions of challenging behaviors. The hypotheses are confirmed or refuted by direct manipulation of variables in analogue environments, a set of pro-cedures often referred to as *functional analysis* (Halle & Spradlin, 1993; Iwata et al., 1990).

Information is gathered from others through interviews and written questionnaires. This information assists in the initial identification of variables that may be controlling the challenging behaviors and narrows the range of natural environments targeted for direct observation. Interviews and questionnaires are focused on describing the challenging behaviors and identifying their antecedents (i.e., social context) and consequences (i.e., social reactions). Written questionnaires or interview formats include the Functional Analysis Interview (O'Neill, 1990) and the Motivational Assessment Scale (Durand & Crimmins, 1988). Carr and colleagues (1994) provide general guidelines for conducting interviews. Taylor and Bailey (1996) also have developed a form for interviewing teachers.

Like interviews and questionnaires, the purpose of direct observation is to determine possible relationships between challenging behaviors and naturally occurring environmental events (Carr et al., 1994; Iwata et al., 1990; Lalli & Goh, 1993). This approach to direct observation is sometimes called descriptive analysis (Bijou, Peterson, & Ault, 1968) because it identifies the conditions in the environment that temporally surround the challenging behaviors and provides an empirical basis for generating hypotheses about the functions of challenging behaviors. Through direct manipulation of variables associated with the behavior in the natural environment (i.e., functional analysis), the hypotheses then are tested and functional relationships can be established. Data are collected in home, school, and community environments in which the challenging behaviors are likely to be displayed. If results from interviews and questionnaires do not reveal useful information for selecting direct observation environments, scatter plot assessment (Touchette, MacDonald, & Langer, 1985) can be used to identify generally the times and situations in which the challenging behaviors occur most frequently.

A variety of descriptive assessment strategies and techniques have been developed to assist in identifying the events and conditions occurring before, after, and concurrently with challenging behaviors. Strategies have included specially designed forms that identify possible antecedent and subsequent events (Koegel, Koegel, Kellegrew, & Mullen, 1996; O'Neill et al., 1990), narrative recording (e.g., Bijou et al., 1968; Pettit & Bates, 1989), and checklists to be completed following episodes of challenging behaviors (Taylor & Bailey, 1996). Forms have been developed especially for parents (e.g., Koegel et al., 1996) and teachers (Taylor & Bailey, 1996). In addition, computer programs have been developed to assist in generating conditional probabilities that a specific antecedent is followed by the target behavior or that the target behavior is followed by a specific consequence (e.g., Repp & Karsh, 1990).

Following the identification of hypotheses about the function of challenging behaviors, analogue environments are constructed for a functional analysis to test the hypotheses and to verify the specific antecedent and consequent stimuli that control the behavior. Some researchers have indicated that this verification step is critical in the development of an intervention strategy (e.g., Carr et al., 1994; Iwata et al., 1990). Others suggest that the functional relationship will be verified indirectly through the development and success of an intervention program (e.g., Koegel et al., 1996; O'Neill et al., 1990). The use of analogue environments to confirm hypotheses seems especially critical if relationships between behaviors and environmental events and conditions appear complex, although the construction of analogue situations may require careful planning so that they resemble the circumstances present in the natural environment (Halle & Spradlin, 1993).

There are two methods to constructing analogue situations (Iwata et al., 1990). The first is to assess the effects of a single variable on the behavior. Carr and colleagues (1994) described multiple examples of this method. One hypothesis is that a child's screaming in independent work environments is an attention-seeking behavior. The antecedent conditions suspected of occasioning the behavior are set up in the analogue environment (e.g., independent work). On some days, the child receives the teacher's attention only after starting to scream. On other days, the child receives the teacher's attention for engaging in her independent work. If screaming continues on those days when she receives the teacher's attention following screaming but does not occur on those days when attention is received for independent work, the hypothesis is confirmed. An intervention can now be developed in which the child is given attention while engaged in independent work. In addition, the child can be taught appropriate strategies for gaining the teacher's attention during independent work tasks, such as raising her hand or calling the teacher by name.

The second method is a general model for determining the extent to which different environmental variables may be maintaining a given challenging behavior (Iwata, Dorsey, Slifer, Bauman, & Richman, 1982). The strategy is particularly appropriate to use when it is suspected that a given challenging behavior may have multiple functions. In this model, multiple hypotheses are tested by exposing children to a series of conditions. For example, Wickstrom-Kane and Goldstein (1999) reported having a child engage in three testing conditions (i.e., solitary play, limited toy access, directed play) contrasted with a free play control condition to determine whether a child's screaming was related to gaining attention, getting materials, or escaping social and task demands. This method may be considered in lieu of limited direct observations, because it investigates a broader range of hypotheses. Following descriptive analysis but before functional analysis, Wacker, Peck, Derby, Berg, and Harding (1996) recommended the use of structural analysis in which a child is exposed to a series of short analogue environments over several days. Each environment tests one hypothesis (e.g., attention) while holding other possible hypotheses constant (e.g., demand, preference).

ASSESSING SOCIAL-COMMUNICATIVE TASKS

Like the assessment of social-communicative skills, direct observation and the acquisition of information from others are important methods of assessing children's social-communicative tasks. The focus in this area, however, is on the sequencing of skills that address the task rather than on the individual social-communicative behaviors themselves. In assessing communicative appropriateness, emphasis is placed on discourse analysis, which is examined through direct observation. Although direct observation in analogue situations is well suited for analyzing successful social task performance (Foster et al., 1993), the assessment of social appropriateness focuses on children's social cognition, which is the thinking processes involved in responding to social situations. Social cognition is typically evaluated using hypothetical reflective reasoning assessments.

The Social Appropriateness
of Social-Communicative Tasks

In hypothetical reflective reasoning assessments, evaluators describe social problems focused on specific social goals (e.g., object acquisition, peer entry, helping someone in need, initiating friendships), and children are asked a variety of questions about the situations (e.g., identifying possible response strategies, describing what happened in the vignette) to gain an understanding of their social cognition (Rubin & Krasnor, 1986). Behavioral role plays, which were described previously, may be a component of the question set (e.g., Dodge & Price, 1994). Pictures or drawings may be used to enhance verbal descriptions of the social situations (e.g., Rubin & Krasnor, 1986). Videotaped vignettes performed by child actors to replace verbal descriptions (e.g., Dodge et al., 1986; Dodge & Price, 1994) improve the validity of hypothetical reasoning techniques (Hughes et al., 1989; Vaughn & Haager, 1994). These techniques also have been used to test the effects of partner characteristics, such as age and gender, on the production of strategies (e.g., Rubin & Krasnor, 1986). A number of tests have been developed based on hypothetical reasoning techniques, for example, the Preschool Interpersonal Problem-Solving test (PIPS; Spivak & Shure, 1974), the Social Problem-Solving Test (SPST; Rubin & Krasnor, 1986), and the What Happens Next Game (WHNG; Spivak, Platt, & Shure, 1976).

The validity of early hypothetical reflective reasoning techniques was questionable (Rubin & Krasnor, 1986). Validity has been improved by selecting social situations that have been shown to be important (e.g., Dodge et al., 1985) and by demonstrating that children's responses to hypothetical situations correlate with measures of behavior in the natural environment and measures of peer acceptance (see Crick & Dodge, 1994; Dodge, 1986; Rubin & Krasnor, 1986). Because many hypothetical reflective reasoning techniques are highly dependent on abstract thinking, taking the perspective of another, and fairly sophisticated language skills, they may not be valid for children who have significant cognitive and language impairments.

The Communicative Appropriateness of Social-Communicative Tasks

At the social-communicative task level, the assessment of communicative appropriateness focuses on the analysis of discourse, or multiple utterances that are connected by a common topic and sequenced according to a prescribed set of rules. The analysis of discourse goes beyond the analysis of speech acts (Carrow-Woolfolk & Lynch, 1982) and adjacency pairs (e.g., questions-responses; directives-compliance; requests-responses). Because of the emphasis on social communication, this chapter focuses on conversational rather than narrative discourse. Three areas of discourse analysis relevant to conversations are 1) topic management, 2) semantic/syntactic cohesion, and 3) turn taking. Although aspects of topic management, cohesion, and turn taking appear in children by the age of 5 (Prutting & Kirchner, 1987), many of these skills are not fully developed until later childhood and adolescence (Mentis, 1991). The Pragmatic Protocol (Prutting & Kirchner, 1983, 1987) discussed previously includes these three aspects of discourse analysis.

Topic Management

Topic management consists of the appropriate selection, introduction and change, and maintenance of topics within conversations (Mentis,

1994; Prutting & Kirchner, 1983, 1987). The selection of topics refers to the speaker's ability to select topics for conversation that are appropriate to the dimensions of interpersonal, physical, and cultural context. For example, it would be considered inappropriate to discuss the outcome of a major league baseball game during a reading lesson focused on a story about a child's pet.

Introducing new topics and shifting conversational topics are critical discourse skills. Younger children introduce more topics than older children and adults (Brinton & Fujiki, 1984). As children develop more sophisticated language skills, they become less dependent on adults for structuring conversations (Foster, 1985). Their topics are explored in greater depth and become increasingly less dependent on the here and now (Brinton & Fujiki, 1984; Mentis, 1994; Wanska & Bedrosian, 1985), and the linguistic skills required for polite shifting, shading, and changing of topics are acquired (Mentis, 1994). The Mentis analysis of topic introduction and change includes the parameters of the number of topics and subtopics introduced, the manner of introduction (i.e., change, shift, inappropriate tangential shift, noncoherent change), the type of introduction (i.e., new, related, reintroduced), and the nature of the content (i.e., abstract versus concrete; here and now versus displaced in time and space).

Maintaining a topic through extended conversation is another major parameter of topic management. An important aspect of maintaining a topic is learning how to extend the content of conversations by introducing new information (Mentis, 1991, 1994). Mentis' (1994) analysis of topic maintenance includes the length of the topic/subtopic sequence and the type of topic maintenance contribution, which has been referred to as Topic Coherence Analysis (Mentis, 1991; Mentis & Lundgren, 1995; Mentis & Prutting, 1991). Topic Coherence Analysis is a coding system designed to investigate how a child contributes new information to the conversation (i.e., unsolicited novel information, requests for novel information, requests for actions or objects, requested information provided); how a child maintains the conversation without contributing new information (i.e., acknowledgements, discourse markers, and various types of repetitions); and the problematic utterances that disrupt topic coherence (i.e., inappropriate responses, perseverations).

Although the refined aspects of introducing and maintaining a topic within conversation are not fully developed until adolescence, the process of learning how to introduce, maintain, and extend conversational topics begins in the early stages of language development (Foster, 1985; Mentis, 1991). Studies have shown how caregivers contribute to children's acquisition of topic coherence (e.g., Bloom, Rocissano, & Hood, 1976; Yoder et al., 1994). Yoder and colleagues (1994) utilized a coding

scheme in which adult and child utterances were coded as topic continuations and topic initiations. Adult topic continuations and initiations consisted of additional subcodes to determine the extent to which
nonquestions and various types of questions set the occasion for child
topic maintenance. Their research demonstrated that young children
with developmental delays were more likely to continue the topic when
adults employed topic-continuing questions rather than other types of
utterances. The coding system could be applied to adult–child interactions to assist teachers and caregivers in understanding how they might
interact to increase children's acquisition of topic coherence.

Semantic/Syntactic Cohesion

A functional approach to pragmatics perceives topic management as
dependent on the acquisition and use of certain semantic relations and
syntactic structures (Mentis, 1994; Ninio & Snow, 1999; Prutting &
Kirchner, 1983, 1987). The use of these linguistic devices produces
"cohesion" in connected discourse; that is, the utterances within a conversation function as a meaningful unit in which many of the component utterances can only be fully understood in reference to others
(Halliday & Hasan, 1976). VanDijk (1980) referred to local and global
cohesion. Local cohesion focuses on the common content and logical
relationships between adjacent utterances; global cohesion addresses
the overall connectedness of the discourse to the topic under discussion. An important aspect of cohesion requires that speakers provide
sufficient information to the listener without repeating information
that has already been conveyed within the conversation or exists as
part of a shared background. Clark (1996) described this as grounding.
Halliday and Hasan (1976) identified five syntactic and semantic
devices that assist in the achievement of cohesion: 1) reference, 2) sub-
stitution, 3) ellipsis, 4) conjunction, and 5) lexical cohesion. As part of
her assessment paradigm, Mentis (1994) described in detail these semantic and syntactic forms that function within discourse to introduce
and maintain topics. Although acquisition of some of these linguistic
devices occurs in a child's early years, most are not mastered fully until
adolescence. The reader is directed to the primary sources for the definitions and detailed procedures for conducting analyses of cohesion.

Turn Taking

Turn taking refers to smooth interchanges between communicative
partners. Children begin to learn turn taking during infancy. By the time
they say their first words, children sustain long episodes of turn taking
that are well timed (Kaye & Charney, 1981). As children grow older,

they display similar skills with peers (Ervin-Tripp, 1979; Martinez, 1987). Prutting and Kirchner (1983, 1987) devote one section of their Pragmatic Protocol to turn taking. Under this category, they have included initiation, response, repair and revision, pause time, interruption and overlap, feedback to listener, adjacency, and contingency. "Initiation" and "response" as aspects of turn taking are similar in meaning to the same terms discussed previously in the effectiveness of social-communicative skills. "Feedback to listener" reflects the use of verbal and nonverbal acknowledgements such as "yeah" or head nods; these aspects are treated as communicative functions also considered under the effectiveness of social-communicative skills. Finally, "adjacency" (i.e., an utterance that follows immediately after a partner's utterance) and "contingency" (i.e., utterances that have the same topic and add new information to a partner's immediately preceding utterance) refer to aspects of topic management.

The aspects that have not been considered previously are repair and revision, pause time, and interruption and overlap. Repair and revision refer to the child's ability to respond to communication breakdowns during conversation from both the speaker and listener perspectives. Children must be able to respond to conversational partners who request clarification so that the conversation remains on track. They also must request clarification when they do not understand or hear their communicative partners. Pause time focuses on the timing between conversational turns, which should be neither too long nor too short. Finally, interruption and overlap considers when one partner interrupts another or when two people talk at the same time.

The Effectiveness of Social-Communicative Tasks

At the social task level, this chapter considers three measures of social-communicative effectiveness: 1) length of interactions, 2) accomplishment of social tasks, and 3) ecological inventories.

Length of Interactions

Initiations and responses are the building blocks of interaction. The length of a child's interactions with others is a gross evaluation of social-communicative sophistication. The length of interactions is best measured through direct observation. Minimally, an interaction represents one initiation-response unit (e.g., Brown et al., 1996; Kamps et al., 1992). Others have defined interaction as an exchange of social behaviors beyond the original initiation-response unit (e.g., Brady, 1997; Reike & Lewis, 1984), often with a minimum time criterion of 3–4 seconds (e.g., Davis et al., 1994; McEvoy et al., 1988). The length of inter-actions may be measured by counting the number of turns or timing the duration of exchanges until the interaction stops or is discontinued for a period of time. In some observational codes, if there is no hiatus in the interaction, a reply to a response (e.g., the third turn following an initiation and first response) is called a "response" as are all subse-quent turns taken by the individuals involved in the interaction (e.g., Strain, 1983; Strain, Shores, & Timm, 1977). In other codes, interaction beyond the initial initiation-response unit is more specifically defined as ongoing interactions (Davis et al., 1994), extended interactions (Hec-imovic et al., 1985), social concurrents/responses (Kohler & Strain, 1997), reciprocal interactions (McEvoy et al., 1988), and continuing ini-tiations/responses (Roeyers, 1996).

Achievement of Social Tasks

The assessment of social tasks is not as well developed as the assess-ment methodologies for social-communicative skills. Social tasks may range from simple situations, such as obtaining another's attention or seeking information, to more complex social situations, such as enter-ing an ongoing play interaction or resolving a conflict that arises dur-ing play. At the simple end, there may be little difference between social-communicative skills and social tasks except to acknowledge that a goal can be accomplished using different social-communicative be-haviors. At the more complex end, however, social tasks often require the successful sequencing of social-communicative skills to accomplish the intended goal. Measurement of the accomplishment of social tasks focuses on the sequence of skills used to accomplish the task, the suc-cessful or unsuccessful outcome of the sequence of skills, and the alternative sequence(s) of skills used if faced with initial failure in ac-complishing the task.

As mentioned previously, some observational codes differentiate social goals from the individual behaviors used to accomplish them (e.g., Brown et al., 1996; Rubin & Krasnor, 1986). Table 3.2 lists the 12 social goals in the Brown and colleagues' observation system. Observa-tion systems such as these are useful in determining the types of social goals a child displays and the behavioral forms typically used to accom-plish them. As with social-communicative skills, the measurement of success of a child's interpersonal goals must be viewed from the child's perspective rather than from the perspective of appropriateness, which is a judgment from the societal perspective.

Research on specific social tasks might be used as the basis for eval-uating the strategies that given children employ when confronted with such tasks. For example, there has been significant research focused on how children of various ages enter into the ongoing play of others (Corsaro, 1979a, 1981; Putallaz & Wasserman, 1989) and how they resolve conflicts that arise during play (Guralnick et al., 1998; Laursen & Hartup, 1989; Shantz, 1987). This research reveals the successful and unsuccessful patterns of social-communicative skills that children use in their interactions with other children. Specific research studies typically offer a complete observation system inclusive of a taxonomy of possible behaviors for accomplishing the specified task as well as definitions of effectiveness. An example of taxonomies specific to peer entry and conflict resolution can be found in Table 3.2.

Ecological Inventories

Taxonomies are not available for all social tasks that a child faces. The use of ecological inventories represents one strategy for determining the sequence of social-communicative skills required for completion of a particular social task. Ecological inventories (Browder, 1991; Brown et al., 1979; Gage & Falvey, 1995) were designed to develop functional curricular content for students with severe disabilities. Children without disabilities are observed performing the designated social task in the natural environment. The skills they display, including the range of variations, are delineated. The target child is then placed in the same environment and observed. A record is kept of the skills the child displays. The child's performance is then analyzed against the list of skills that the children without disabilities displayed. Skills that the child does not display are then targeted as part of the child's instructional program. Alternatively, adaptations and accommodations for specific skills may also be identified.

ASSESSING OVERALL SOCIAL-COMMUNICATIVE PERFORMANCE AND OUTCOMES

In this section, global social measures and the outcomes of peer acceptance, friendships, and social networks are considered.

Global Social Measures

There are a variety of available formal, norm-referenced instruments for measuring children's social competence. Some developmental and adaptive behavior scales also include a social domain (e.g., Battelle Developmental Inventory [BDI], Newborg, Stock, Wnek, Guidubaldi, &

Svinicki, 1984; Vineland Adaptive Behavior Scales [VABS], Sparrow, Balla, & Cicchetti, 1984). Although many of these instruments include items that relate to social communication, they also contain a variety of items that address other aspects of social competence. For example, the Social Skills Rating System (SSRS; Gresham & Elliott, 1990), a tool designed for preschool, elementary, and secondary school children, samples behaviors in the domains of social skills, problem behaviors, and academic competence. The tool consists of subscales focused on cooperation, assertion, responsibility, empathy, and self-control and includes such items as "finishes class assignments within time limits," "keeps room clean and neat without being reminded," and "reports accidents to appropriate persons."

Most tools are like the SSRS in that they address both positive and negative behaviors (e.g., Matson Evaluation of Social Skills with Youngsters [MESSY], Matson, 1989; Preschool and Kindergarten Behavior Scales [PKBS], Merrell, 1994; Early Screening Project [ESP], Walker, Severson, & Feil, 1995). Other tools, however, focus primarily on negative behaviors (e.g., Revised Behavior Problems Checklist, Quay & Peterson, 1983; Child Behavior Checklist, Achenbach, 1991). Some tools have subscales that focus specifically on social interaction (e.g., PKBS, ESP). Readers are referred to Wittmer, Doll, and Strain (1996) for a review of preschool measures and Merrell (1993) for a review of school-age measures. In keeping with their multiple measure approach to evaluating social competence, McConnell and Odom (1999) proposed a performance-based approach that uses direct observation, observer impressions, teacher rating, and peer ratings.

Global Communication Measures

Although there are many norm-referenced instruments that measure children's language development, few include a focus on pragmatic abilities. For example, in a review of eight instruments focusing on early communication development, only three included consideration of pragmatic functions (McCathren, Warren, & Yoder, 1996): Assessing Prelinguistic and Early Linguistic Behaviors in Developmentally Young Children (Olswang, Stoel-Gammon, Coggins, & Carpenter, 1987), the Communication and Symbolic Behavior Scales (CSBS; Wetherby & Prizant, 1993), and the Sequenced Inventory of Communication Development–Revised (Hedrick, Prather, & Tobin, 1975). (See Chapter 4 for a detailed review of the CSBS.) Some of the newer comprehensive language instruments have included more of an emphasis on pragmatics. For example, the Comprehensive Assessment of Spoken Language

(CASL; Carrow-Woolfolk, 1999), which is a relatively new instrument for ages 3 through 21, includes a pragmatic subscale that focuses on the use of appropriate language in situational contexts. Children are asked to respond with utterances that are appropriate to specific contexts (e.g., expressing gratitude, offering sympathetic support, politely declining an unwanted invitation). A number of other aspects of pragmatics (e.g., inference, perspective taking) are incorporated into the other subscales. In addition to comprehensive instruments, there are formal measures devoted exclusively to pragmatics (e.g., Test of Pragmatic Skills–Revised, Shulman, 1986; Interpersonal Language Skills Assessment, Blagden & McConnell, 1985; Test of Pragmatic Language, Phelps-Terasaki & Phelps-Gunn, 1992).

Social-Communicative Outcomes

Social competence research has focused primarily on three outcome measures, which we extend to the concept of social-communicative competence: 1) Is the child liked by peers? 2) Does the child have friends? and 3) Is the child a member of one or more social networks? Unlike the measurement strategies discussed previously, measurements of these outcomes do not assess child behavior directly. Rather, they assess the benefits one hopes a child experiences as an outgrowth of social-communicative competence.

Peer Acceptance

Peer acceptance is assessed through sociometric measures, which are the most widely used research methods for evaluating children's social competence (see Bukowski & Hoza, 1989; Coie, Dodge, & Kupersmidt, 1990; McConnell & Odom, 1986, for reviews). Sociometric measures assess peers' feelings of attraction for other children (Foster et al., 1993) and focus on the degree to which a child is valued, liked, or accepted by his or her peer group. Research has shown that socially skilled behavior is related to peer acceptance and socially unskilled behavior to peer rejection and peer neglect (see Coie et al., 1990; Dodge & Feldman, 1990; Hymel & Rubin, 1985); however, there is evidence that other factors may mitigate the relationship between behavior and peer acceptance or rejection. For example, Crick and Dodge (1994) pointed out that age affects the relationship between peers' perceptions of social competence and peer acceptance. From preschool to second grade, there is no relationship between peers' perceptions of a child's social competence and peer acceptance. By third grade, they are positively related and become increasingly so for fifth graders. Hymel, Wagner, and Butler (1990) proposed that a child's established reputation can bias how a child's behavior is perceived, thus preserving social status even when behavior changes. There is some evidence to suggest that peer sociometrics actually measure a unique aspect of social competence that is distinct from teacher ratings and direct observational measures such as initiations and responses (Guralnick, Connor, Hammond, et al., 1995; McConnell & Odom, 1999).

Sociometric measures, specifically peer ratings and peer nominations, are commonly used to determine the status of a child within a peer group (Gresham, 1986; McConnell & Odom, 1986). Although some have suggested that peer ratings and nominations measure different aspects of social behavior (Asher & Taylor, 1981; McConnell & Odom, 1986), others have provided evidence that they measure the same conceptual construct (Bukowski & Hoza, 1989; Coie et al., 1990). The term *peer acceptance* refers to that construct.

In peer nominations, children are asked to name other children based on specific criteria. The criteria may be quite general (e.g., name three children you like to play with) or more specific (e.g., name three children you would like to play outside with or go on a trip with). Younger children usually are asked to select from photographs of classmates. A child's score is the number of positive nominations a child receives. Some peer nomination procedures also require children to make negative nominations (e.g., pick three children you would not want to read a story with). When negative nominations are used, negative nominations are subtracted from positive nominations to determine a child's score.

Peer ratings involve having a child rate each peer on a Likert-type scale using criteria similar to peer nominations (e.g., like to play with this person a lot, kind of like to play with this person, do not like to play with this person). Children have been asked to rate peers on scales that have ranged from two to seven points (see McConnell & Odom, 1986). For young children, the categories are fewer in number and typically depicted with faces (e.g., happy, neutral, sad) or other pictures that convey the meaning of the categories. Summing or averaging the ratings received determines a child's score.

Although there appears to be no empirical evidence to support the position (see Foster et al., 1993; McConnell & Odom, 1986, for reviews; Iverson, Barton, & Iverson, 1997), negative nominations and ratings are controversial because some believe that asking children to articulate peer rejection may further enhance that rejection. Furthermore, the act of asking children to express negative feelings about other children runs contrary to the philosophies espoused in educational and other environments in which children interact socially. The extent to which teachers and other direct service personnel use sociometric measures is unclear, but it would seem that the controversy surrounding them in the research community would make them poor choices as tools for the everyday practitioner. In the least, practitioners who wish to use sociometric measures, especially those using negative nominations, should obtain parental permission explicitly. To minimize risk of harm, some have suggested engaging children in an activity following peer rating and nomination procedures, so children are less likely to discuss their ratings with other children (Doll, 1996; Fujiki, Brinton, Hart, & Fitzgerald, 1999). Practitioners may also find those measures that avoid negative nominations to be more acceptable. For example, Goldstein and colleagues (English, Goldstein, et al., 1997; Goldstein et al., 1997) described the "friendship train" in which children selected photographs of classmates with whom they wished to take a ride to a desirable location. The rater's photo was placed in the engineer's compartment. The rater was then instructed to select three friends for the first ride. After the first three were chosen, those photographs were set aside and the child was instructed to select another set of three. The procedure continued until all children in the class were selected for rides. Children's status in the group was determined by their average rank order.

Friendships

Friendships are desirable for all children. Friendships, however, are a distinctly different social construct from peer acceptance (Asher, Parker, & Walker, 1996; Bukowski & Hoza, 1989). Peer acceptance involves general, unilateral judgments of individuals within a group about an individual child whereas friendship focuses on a dyad and their bilateral judgments about each other on specific relational characteristics (e.g., loyalty, intimacy). The features of friendship include such characteristics as self-esteem enhancement and self-evaluation, emotional security, intimacy and affection, informational or instrumental assistance, and companionship and stimulation (Parker et al., 1995). Measures of friendship have been used less frequently in the literature than measures of peer acceptance (Bukowski & Hoza, 1989).

As with peer acceptance, sociometric measures are among the most common determinants of friendships (Bukowski & Hoza, 1989). A friendship is defined when two children nominate each other or rate each other highly. Friendships may be determined directly by asking children to identify their best or closest friends from memory or from lists and/or photos. The number of nominations can be restricted to a certain number (e.g., Urberg, Degirmencioglu, Tolson, & Halliday-Scher,

1995), limited by a defined list, such as a list of classmates (e.g., Ray, Cohen, & Secrist, 1995), or not restricted at all (e.g., George & Hartmann, 1996). Mutually high rankings on any sociometric rating or nomination may also define friendship. Some researchers (e.g., Buysse, 1993; Guralnick, Gottman, & Hammond, 1996; Guralnick & Groom, 1988) have used the terminology "reciprocal" or "mutual" friendships to highlight the bidirectional nature of friendship and to distinguish it from "unilateral" friendships when positive nominations or high ratings are made by only one child in the dyad.

There are a variety of other methods for defining friendships among children. Some have determined friendships based on direct observational measures (e.g., Guralnick & Groom, 1988; Howes, 1983; Roopnarine & Field, 1984). Guralnick and colleagues (1996), for example, based the definition of "reciprocal friendship" on mutually high levels of interaction between two children (i.e., 33% of each child's total positive interactions were with each other). Others have identified friendships among children by asking parents, teachers, or the children themselves through written or verbal questionnaires, rating scales, or interviews (e.g., Berndt, 1986; Furman & Buhrmester, 1985; Guralnick, Connor, & Hammond, 1995). Friendships of infants, toddlers, and preschoolers are best assessed by asking parents or by observing children directly (see Howes, 1996). Buysse (1993), for example, developed the Early Childhood Friendship Survey for teachers and parents that focuses on children's mutual friendships and unilateral relationships through a set of closed and open-ended questions.

A child's friendships are most commonly described by counting a child's mutual (and sometimes unilateral) friendships (e.g., Farver, 1996; Ray et al., 1995). This has sometimes been referred to as a child's friendship network (e.g., George & Hartmann, 1996; Ray et al., 1995). Bukowski and Hoza (1989) proposed a three-level assessment scheme for measuring children's friendships. Level 1 involves determining whether a child has a friendship with at least one child (i.e., reciprocally high positive feelings between two children). Level 2 focuses on the number of reciprocal, positive relationships that a child has (i.e., counting the number of mutually positive nominations or ratings for a particular child). Level 3 focuses an analysis of the qualitative characteristics of a child's friendships through closed or open questionnaires. A number of questionnaires are available for assessing the quality of school-age and adolescent friendships (e.g., Berndt & Perry, 1986; Bukowski, Boivin, & Hoza, 1994; Furman & Buhrmester, 1985; Parker & Asher, 1993). These and other measures of the multidimensional features of friendships are reviewed by Furman (1996).

Social Networks

Social networks are an extension of the investigation of friendships. A social network is:

> The social position of individuals and their peer groups relative to other individuals and peer groups within a broader social system (e.g., classroom, school). It describes who affiliates with whom and how salient the various groupings and individuals are within the social system. (Farmer & Farmer, 1996, p. 433)

A social network describes the interconnections among members of social groups. Although considerable research has shown that children with disabilities tend to have lower levels of social acceptance than typical children (e.g., Fujiki et al., 1999; Guralnick & Groom, 1988; Nabors, 1997; Sabornie, 1987), this may not be a complete picture. It overlooks the role that social networks play in supporting the establishment and maintenance of social behaviors in children with disabilities. Farmer and Farmer (1996), for example, demonstrated that children with disabilities in mainstreamed classrooms were not isolated but rather were members of peer groups with varying degrees of inclusion. As with other research (e.g., Berndt, 1982; Farver, 1996; Johnson et al., 1997), this study revealed that children form social groups based on common characteristics such as gender and behavioral style. By examining peer social networks, a broader picture of a child's social ecology is explored.

To determine social networks, individuals in the group are asked to identify their friends or the people they hang out with, often stratifying the strength of those relationships by using such designations as "very best friend," "best friends," and "other friends" (e.g., George & Hartmann, 1996; Parker & Asher, 1993; Ray et al., 1995). Parents or teachers may be asked to make these determinations for younger children (e.g., Farver, 1996). Another approach to gathering data asks all children to identify who hangs out with whom (e.g., Cairns, Perrin, & Cairns, 1985; Farmer & Farmer, 1996; Kindermann, 1995). This composite approach to mapping social networks views children as expert observers and provides an empirical determination of consensus among group members (Kindermann, 1995). Occasionally, data from direct observation is combined with sociometric data to examine friendship networks (e.g., Johnson et al., 1997).

A basic analysis of children's social networks may simply mean the number and type of child social contacts (e.g., Guralnick, 1997; Lewis, Feiring, & Brooks-Gunn, 1987) or friends (e.g., Ray et al., 1995). More commonly, the investigation of children's networks is based on an elab-

TOURO COLLEGE LIBRARY

orate analysis of the friendship nominations of a group designed to assign children to groups (sometimes referred to as cliques), determine linkages among individuals and groups, and assess the strength of an individual's connections to the network. Sociograms are often developed to depict these relationships (e.g., Farver, 1996; Jansson, 1997; Johnson et al., 1997; Kindermann, 1995). Computer programs are available to assist in these processes (e.g., Kindermann, 1995; Urberg et al., 1995). A variety of statistical methods have been used in investigating children's social networks, including binomial z-tests of conditional probabilities (Kindermann, 1995), logit models (Anderson, Wasserman, & Crouch, 1999), maximum likelihood and Bayesian approaches (Jansson, 1997), and matrix techniques (Johnson et al., 1997).

CONCLUSION

This chapter provides an interdisciplinary framework for assessing social communication in children. It weds the assessment practices of social and communicative competence in a 3×3 matrix. The model examines social communication at three increasingly complex levels of performance from basic social-communicative skills to overall performance and its related outcomes. Each level may be evaluated in terms of the divergent conceptualizations of social and communicative competence and the convergent conceptualizations of function. Although all aspects of the model may not be relevant to all children at all times, the framework provides an overview of measures and how they relate to one another.

The assessment of social communication is complex, and this complexity obviously affects how assessments are implemented. Expertise is needed that goes well beyond a single discipline, especially at more sophisticated levels of social communication. To acquire a comprehensive picture of a child's competence, collaboration among evaluators is critical. Speech-language pathologists, psychologists, teachers, and other related services providers all play a role in the evaluation of social communication. Parents and other family members also must be an integral part of the assessment process. They provide important information about a child's behavior in environments that are generally not accessible to professionals, give insight into the family's cultural background and its intersection with social-communicative behaviors, and supply essential input into the development of a viable intervention program. Although decisions about appropriateness consider a child's family, decisions about function must focus specifically on the child. Judgments about effectiveness require that practitioners determine the

TOURO COLLEGE LIBRARY

extent to which children are achieving their interpersonal social and communicative goals, the impact that children have on the peers and adults around them, and the barriers that impede their success. By gathering this information, they can design intervention programs that focus on ensuring successful interactions and rewarding relationships with others.

REFERENCES

Achenbach, T.M. (1991). *Manual for the Child Behavior Checklist/4–18 and 1991 Profile*. Burlington: University of Vermont, Department of Psychiatry.

Achenbach, T.M., & Edelbrock, C.S. (1978). The classification of child psychopathology: A review and analysis of empirical efforts. *Psychological Bulletin, 85,* 1275–1301.

Adams, C., & Bishop, D.V.M. (1989). Conversational characteristics of children with semantic-pragmatic disorder: I. Exchange structure, turntaking, repairs and cohesion. *British Journal of Disorders of Communication, 24,* 211–239.

Anderson, C.J., Wasserman, S., & Crouch, B. (1999). A p* primer: Logit models of social networks. *Social Networks, 21,* 37–66.

Asante, M.K., & Davis, A. (1989). Encounters in the interracial workplace. In M.K. Asante & W.B. Gudykunst (Eds.), *Handbook of international and intercultural communication* (pp. 374–391). Thousand Oaks, CA: Sage Publications.

Asher, S.R., Markell, R.A., & Hymel, S. (1981). Identifying children at risk in peer relations: A critique of the rate of interaction approach to assessment. *Child Development, 52,* 1239–1245.

Asher, S.R., & Parker, J.G. (1989). Significance of peer relationship problems in childhood. In B. Schnieder, G. Attili, J. Nadel, & R. Weisberg (Eds.), *Social competence in developmental perspective* (pp. 5–23). Norwell, MA: Kluwer Academic/Plenum Publishers.

Asher, S.R., Parker, J.G., & Walker, D.L. (1996). Distinguishing friendship from peer acceptance: Implications for intervention and assessment. In W.M. Bukowski, A.F. Newcomb, & W.W. Hartup (Eds.), *The company they keep: Friendship in childhood and adolescence* (pp. 366–405). Cambridge, England: Cambridge University Press.

Asher, S.R., & Taylor, A.R. (1981). Social outcomes of mainstreaming: Sociometric assessment and beyond. *Exceptional Education Quarterly, 1,* 13–30.

Baker, L., & Cantwell, D.P. (1982) Developmental, social and behavioral characteristics of speech and language disordered children. In S. Chess & A. Thomas (Eds.), *Annual progress in child psychiatry and child development* (pp. 205–216). Levittown, PA: Brunner/Mazel Publishing.

Baltaxe, C.A. (1977). Pragmatic deficits in the language of autistic adolescents. *Journal of Pediatric Psychology, 2,* 176–180.

Baltaxe, C.A., & Simmons, J.Q. (1988). Communication deficits in preschool children with psychiatric disorders. *Seminars in Speech and Language, 9,* 81–91.

Bates, E. (1976). *Language and context: The acquisition of pragmatics.* San Diego: Academic Press.

Beckman, P.J., & Lieber, J. (1994). The social strategy rating scale: An approach to evaluating social competence. *Journal of Early Intervention, 18,* 1–11.

Berg, C. (1989). Knowledge of strategies for dealing with everyday problems. *Developmental Psychology, 25,* 607–618.

Berndt, T. (1982). The features and effects of friendships in early adolescence. *Child Development, 53,* 1447–1460.

Berndt, T. (1986). Children's comments about friendships. In M. Perlmutter (Ed.), *Minnesota Symposia on Child Psychology: Vol. 18. Cognitive perspectives on children's social and behavioral development* (pp. 189–212). Mahwah, NJ: Lawrence Erlbaum Associates.

Berndt, T.J., & Perry, T.B. (1986). Children's perceptions of friendships as supportive relationships. *Developmental Psychology, 22,* 640–648.

Betancourt, H., & Lopez, S.R. (1993). The study of culture, ethnicity, and race in American psychology. *American Psychologist, 48,* 629–637.

Bierman, K.L., & Montminy, H.P. (1993). Developmental issues in social-skills assessment and intervention with children and adolescents. *Behavior Modification, 17,* 229–254.

Bijou, S.W., Peterson, R.F., & Ault, M.H. (1968). A method to integrate descriptive and experimental field studies at the level of data and empirical concepts. *Journal of Applied Behavior Analysis, 1,* 175–191.

Bishop, D.V.M. (1998). Development of the children's communicative checklist (CCC): A method for assessing qualitative aspects of communicative impairment in children. *Journal of Child Psychology and Psychiatry and Applied Disciplines, 39,* 879–891.

Bishop, D.V.M., & Adams, C. (1989). Conversational characteristics of children with semantic-pragmatic disorder: II. What features lead to a judgement of inappropriacy? *British Journal of Disorders of Communication, 24,* 241–263.

Bishop, D.V.M., Hartley, J., & Weir, F. (1994). Why and when do some language-impaired children seem talkative?: A study of initiation in conversations with children with semantic-pragmatic disorder. *Journal of Autism and Developmental Disorders, 24,* 177–197.

Blagden, C.M., & McConnell, N.L. (1985). *Interpersonal Language Skills Assessment.* East Moline, IL: LinguiSystems.

Bloom, L., Rocissano, L., & Hood, L. (1976). Adult-child discourse: Developmental interaction between information processing and linguistic knowledge. *Cognitive Psychology, 8,* 521–552.

Brady, N.C. (1997). The teaching game: A reciprocal peer tutoring program for preschool children. *Education and Treatment of Children, 20,* 123–149.

Brinton, B., & Fujiki, M. (1984). Development of topic manipulation skills in discourse. *Journal of Speech and Hearing Research, 27,* 350–358.

Brody, G.H., Stoneman, G., & Wheatley, P. (1984). Peer interaction in the presence and absence of observers. *Child Development, 55,* 1425–1428.

Browder, D.M. (1991). *Assessment of individuals with severe disabilities: An applied behavior approach to life skills assessment* (2nd ed.). Baltimore: Paul H. Brookes Publishing Co.

Brown, L., Branston, M.B., Hamre-Nietupski, S., Pumpian, I., Certo, N., & Gruenewald, L. (1979). A strategy for developing chronological age appropriate and functional curricular content for severely handicapped adolescents and young adults. *Journal of Special Education, 13*(1), 81–90.

Brown, W.H., Odom, S.L., & Holcombe, A. (1996). Observational assessment of young children's social behavior with peers. *Early Childhood Research Quarterly, 11,* 19–40.

Brown, W.H., Ragland, E.U., & Fox, J.J. (1988). Effects of group socialization procedures on the social interactions of preschool children. *Research in Developmental Disabilities, 9,* 359–376.

Bruner, J.S. (1975). From communication to language: A psychological perspective. *Cognition, 3*(3), 255–287.

Bukowski, W.M., Boivin, M., & Hoza, B. (1994). Measuring friendship quality in pre- and early adolescence: The development and psychometric properties of the friendship qualities scale. *Journal of Social and Personal Relationships, 2,* 471–484.

Bukowski, W.M., & Hoza, B. (1989). Popularity and friendship: Issues in theory, measurement, and outcome. In T.J. Berndt & G.W. Ladd (Eds.), *Peer relationships in child development* (pp. 15–45). New York: John Wiley & Sons.

Buysse, V. (1993). Friendships of preschoolers with disabilities in community-based child care settings. *Journal of Early Intervention, 17,* 380–395.

Cairns, R.B., Perrin, J.E., & Cairns, B.D. (1985). Social structure and social cognition in early adolescence: Affiliative patterns. *Journal of Early Adolescence, 5,* 339–355.

Carr, E.G., Levin, L., McConnachie, G., Carlson, J.I., Kemp, D.C., & Smith, C.E. (1994). *Communication-based intervention for problem behavior: A user's guide for producing positive change.* Baltimore: Paul H. Brookes Publishing Co.

Carr, E.G., & Newsom, C.D. (1985). Demand-related tantrums: Conceptualization and treatment. *Behavior Modification, 9,* 403–426.

Carr, E.G., Taylor, J.C., & Robinson, S. (1991). The effects of severe behavior problems in children on the teaching behavior of adults. *Journal of Applied Behavior Analysis, 24,* 523–535.

Carrow-Woolfolk, E. (1999). *Comprehensive Assessment of Spoken Language.* Circle Pines, MN: American Guidance Service.

Carrow-Woolfolk, E., & Lynch, J.I. (1982). *An integrative approach to language disorders in children.* New York: Grune & Stratton.

Chandler, L.K., Fowler, S.A., & Lubeck, R.C. (1992). An analysis of the effects of multiple setting events on the social behavior of preschool children with special needs. *Journal of Applied Behavior Analysis, 25*(2), 249–263.

Clancy, P.M. (1986). The acquisition of communicative style in Japanese. In B.B. Schieffelin & E. Ochs (Eds.), *Language socialization across cultures* (pp. 213–250). Cambridge, England: Cambridge University Press.

Clark, H. (1996). *Using language.* Cambridge, England: Cambridge University Press.

Clark, H., & Bly, B. (1995). Pragmatics and discourse. In J.L. Miller & P.D. Eimas (Eds.), *Speech, language, and communication* (pp. 371–410). San Diego: Academic Press.

Coie, J.D., Dodge, K.A., & Kupersmidt, J.B. (1990). Peer group behavior and social status. In S.R. Asher & J.D. Coie (Eds.), *Peer rejection in childhood* (pp. 17–59). New York: Cambridge University Press.

Corsaro, W.A. (1979a). "We're friends, right?": Children's use of access rituals in a nursery school. *Language in Society, 8,* 315–336.

Corsaro, W.A. (1979b). Young children's conception of status and role. *Sociology of Education, 52,* 46–59.

Corsaro, W.A. (1981). Friendship in the nursey school: Social organization in a peer environment. In S.R. Asher & J.M. Gottman (Eds.), *The development of children's friendships* (pp. 207–241). New York: Cambridge University Press.

Craig, H.K. (1995). Pragmatic impairments. In P. Fletcher & B. MacWhinney (Eds.), *The handbook of child language* (pp. 623–640). St. Louis: Blackwell Mosby.

Craig, H.K., & Washington, J.A. (1993). Access behaviors of children with specific language impairment. *Journal of Speech and Hearing Research, 36,* 322–337.

Crick, N., & Dodge, K.A. (1994). A review and reformulation of social infor-
mation-processing mechanisms in children's social adjustment. *Psychological
Bulletin, 115*(1), 74–101.

Dale, P.S. (1996). Parent report assessment of language and communication. In
S.F. Warren & J. Reichle (Series Eds.) & K.N. Cole, P.S. Dale, & D.J. Thal (Vol.
Eds.), *Communication and language intervention series: Vol. 6. Assessment of communication and language* (pp. 161–182). Baltimore: Paul H. Brookes Publishing Co.

Davis, C.A., Brady, M.P., Hamilton, R., McEvoy, M.A., & Williams, R.E. (1994).
Effects of high probability requests on the social interactions of young children with severe disabilities. *Journal of Applied Behavior Analysis, 27,* 619–637.

Day, R.M., Rea, J.A., Schussler, N.G., Larsen, S.E., & Johnson, W.L. (1988). A
functionally-based approach to the treatment of self-injurious behavior. *Behavior Modification, 12,* 565–589.

Dodge, K.A. (1986). A social information processing model of social competence in children. In M. Perlmutter (Ed.), *Minnesota Symposia on Child
Psychology: Vol. 18. Cognitive perspectives on children's social and behavioral development* (pp. 77–125). Mahwah, NJ: Lawrence Erlbaum Associates.

Dodge, K.A., & Feldman, E. (1990). Issues in social cognition and sociometric
status. In S.R. Asher & J.D. Coie (Eds.), *Peer rejection in childhood* (pp. 119–155).
New York: Cambridge University Press.

Dodge, K.A., McClaskey, C.L., & Feldman, E. (1985). Situational approach to
the assessment of social competence in children. *Journal of Consulting and
Clinical Psychology, 53,* 344–353.

Dodge, K.A., Pettit, G.S., McClaskey, C.L., & Brown, M.M. (1986). Social competence in children. *Monographs of the Society for Research in Children Development, 51*(2, Serial No. 213).

Dodge, K.A., & Price, J.M. (1994). On the relation between social information
processing and social competent behavior in early school-aged children.
Child Development, 65, 1385–1397.

Doll, B. (1996). Children without friends: Implications for practice and policy.
School Psychology Review, 25, 165–183.

Dore, J. (1975). Holophrases, speech acts, and language universals. *Journal of
Child Language, 2,* 21–40.

Dore, J. (1978). Requestive systems in nursery school conversations: Analysis
of talk in its social context. In R. Campbell & P. Smith (Eds.), *Recent advances
in the psychology of language: Language development and mother–child interaction*
(pp. 271–292). New York: Kluwer Academic/Plenum Publishers.

Durand, V.M., & Crimmins, D.B. (1988). Identifying the variables maintaining
self-injurious behavior. *Journal of Autism and Developmental Disorders, 18,*
99–117.

Durand, V.M., Crimmins, D.B., Caulfield, M., & Taylor, J. (1989). Reinforcer
assessment: I. Using problem behaviors to select reinforcers. *Journal of The
Association for Persons with Severe Handicaps, 14,* 113–126.

English, K., Goldstein, H., Shafer, K., & Kaczmarek, L. (1997). Promoting interactions among preschoolers with and without disabilities: Effects of a buddy
system skills-training program. *Exceptional Children, 63,* 229–243.

English, K., Shafer, K., Goldstein, H., & Kaczmarek, L. (1997). *Innovations: Teaching buddy skills to preschoolers* (Monograph No. 9). Washington, DC: American
Association on Mental Retardation.

Ervin-Tripp, S. (1979). Children's verbal turn-taking. In E. Ochs & B. Schieffelin (Eds.), *Developmental pragmatics* (pp. 391–414). San Diego: Academic Press.

Farmer, T.W., & Farmer, E.M.Z. (1996). Social relationships of students with exceptionalities in mainstream classrooms: Social networks and homophily. *Exceptional Children, 62*(5), 431–450.

Farver, J.M. (1996). Aggressive behavior in preschoolers: Do birds of a feather flock together? *Early Childhood Research Quarterly, 11,* 333–350.

Ferrell, D. (1990). *Communicative interaction between handicapped and nonhandicapped preschool children: Identifying facilitative strategies.* Unpublished doctoral dissertation, University of Pittsburgh.

Fey, M.E. (1986). *Language intervention with children.* San Diego: College-Hill Press.

Fogel, A., Toda, S., & Kawai, M. (1988). Development of early expressive and communicative action: Reinterpreting the evidence from a dynamic systems perspective. *Developmental Psychology, 34,* 398–406.

Folger, J.P., & Chapman, R.S. (1978). A pragmatic analysis of spontaneous imitations. *Journal of Child Language, 5*(1), 25–38.

Foster, S. (1985). Development of discourse topic skills by infants and young children. *Topics in Language Disorders, 5*(2), 31–45.

Foster, S.L., Inderbitzen, H.M., & Nangle, D.W. (1993). Assessing acceptance and social skills with peers in childhood. *Behavior Modification, 17,* 255–286.

Freedman, B.J., Rosenthal, L., Donahoe, C.P., Schlundt, D.G., & McFall, R.M. (1978). A social behavioral analysis of social skills deficits in delinquent and nondelinquent adolescent boys. *Journal of Counseling and Clinical Psychology, 46,* 1448–1462.

Fujiki, M., & Brinton, B. (1994). Social competence and language impairment in children. In S.F. Warren & J. Reichle (Series Eds.) & R.V. Watkins & M.L. Rice (Vol. Eds.), *Communication and language intervention series: Vol. 4. Specific language impairments in children* (pp. 123–143). Baltimore: Paul H. Brookes Publishing Co.

Fujiki, M., Brinton, B., Hart, C.H., & Fitzgerald, A.H. (1999). Peer acceptance and friendship in children with specific language impairment. *Topics in Language Disorders, 19*(2), 34–48.

Furman, W. (1996). The measurement of friendship perceptions: Conceptual and methodological issues. In W.M. Bukowski, A.F. Newcomb, & W.W. Hartup (Eds.), *The company they keep: Friendship in childhood and adolescence* (pp. 41–86). Cambridge, England: Cambridge University Press.

Furman, W., & Buhrmester, D. (1985). Children's perceptions of the personal relationships in their social networks. *Developmental Psychology, 21,* 1016–1024.

Gage, S.T., & Falvey, M.A. (1995). Assessment strategies to develop appropriate curricula and education programs. In M.A. Falvey (Ed.), *Inclusive and heterogeneous schooling: Assessment, curriculum, and instruction* (pp. 59–86). Baltimore: Paul H. Brookes Publishing Co.

Gallagher, T.M. (1991). Language and social skills: Implications for clinical assessment and intervention of school-aged children. In T.M. Gallagher (Ed.), *Pragmatics of language: Clinical practice issues.* San Diego: Singular Publishing Group.

Gallagher, T.M., & Craig, H.K. (1984). Pragmatic assessment: Analysis of a highly frequent repeated utterance. *Journal of Speech and Hearing Disorders, 49,* 368–377.

Garcia Coll, C.T. (1990). Developmental outcome of minority infants: A process oriented look into our beginnings. *Child Development, 61,* 270–289.

George, T.P., & Hartmann, D.P. (1996). Friendship networks of unpopular, average, and popular children. *Child Development, 67,* 2301–2316.

Ghuman, J.K., Freund, L., Reiss, A., Serwint, J., & Folstein, S. (1998). Early detection of social interaction problems: Development of a social interaction instrument in young children. *Developmental and Behavioral Pediatrics, 19,* 411–419.

Gnepp, J. (1989a). Children's use of personal information to understand other people's feelings. In C. Saarni & P. Harris (Eds.), *Children's understanding of emotions* (pp. 151–177). Cambridge, England: Cambridge University Press.

Gnepp, J. (1989b). Personalized inferences of emotions and appraisals: Component processes and correlates. *Developmental Psychology, 25,* 277–288.

Goldfried, M.R., & D'Zurilla, T.J. (1969). A behavioral analytic model for assessing competence. In C.D. Spielberger (Ed.), *Current topics in clinical and community psychology* (Vol. 1, pp. 151–196). San Diego: Academic Press.

Goldstein, H., English, K., Shafer, K., & Kaczmarek, L. (1997). Interaction among preschoolers with and without disabilities: Effects of across-the-day peer intervention. *Journal of Speech, Language, & Hearing Research, 40,* 33–48.

Goldstein, H., & Kaczmarek, L. (1992). Promoting communicative interaction among children in integrated intervention settings. In S.F. Warren & J. Reichle (Series & Vol. Eds.), *Communication and language intervention series: Vol. 1. Causes and effects in communication and language intervention* (pp. 81–111). Baltimore: Paul H. Brookes Publishing Co.

Goldstein, H., Kaczmarek, L., Pennington, R., & Shafer, K. (1992). Peer-mediated intervention: Attending to, commenting on, and acknowledging the behavior of preschoolers with autism. *Journal of Applied Behavior Analysis, 25,* 289–305.

Greenwood, C.R., Walker, H.M., Todd, N.M., & Hops, H. (1981). Normative and descriptive analysis of preschool free play social interaction rates. *Journal of Pediatric Psychology, 6,* 343–367.

Gresham, F.M. (1986). Conceptual issues in the assessment of social competence in children. In P.S. Strain, M.J. Guralnick, & H.M. Walker (Eds.), *Children's social behavior: Development, assessment, and modification* (pp. 143–179). San Diego: Academic Press.

Gresham, F.M., & Elliott, S.N. (1990). *Social skills rating system.* Circle Pines, MN: American Guidance Service.

Guralnick, M.J. (1992). A hierarchical model for understanding children's peer-related social competence. In S.L. Odom, S.R. McConnell, & M.A. McEvoy (Eds.), *Social competence in young children with disabilities: Issues and strategies for intervention* (pp. 37–64). Baltimore: Paul H. Brookes Publishing Co.

Guralnick, M.J. (1997). Peer social networks of young boys with developmental delays. *American Journal on Mental Retardation, 101,* 595–612.

Guralnick, M.J., Connor, R.T., & Hammond, M. (1995). Parent perspectives of peer relationships and friendships in integrated and specialized programs. *American Journal on Mental Retardation, 99,* 457–476.

Guralnick, M.J., Connor, R.T., Hammond, M., Gottman, J.M., & Kinnish, K. (1995). Immediate effects of mainstreamed settings on the social interactions and social integration of preschool children. *American Journal on Mental Retardation, 100,* 359–377.

Guralnick, M.J., Gottman, J.M., & Hammond, M.A. (1996). Effects of social setting on the friendship formation of young children differing in developmental status. *Journal of Applied Developmental Psychology, 17,* 625–651.

Guralnick, M.J., & Groom, J.M. (1985). Correlates of peer-related social competence of developmentally delayed preschool children. *American Journal of Mental Deficiency, 90,* 140–150.

Guralnick, M.J., & Groom, J.M. (1988). Friendships of preschool children in mainstreamed playgroups. *Developmental Psychology, 24,* 595–604.

Guralnick, M.J., & Paul-Brown, D. (1986). Communicative interactions of mildly delayed and normally developing preschool children: Effects of listener's developmental level. *Journal of Speech and Hearing Research, 29,* 2–10.

Guralnick, M.J., & Paul-Brown, D. (1989). Peer-related communicative competence of preschool children: Developmental and adaptive characteristics. *Journal of Speech and Hearing Research, 32,* 930–943.

Guralnick, M.J., Paul-Brown, D., Groom, J.M., Booth, C.L., Hammond, M.A., Tupper, D.B., & Gelenter, A. (1998). Conflict resolution patterns of preschool children with and without developmental delays in heterogeneous playgroups. *Early Education and Development, 9*(1), 49–77.

Guralnick, M.J., & Weinhouse, E. (1984). Peer-related social interactions of developmentally delayed young children: Development and characteristics. *Developmental Psychology, 20,* 815–827.

Halle, J.W., & Spradlin, J.E. (1993). Identifying stimulus control of challenging behavior: Extending the analysis. In S.F. Warren & J. Reichle (Series Eds.) & J. Reichle & D. Wacker (Vol. Eds.), *Communication and language intervention series: Vol. 3. Communicative alternatives to challenging behavior: Integrating functional assessment and intervention strategies* (pp. 83–109). Baltimore: Paul H. Brookes Publishing Co.

Halliday, M.A.K. (1975). *Learning how to mean: Explorations in the development of language.* New York: Elsevier/North Holland.

Halliday, M.A.K., & Hasan, R. (1976). *Cohesion in English.* London: Longman Publishing.

Harkness, S., & Super, C.M. (1995). Culture and parenting. In M. Bornstein (Ed.), *Handbook of parenting* (Vol. 2, pp. 211–234). Mahwah, NJ: Lawrence Erlbaum Associates.

Hecht, M.L., Andersen, P.A., & Ribeau, S.A. (1989). The cultural dimensions of nonverbal communication. In M.K. Asante & W.B. Gudykunst (Eds.), *Handbook of international and intercultural communication* (pp. 163–185). Thousand Oaks, CA: Sage Publications.

Hecimovic, A., Fox, J.J., Shores, R.E., & Strain, P.S. (1985). An analysis of developmentally integrated and segregated free play settings and the generalization of newly-acquired social behaviors of socially withdrawn preschoolers. *Behavioral Assessment, 7,* 367–388.

Hedrick, D.L., Prather, E.M., & Tobin, A.R. (1975). *Sequenced Inventory of Communication Development* (Rev. ed.). Seattle: University of Washington Press.

Howes, C. (1983). Patterns of friendship. *Child Development, 54,* 1041–1053.

Howes, C. (1996). The earliest friendships. In W.M. Bukowski, A.F. Newcomb, & W.W. Hartup (Eds.), *The company they keep: Friendship in childhood and adolescence* (pp. 66–86). Cambridge, England: Cambridge University Press.

Hughes, J.N., Boodoo, G., Alcala, J., Maggio, M.C., Moore, L., & Villapando, R. (1989). Validation of a role play measure of children's social skills. *Journal of Abnormal Child Psychology, 17,* 633–646.

Hymel, S., & Rubin, K. (1985). Children with peer relationships and social skills problems: Conceptual, methodological, and developmental issues. In G. Whitehurst (Ed.), *Annals of child development* (Vol. 2, pp. 251–297). Stamford, CT: JAI Press.

Hymel, S., Wagner, E., & Butler, L. (1990). Reputational bias: View from the peer group. In S.R. Asher & J.D. Coie (Eds.), *Peer rejection in childhood* (pp. 156–186). New York: Cambridge University Press.

Iverson, A.M., Barton, E.A., & Iverson, G.L. (1997). Analysis of risk to children participating in a sociometric task. *Developmental Psychology, 33,* 104–112.

Iwata, B.A., Dorsey, M.F., Slifer, K.J., Bauman, K.E., & Richman, G.S. (1982). Toward a functional analysis of self-injury. *Analysis and Intervention in Developmental Disabilities, 2,* 1–20.

Iwata, B.A., Vollmer, T.R., & Zarcone, J.R. (1990). The experimental (functional) analysis of behavior disorders: Methodology, applications, and limitations. In A.C. Repp & N.N. Singh (Eds.), *Perspectives on the use of aversive and nonaversive interventions for persons with developmental disabilities* (pp. 301–330). Sycamore, IL: Sycamore Publishing Co.

Jacobson, J.L., Tianen, R.L., Willie, D.E., & Aytch, D.M. (1986). Infant–mother attachment and early peer relations: The assessment of behavior in an interaction context. In E.C. Mueller & C.R. Cooper (Eds.), *Process and outcome in peer relationships* (pp. 57–77). San Diego: Academic Press.

Jansson, I. (1997). Clique structure in school class data. *Social Networks, 19,* 285–301.

Johnson, J.C., Ironsmith, M., Whitcher, A.L., Poteat, G.M., Snow, C.W., & Mumford, S. (1997). The development of social networks in preschool children. *Early Education and Development, 8,* 389–405.

Kaczmarek, L. (1990). Teaching spontaneous language to individuals with severe handicaps: A matrix model. *Journal of The Association for Persons with Severe Handicaps, 15,* 160–169.

Kaczmarek, L.A., Evans, B.C., & Stever, N.M. (1995). Initiating expressive communication: An analysis of the listener preparatory behaviors of preschools with developmental disabilities in center-based programs. *Journal of The Association for Persons with Severe Handicaps, 20,* 66–79.

Kamps, D.M., Leonard, B.R., Vernon, S., Dugan, E.P., Delquadri, J.C., Gershon, B., Wade, L., & Folk, L. (1992). Teaching social skills to students with autism to increase peer interactions in an integrated first-grade classroom. *Journal of Applied Behavior Analysis, 25,* 281–288.

Kaye, K., & Charney, R. (1981). Conversational asymmetry between mothers and children. *Journal of Child Language, 8,* 35–50.

Kazdin, A.E., Matson, J.L., & Esveldt-Dawson, K. (1984). The relationship of role-play assessment of children's social skills to multiple measures of social competence. *Behaviour Research and Therapy, 22,* 129–139.

Kindermann, T.A. (1995). Distinguishing "buddies" from "bystanders": The study of children's development within natural peer contexts. In T.A. Kindermann & J. Valsiner (Eds.), *Development of person-context relations* (pp. 205–226). Mahwah, NJ: Lawrence Erlbaum Associates.

Koegel, L.K., Koegel, R.L., Kellegrew, D., & Mullen, K. (1996). Parent education for prevention and reduction of severe problem behaviors. In L.K. Koegel, R.L. Koegel, & G. Dunlap (Eds.), *Positive behavioral support: Including people with difficult behavior in the community* (pp. 3–30). Baltimore: Paul H. Brookes Publishing Co.

Kohler, F.W., & Strain, P.S. (1997). Procedures for assessing and increasing social interaction. In N.N. Singh (Ed.), *Prevention and treatment of severe behavior problems: Models and methods in developmental disabilities.* Pacific Grove, CA: Brooks/Cole Thomson Learning.

Kohler, F.W., Strain, P.S., Hoyson, M., Davis, L., Donina, W., & Rapp, N. (1995). Using a group-oriented contingency to increase social interactions between children with autism and their peers: A preliminary analysis of corollary supportive behaviors. *Behavior Modification, 19*(1), 10–32.

Krasnor, L.R. (1982). An observational study of social problem solving young children. In K.H. Rubin & H.S. Ross (Eds.), *Peer relations and social skills in childhood* (pp. 113–132). New York: Springer-Verlag.

Krasnor, L.R., & Rubin, K.H. (1983). Preschool social problem-solving: Attempts and outcomes in naturalistic observations. *Child Development, 54,* 1545–1558.

LaGreca, A.M., & Stark, P. (1986). Naturalistic observations of children's social behavior. In P.S. Strain, M.J. Guralnick, & H.M. Walker (Eds.), *Children's social behavior: Development, assessment, and modification* (pp. 181–213). San Diego: Academic Press.

Lalli, J.S., & Goh, H.-L. (1993). Naturalistic observations in community settings. In S.F. Warren & J. Reichle (Series Eds.) & J. Reichle & D.P. Wacker (Vol. Eds.), *Communication and language intervention series: Vol. 3. Communicative alternatives to challenging behavior: Integrating functional assessment and intervention strategies* (pp. 11–39). Baltimore: Paul H. Brookes Publishing Co.

Laursen, B., & Hartup, W.W. (1989). The dynamics of preschool children's conflicts. *Merrill-Palmer Quarterly, 35,* 281–297.

Leinonen, E., & Smith, B.R. (1994). Appropriacy judgements and pragmatic performance. *European Journal of Disorders of Communication, 29,* 77–84.

Levin, E., & Rubin, K.H. (1983). Getting others to do what you want them to do: The development of children's requestive strategies. In K. Nelson (Ed.), *Children's language* (Vol. 4, pp. 157–186). Mahwah, NJ: Lawrence Erlbaum Associates.

Lewis, M., Feiring, C., & Brooks-Gunn, J. (1987). The social networks of children with and without handicaps: A developmental perspective. In S. Landesman, P.M. Vietze, & M.J. Begab (Eds.), *Living environments and mental retardation* (pp. 377–400). Washington, DC: American Association on Mental Retardation.

Linder, T.W. (1993). *Transdisciplinary play-based assessment: A functional approach to working with young children* (Rev. ed.). Baltimore: Paul H. Brookes Publishing Co.

Lynch, E.W. (1998). Developing cross-cultural competence. In E.W. Lynch & M.J. Hanson (Eds.), *Developing cross-cultural competence: A guide for working with children and their families* (2nd ed., pp. 47–89). Baltimore: Paul H. Brookes Publishing Co.

Mack, A.E., & Warr-Leeper, G.A. (1992). Language abilities of boys with chronic behavior disorders. *Language, Speech, and Hearing Services in the Schools, 23,* 214–223.

MacWhinney, B. (1999). The CHILDES System. In W.C. Ritchie & T.K. Bhatia (Eds.), *Handbook of child language acquisition* (pp. 457–494). San Diego: Academic Press.

Martinez, M.A. (1987). Dialogues among children and between children and their mothers. *Child Development, 58,* 1035–1043.

Matson, J.L. (1989). *The Matson evaluation of social skills with youngsters.* Orland Park, IL: International Diagnostic Systems.

McCathren, R.B., Warren, S.F., & Yoder, P.J. (1996). Prelinguistic predictors of later language development. In S.F. Warren & J. Reichle (Series Eds.) & K.N. Cole, P.S. Dale, & D.J. Thal (Vol. Eds.), *Communication and language intervention series: Vol. 6. Assessment of communication and language* (pp. 57–75). Baltimore: Paul H. Brookes Publishing Co.

McCollum, J.A., & McBride, S.L. (1997). Ratings of parent–infant interaction: Raising questions of cultural validity. *Topics in Early Childhood Special Education, 17,* 494–519.

McConnell, S., & Odom, S.L. (1986). Sociometrics: Peer-referenced measures and the assessment of social competence. In P.S. Strain, M.J. Guralnick, & H.M. Walker (Eds.), *Children's social behavior: Development, assessment, and modification* (pp. 215–284). San Diego: Academic Press.

McConnell, S.R., & Odom, S.L. (1999). A multimeasure performance-based assessment of social competence in young children with disabilities. *Topics in Early Childhood Special Education, 19,* 67–74.

McConnell, S.R., Sisson, L.A., Cort, C.A., & Strain, P.S. (1991). Effects of social skills training and contingency management on reciprocal interaction of preschool children with behavioral handicaps. *Journal of Special Education, 24,* 473–495.

McEvoy, M.A., Nordquist, V.M., Twardosz, S., Heckaman, K.A., Wehby, J.H., & Denny, R.K. (1988). Promoting autistic children's peer interaction in an integrated early childhood setting using affection activities. *Journal of Applied Behavior Analysis, 21,* 193–200.

McFall, R.M. (1982). A review and reformulation of the concept of social skills. *Behavioral Assessment, 4,* 1–33.

Mentis, M. (1991). Topic management in the discourse of normal and language impaired children. *Journal of Child Communication Disorders, 14,* 45–56.

Mentis, M. (1994). Topic management in discourse: Assessment and intervention. *Topics in Language Disorders, 14*(3), 29–54.

Mentis, M., & Lundgren, K. (1995). Effects of prenatal exposure to cocaine and associated risk factors on language development. *Journal of Speech and Hearing Research, 38,* 1303–1318.

Mentis, M., & Prutting, C.A. (1991). Analysis of topic as illustrated in a head injured and normal adult. *Journal of Speech and Hearing Research, 34,* 583–595.

Merrell, K.W. (1993). Assessment of social skills and peer relations. In H.B. Vance (Ed.), *Best practices in assessment for school and clinical settings* (pp. 307–340). Brandon, VT: Clinical Psychology Publishing Co.

Merrell, K.W. (1994). *Preschool and Kindergarten Behavior Scales.* Brandon, VT: Clinical Psychology Publishing Co.

Miller, J.F. (1981). *Assessing language production in children: Experimental procedures.* Baltimore: University Park Press.

Miller, J.F. (1996). Progress in assessing, describing, and defining child language disorder. In S.F. Warren & J. Reichle (Series Eds.) & K.N. Cole, P.S. Dale, & D.J. Thal (Vol. Eds.), *Communication and language intervention series: Vol. 6. Assessment of communication and language* (pp. 309–324). Baltimore: Paul H. Brookes Publishing Co.

Miniutti, A.M. (1991). Language deficiencies in inner-city children with learning and behavioral problems. *Language, Speech, and Hearing Services in the Schools, 22,* 31–38.

Nabors, L. (1997). Playmate preferences of children who are typically developing for their classmates with special needs. *Mental Retardation, 35,* 107–113.

Newborg, J., Stock, J., Wnek, L. (Initial Development), Guidubaldi, J. (Pilot Norming Study), & Svinicki, J. (Completion and Standardization). (1984). *Battelle Developmental Inventory (BDI).* Itasca, IL: The Riverside Publishing Co.

Ninio, A., & Snow, C.E. (1999). The development of pragmatics: Learning to use language appropriately. In W.C. Ritchie & T.K. Bhatia (Eds.), *Handbook of child language acquisition* (pp. 347–383). San Diego: Academic Press.

Ochs, E., & Schieffelin, B.B. (1984). Language acquisition and socialization: Three developmental stories and their implications. In R. Shweder & R. Le-

Vine (Eds.), *Culture theory: Essays on mind, self, and emotion* (pp. 276–320). Cambridge, England: Cambridge University Press.

Odom, S., McConnell, S., & McEvoy, M.A. (1992). Peer-related social competence and its significance for young children with disabilities. In S.L. Odom, S.R. McConnell, & M.A. McEvoy (Eds.), *Social competence of young children with disabilities: Issues and strategies for intervention* (pp. 3–35). Baltimore: Paul H. Brookes Publishing Co.

Odom, S.L., & Ogawa, I. (1992). Direct observations of young children's social interaction with peers: A review of methodology. *Behaviour Assessment, 14,* 407–441.

Olswang, L., Stoel-Gammon, C., Coggins, T., & Carpenter, R. (1987). *Assessing prelinguistic and early linguistic behaviors in developmentally young children.* Seattle: University of Washington Press.

O'Neill, R.E. (1990). Establishing verbal repertoires: Toward the application of general case analysis and programming. *The Analysis of Verbal Behavior, 8,* 113–126.

O'Neill, R.E., Horner, R.H., Albin, R.W., Storey, K., & Sprague, J.R. (1990). *Functional analysis: A practical assessment guide.* Sycamore, IL: Sycamore Publishing Co.

O'Neill, R., & Reichle, J. (1993). Addressing socially motivated challenging behaviors by establishing communicative alternatives: Basics of a general-case approach. In S.F. Warren & J. Reichle (Series Eds.) & J. Reichle & D.P. Wacker (Vol. Eds.), *Communication and language intervention series: Vol. 3. Communicative alternatives to challenging behavior: Integrating functional assessment and intervention strategies* (pp. 205–235). Baltimore: Paul H. Brookes Publishing Co.

Parker, J.G., & Asher, S.R. (1993). Friendship and friendship quality in middle school: Links with peer group acceptance and feelings of loneliness and social dissatisfaction. *Developmental Psychology, 29,* 611–621.

Parker, J.G., Rubin, K.H., Price, J.M., & DeRosier, M.E. (1995). Peer relationships, child development, and adjustment: A developmental psychopathology perspective. In D. Cicchetti & D.J. Cohen (Eds.), *Developmental psychopathology: Vol. 2. Risk, disorder, and adaptation* (pp. 96–161). New York: John Wiley & Sons.

Pennycook, A. (1985). Actions speak louder than words: Paralanguage, communication, and education. *TESOL Quarterly, 19,* 259–282.

Pettit, G.S., & Bates, J.E. (1989). Family interaction patterns and children's behavior problems from infancy to 4 years. *Developmental Psychology, 25,* 413–420.

Pettit, G.S., McClaskey, C.L., Brown, M.M., and Dodge, K.A. (1987). The generalizability of laboratory assessments of children's socially competent behavior in specific situations. *Behaviour Assessment, 9,* 81–96.

Phelps-Terasaki, D., & Phelps-Gunn, T. (1992). *Test of Pragmatic Language.* Austin, TX: PRO-ED.

Piche, G., Rubin, D., & Michlin, M. (1978). Age and social class in children's use of persuasive communicative appeals. *Child Development, 49,* 773–780.

Pope, A., & Bierman, K.L. (1991). Play assessment of peer interactions in children. In C. Schaefer, K. Gitlin, & A. Sandgrun (Eds.), *Play diagnosis and assessment* (pp. 553–577). New York: John Wiley & Sons.

Prizant, B.M., & Duchan, J. (1981). The functions of immediate echolalia in autistic children. *Journal of Speech and Hearing Disorders, 46,* 241–249.

Prizant, B.M., & Rydell, P.J. (1984). Analysis of functions of delayed echolalia in autistic children. *Journal of Speech and Hearing Research, 27,* 183–192.

Prizant, B.M., & Wetherby, A.M. (1990). Toward an integrated view of early language and communication development and socioemotional development. *Topics in Language Disorders, 10*(4), 1–16.

Prutting, C.A. (1982). Pragmatics as social competence. *Journal of Speech and Hearing Disorders, 47,* 123–134.

Prutting, C.A., & Kirchner, D.M. (1983). Applied pragmatics. In T. Gallagher & C.A. Prutting (Eds.), *Pragmatic assessment and intervention issues in language* (pp. 29–64). San Diego: College-Hill.

Prutting, C.A., & Kirchner, D.M. (1987). A clinical appraisal of the pragmatic aspects of language. *Journal of Speech and Hearing Disorders, 52,* 105–119.

Putallaz, M. (1983). Predicting children's sociometric status from their behavior. *Child Development, 54,* 1417–1426.

Putallaz, M., & Gottman, J.M. (1981). An interactional model of children's entry into peer groups. *Child Development, 52,* 986–994.

Putallaz, M., & Wasserman, A. (1989). Children's naturalistic entry behavior and sociometric status: A developmental perspective. *Developmental Psychology, 25,* 793–796.

Quay, H.C., & Peterson, D.R. (1983). *Revised behavior problems checklist.* Los Angeles: Western Psychological Services.

Ray, G.E., Cohen, R., & Secrist, M.E. (1995). Best friend networks of children across settings. *Child Study Journal, 25*(3) 169–188.

Reike, J.A., & Lewis, J. (1984). Preschool intervention strategies: The communication base. *Topics in Language Disorders, 5*(1), 41–57.

Repp, A.C., Barton, L., & Brulle, A. (1987). An applied behavior analysis perspective on naturalistic observation and adjustment to new settings. In S. Landesman, P.M. Vietze, & M.J. Begab (Eds.), *Living environments and mental retardation* (pp. 151–171). Washington, DC: American Association on Mental Retardation.

Repp, A.C., & Karsh, K.G. (1990). A taxonomic approach to the nonaversive treatment of maladaptive behavior of persons with developmental disabilities. In A.C. Repp & N.N. Singh (Eds.), *Perspectives on the use of aversive and nonaversive interventions for persons with developmental disabilities* (pp. 331–347). Sycamore, IL: Sycamore Publishing Co.

Rice, M., Sell, M., & Hadley, P. (1991). Social interactions of speech and language impaired children. *Journal of Speech and Hearing Research, 34,* 1299–1307.

Roberts, J.E., Prizant, B., & McWilliam, R.A. (1995). Out-of-class versus in-class service delivery in language intervention: Effects on communication interactions with young children. *American Journal of Speech Language Pathology, 4,* 87–94.

Roeyers, H. (1996). The influence of nonhandicapped peers on the social interactions of children with pervasive developmental disorder. *Journal of Autism and Developmental Disorders, 26,* 303–320.

Roopnarine, L., & Field, T.M. (1984). Play interactions of friends and acquaintances in nursery school. In T. Field, J.L. Roopnarine, & M. Segal (Eds.), *Friendships in normal and handicapped children* (pp. 89–98). Stamford, CT: Ablex Publishing Co.

Rubin, K.H. (1998). Social and emotional development from a cultural perspective. *Developmental Psychology, 34,* 611–615.

Rubin, K.H., & Borwick, D. (1984). Communication skills and sociability. In H. Sypher & J. Applegate (Eds.), *Communication by children and adults: Social cognition and strategic processes* (pp. 152–170). Thousand Oaks, CA: Sage Publications.

Rubin, K.H., Bream, L., & Rose-Krasnor, L. (1991). Social problem solving and aggression in childhood. In D.J. Pepler & K.H. Rubin (Eds.), *The development and treatment of childhood aggression* (pp. 219–248). Mahwah, NJ: Lawrence Erlbaum Associates.

Rubin, K.H., & Krasnor, L.R. (1983). Age and gender differences in the development of a representative social problem solving skill. *Journal of Applied Developmental Psychology, 4,* 263–275.

Rubin, K.H., & Krasnor, L.R. (1986). Social-cognitive and social behavioral perspectives on problem-solving. In M. Perlmutter (Ed.), *Minnesota Symposia on Child Psychology: Vol. 18. Cognitive perspectives on children's social and behavioral development* (pp. 1–68). Mahwah, NJ: Lawrence Erlbaum Associates.

Rubin, K.H., & Moller, L., & Emptage, A. (1987). The preschool behavior questionnaire: A useful index of behavior problems in elementary school-age children. *Canadian Journal of Behavioural Sciences, 19,* 86–100.

Rubin, K.H., & Rose-Krasnor, L. (1992). Interpersonal problem solving and social competence in children. In V.B. Van Hasselt & M. Hersen (Eds.), *Handbook of social development* (pp. 283–323). New York: Kluwer Academic/Plenum Publishers.

Sabornie, E.J. (1987). Bi-directional social status of behaviorally disordered and nonhandicapped elementary school pupils. *Behavior Disorders, 12,* 45–57.

Sachs, J., & Devin, J. (1976). Young children's use of age-appropriate speech styles in social interaction and role playing. *Journal of Child Language, 3,* 81–98.

Sameroff, A.J. (1987). The social context of development. In N. Eisenberg (Ed.), *Contemporary topics in developmental psychology* (pp. 273–291). New York: John Wiley & Sons.

Schegloff, E.A., & Sacks, H. (1973). Opening up closings. *Semiotics, 8,* 289–327.

Searle, J.R. (1969). *Speech acts.* Cambridge, England: Cambridge University Press.

Seibert, J.M., Hogan, A.E., & Mundy, P.C. (1982). Assessing interactional competencies: The Early Social-Communicative Scales. *Infant Mental Health Journal, 3,* 244–259.

Selman, R.L. (1980). *The growth of interpersonal understanding: Clinical and developmental analyses.* San Diego: Academic Press.

Shantz, C.U. (1987). Conflicts between children. *Child Development, 58,* 283–305.

Shatz, M., & Gelman, R. (1973). The development of communication skills: Modifications in the speech of young children as a function of listener. *Monographs of the Society for Research in Child Development, 38*(5), 1–37.

Shulman, B. (1986). *Test of Pragmatic Skills–Revised.* Tucson, AZ: Communication Skill Builders.

Snow, C. (1984). Parent–child interaction and the development of communicative ability. In R.L. Schiefelbusch & J. Pikar (Eds.), *The acquisition of communicative competence* (pp. 69–107). Baltimore: University Park Press.

Sparrow, S.S., Balla, D.A., & Cicchetti, D.V. (1984). *Vineland Adaptive Behavior Scales (VABS).* Circle Pines, MN: American Guidance Service.

Spivak, G., Platt, J., & Shure, M. (1976). *The problem-solving approach to adjustment.* San Francisco: Jossey-Bass.

Spivak, G., & Shure, M. (1974). *Social adjustment of young children.* San Francisco: Jossey-Bass.

Strain, P.S. (1983). Generalization of autistic children's social behavior change: Effects of developmentally integrated and segregated settings. *Analysis and Intervention in Developmental Disabilities, 3,* 23–34.

Strain, P.S. (1984). Social behavior patterns of nonhandicapped and developmentally disabled friend pairs. *Analysis and Intervention in Developmental Disabilities, 4,* 15–28.

Strain, P.S., Shores, R.E., & Timm, M.A. (1977). Effects of peer social initiations on the behavior of withdrawn preschool children. *Journal of Applied Behavior Analysis, 10,* 289–298.

Taylor, C.C., & Bailey, J.S. (1996). Reducing corporal punishment with elementary school students using behavioral diagnostic procedures. In L.K. Koegel, R.L. Koegel, & G. Dunlap (Eds.), *Positive behavioral support: Including people with difficult behavior in the community* (pp. 207–225). Baltimore: Paul H. Brookes Publishing Co.

Taylor, J.C., & Carr, E.G. (1992). Severe problem behaviors related to social interaction: I. Attention seeking and social avoidance. *Behavior Modification, 16,* 305–335.

Thompson, L. (1996). The development of pragmatic competence: Past findings and future directions for research. In L. Thompson (Ed.), *Children talking: The development of pragmatic competence* (pp. 3–21). Philadelphia: Multilingual Matters.

Touchette, P.E., MacDonald, R.F., & Langer, S.N. (1985). A scatter plot for identifying stimulus control of problem behavior. *Journal of Applied Behavior Analysis, 18,* 343–351.

Tough, J. (1977). *The development of meaning.* New York: Halsted Press.

Tremblay, A., Strain, P.S., Hendrickson, J.M., & Shores, R.E. (1981). Social interactions of normally developing preschool children: Using normative data for subject selection and target behavior selection. *Behavior Modification, 5,* 237–253.

Urberg, K.A., Degirmencioglu, S.M., Tolson, J.M., & Halliday-Scher, K. (1995). The structure of adolescent peer networks. *Developmental Psychology, 31,* 540–547.

Van Hasselt, V.B., Hersen, M., & Bellack, A.S. (1981). The validity of role play tests for assessing social skills in children. *Behavior Therapy, 12,* 202–216.

VanDijk, T. (1980). *Macrostructures: An interdisciplinary study of global structures in discourse, interactions, and cognition.* Mahwah, NJ: Lawrence Erlbaum Associates.

Vaughn, S., & Haager, D. (1994). The measurement and assessment of social skills. In G.R. Lyon (Ed.), *Frames of reference for the assessment of the learning disabled: New views on measurement issues* (pp. 555–570). Baltimore: Paul H. Brookes Publishing Co.

Voeller, K.K.S. (1994). Techniques for measuring social competence in children. In G.R. Lyon (Ed.), *Frames of reference for the assessment of the learning disabled: New views on measurement issues* (pp. 523–554). Baltimore: Paul H. Brookes Publishing Co.

Wacker, D.P., Peck, S., Derby, K.M., Berg, W., & Harding, J. (1996). Developing long-term reciprocal interactions between parents and their young children with problematic behavior. In L.K. Koegel, R.L. Koegel, & G. Dunlap (Eds.), *Positive behavioral support: Including people with difficult behavior in the community* (pp. 51–80). Baltimore: Paul H. Brookes Publishing Co.

Walker, H.M., Messinger, D., Fogel, A., & Karns, J. (1992). Social and communicative development in infancy. In V.B. Van Hasselt & M. Hersen (Eds.), *Handbook of social development* (pp. 157–181). New York: Kluwer Academic/ Plenum Publishers.

Walker, H.M., Severson, H., & Feil, E. (1995). *Early screening project.* Longmont, CO: Sopris West.

Wanska, S.K., & Bedrosian, J.L. (1985). Conversational structure and topic performance in mother–child interaction. *Journal of Speech and Hearing Research, 28,* 579–584.

Wetherby, A.M, & Prizant, B.M. (1993). *Communication and Symbolic Behavior Scales (CSBS).* Chicago: Applied Symbolix.

Wetherby, A.M, & Prutting, C. (1984). Profiles of communicative and cognitive-social abilities in autistic children. *Journal of Speech and Hearing Research, 27,* 364–377.

Wickstrom-Kane, S., & Goldstein, H. (1999). Communication assessment and intervention to address challenging behavior in toddlers. *Topics in Language Disorders, 19*(2), 70–89.

Williamson, D.A., Moody, S.C., Granberry, S.W., Lethermon, V.R., & Blouin, D.C. (1983). Criterion-related validity of a role-play social skills test for children. *Behavior Therapy, 14,* 466–481.

Windsor, J. (1995). Language impairment and social competence. In S.F. Warren & J. Reichle (Series Eds.) & M.E. Fey, J. Windsor, & S.F. Warren (Vol. Eds.), *Communication and language intervention series: Vol. 5. Language intervention: Preschool through the elementary years* (pp. 213–238). Baltimore: Paul H. Brookes Publishing Co.

Wittmer, D., Doll, B., & Strain, P. (1996). Social and emotional development in early childhood: The identification of competence and disabilities. *Journal of Early Intervention, 20,* 299–318.

Yoder, P.J., Davies, B., & Bishop, K. (1994). Reciprocal sequential relations in conversations between parents and children with developmental delays. *Journal of Early Intervention, 18,* 362–379.

II

Promoting Social Communication from Infancy Through the School Years

Kristina M. English

The first section of this book describes the complex relationships between communication and social competence and the adverse effects of communication difficulties on the development of social skills. The following section provides meaningful applications of these concepts by taking the reader through a chronological consideration of the communication and social interactions of children who have developmental disabilities. What does a caregiver need to consider when interacting with an infant who is slow to respond to "baby talk" or "motherese"? What can early childhood educators do to promote age-appropriate social skills in the preschool environment? As children progress through school, what strategies have been found to facilitate successful interactions between peers? Do these strategies facilitate friendship development?

In this section of the book, authors contribute two complementary chapters for each of four age groups. First, the authors provide a review of current research and contrast 1) interventions that focus on manipulating the environment to facilitate interaction, 2) interventions that teach social-communicative skills directly to individuals with developmental disabilities, and 3) interventions mediated by communication partners. Second, these authors teamed with practitioners to prepare chapters that describe how the research can be applied. In these chapters, the reader will find case studies designed to highlight and compare intervention strategies. Across chapters, the reader will observe how these interventions change as the settings and communication roles change.

Chapters 4 and 5 start at the beginning of a child's life span by considering the social communication between infants and their caregivers. As with most communicators, the adult–child dyad typically expects reciprocity: The adult talks to the infant, the infant responds, thereby motivating the adult to provide yet more conversation. In Chapter 4, authors Warren, Yoder, and Leew describe how caregivers of infants with disabilities can successfully heighten their own responsiveness to an infant's delayed responses by using a "notice and nurture" scaffolding approach. They also describe a range of strategies to help caregivers increase communication opportunities, such as reducing the amount of directives and teaching intentional communication. To breathe life into this information, they then present two case studies in Chapter 5, taking the reader through the process of assessment, the development of goals and objectives, the implementation of interventions, and the evaluation of outcomes for infant–caregiver social communication.

Brown and Conroy focus on the preschool-age child. Their literature review provides us with an appreciation for a necessary reduction in adult–child interaction to allow for an increase in child–child interaction. In Chapter 6, they demonstrate how an ecological approach can give the interventionist information about the child's physical environment as well as the opportunities to practice the rules of social interaction. Their review of current research describes effective strategies for adults (e.g., coaching with praise and attention to shape peers' social interactions, developing friendship activities), as well as for trained typically developing peers. They conclude this chapter with an outline of ongoing challenges: specifically, the issues of generalization and maintenance of social skills and the identification of behaviors that effectively increase social communication and that contribute to friendship development. Their companion chapter (Chapter 7) applies case studies to the issues of assessment and intervention in the preschool environment.

Chapter 8 targets the school-age child. Kamps, Kravits, and Ross provide an historical perspective on early efforts to promote social communication by directly teaching children with disabilities how to interact and what to say. They then explain current thinking on naturalistic teaching approaches, including the use of playgroups and milieu language interventions. Augmentative and alternative communication strategies are described and include sign language systems, picture pointing systems, scripts, and communication books. Because these strategies cannot be used in isolation, they also provide background on the use of peer networks and the expansion of social interaction beyond the school environment and into the community. The companion case study chapter (Chapter 9) is written by Kamps, Lopez, and Golden, and it provides illuminating examples of how to implement the strategies described in Chapter 8.

Chapters 10 and 11 tackle the often overlooked topics of severe disabilities, adolescence, and social interactions. In Chapter 10, Kennedy expands consideration of social communication into a quality of life issue. Social support relies on social interaction, and adolescents with severe disabilities are at risk for significant loneliness and lack of friends if opportunities for social interaction are not nurtured and supported. He describes the changes that occur in social interactions during this life stage and the incorporation of these changes into a variety of interventions (e.g., replacing dyadic with triadic structures, attempting to influence the quality as well as the quantity of interactions). Ultimately, the goal for humans as social beings is to form durable relationships, but Kennedy shows that research is still needed to describe strategies that maintain those relationships. Chapter 11, the companion chapter by Cushing and Kennedy, provides case studies to demonstrate a set of strategies proven to facilitate communication and relationships between adolescents with and without disabilities.

In Chapter 12, Greenwood, Walker, and Utley provide a broader context for the preceding chapters in this section of the book. They discuss how the social-communicative skills addressed in prior chapters relate to general life achievements and serve as a keystone from which other forms of competence emerge. Greenwood and his colleagues offer an analysis of the interaction patterns and the intervention strategies and policies that promote the social-communicative competence of children with developmental disabilities. They argue that careful scrutiny of the effectiveness and practicality of our instructional technology is needed if implementation is expected to change developmental trajectories, and they remind us of the importance of longitudinal investigations to examine how families, interventionists, and teachers can capitalize on the strategies discussed in previous chapters. Their belief is that throughout the school years, the knowledge presented in the chapters on infants and toddlers should be used to prevent and ameliorate the life course effects of developmental disabilities and to maximize individuals' life achievements associated with social-communicative competence.

4

Promoting Social-Communicative Development in Infants and Toddlers

Steven F. Warren, Paul J. Yoder, and Shirley V. Leew

The process of language acquisition begins in the last trimester of pregnancy when infants begin to learn the sound of their mother's voices (DeCasper & Fifer, 1980). At birth, infants appear to hear and discriminate speech sounds already. They orient toward the sound of their mother's speech and quickly show other signs of social responsiveness to their caregivers (Locke, 1993). In the weeks and months that follow, they move steadily toward their first intentional communications, which typically emerge at about 9 months (Adamson & Bakeman, 1991). A few months later, often somewhere around their first birthday, they may utter their first words. The progression from infant to toddler is accompanied by the development of increasingly complex language. By age 3, this seemingly relentless process may have resulted in the child's having a productive vocabulary of 1,000 words and the ability to speak in elaborate sentences about fictitious events that reside only in his or her imagination (Sachs, 1997).

The pace and complexity of early communication and language development has occasionally led scholars to underestimate the social nature of this extraordinary accomplishment. Certainly the biological side of the language acquisition equation is of fundamental importance. Yet as important as biological endowment may be, to downplay the profoundly social nature of early communication and language development would be pure folly. Communication and language develop in a social context to achieve largely social ends (Carpenter, Nagell, & Tomasello, 1998). After all, language is primarily acquired "in order to interact with someone about something the two of you share" (Bruner, 1976, p. 47).

The social contexts of infants and toddlers—primarily either the parent–child dyad or the more general caregiver–child dyad (e.g., child care workers, early interventionists)—are the focal points for efforts to promote and enhance the development of social communication for children at risk for or with already established developmental delays. The purpose of this chapter is to describe basic intervention approaches to facilitate communication and early language acquisition in children functioning at a developmental age of younger than 24 months. First, we discuss the assumptions and implications of the transactional model of development and intervention and some of the fundamental assumptions of early social communication and language intervention approaches. Second, we explore the nature of social competence and its development in infants and toddlers. This explanation is followed by a discussion of the assessment of early skills related to social competence. The discussion focuses on identifying impairments, generating goals for intervention, and monitoring intervention progress. Next, we describe the basic intervention approaches and their applications. The chapter concludes with a discussion of the implications of these approaches for practitioners and families.

The focus on social competence as it emerges primarily in caregiver–child interaction reflects the view that the roots of social competence lie in the nature of these early interactions and that peer interaction is relatively unimportant until children are capable of engaging in meaningful conversations with their peers (Scheffelin & Ochs, 1986). A developmental as opposed to a chronological age approach is taken in this chapter. Thus, we focus on the birth to 24-month period of development, as this seems most relevant to a consideration to intervention with children younger than age 3 who have developmental delays.

THE TRANSACTIONAL MODEL OF DEVELOPMENT AND INTERVENTION

The fundamental assumption of the transactional model of social-communicative development (McLean & Snyder-McLean, 1978; Sameroff, 1983; Sameroff & Chandler, 1975) is that development is facilitated by bidirectional, reciprocal interactions between the child and his or her environment. For example, a change in the child such as the onset of intentional communication may trigger a change in the social environment, such as increased linguistic mapping by his or her caregivers. These changes then support further development in the child (e.g., increased vocabulary) and subsequently further changes by the caregivers (e.g., more complex language interaction with the child). In this way, both the child and the environment change over time and affect each other in a reciprocal fashion as early achievements pave the way for subsequent development.

A transactional model may be particularly well-suited to understanding social-communicative development in young children because caregiver–child interaction is assumed to play such an important role in this process. The period of early development (from birth to age 3) may represent a unique time during which transactional effects can have a substantial impact on development: The young child's relatively restricted repertoire can make changes in his or her behavior more salient and easily observable to caregivers. This fact in turn can allow adults to be more specifically contingent with their responsiveness than is possible later in development when children's behavioral repertoires are more expansive and complex. This window of opportunity occurs at the same time when the child's behavior and brain development may be the most susceptible to alteration (positively or negatively) by environmental events and social responsiveness (Shore, 1997). During this period, the transactional model may be employed by a clever practitioner to multiply the effects of relatively circumscribed interventions and perhaps alter the very course of the child's development in a significant way, but the actions of the practitioner may need to be swift and intense or they may be muted by the child's steadily accumulating history.

Consideration of the relentless manner in which cumulative advantages and impairments develop during the first few years of life is necessary to appreciate the true potential of transactional effects. For example, an input difference in positive affect expressed by a parent toward his or her child of 10 events per day (a difference of less than 1 event per waking hour on average) will result in a cumulative difference of 10,950 such events over a 3-year period. If a child who experiences less positive affect also experiences cumulatively more negative affect (e.g., "Stop that!" "Get out of there," "Shut your mouth up," "You're a bad baby"), it is easy to conceive of the combination of these qualitative and quantitative experiential differences contributing to impairments in attachment, exploratory behavior, self-concept, language development, school achievement, and so forth.

What evidence is there that such large cumulative impairments occur, and that they play havoc with social and communicative development? Although the evidence is virtually all correlational, it is compelling. There is substantial evidence that typically developing young children experience large differences in terms of the quantity and quality of language input they receive. Furthermore, these differences correlate with important indicators of development later in childhood, such as vocabulary size, IQ score, reading ability, and school achievement (Feagans & Farran, 1982; Gottfried, 1984; Hart & Risley, 1992; Prizant & Wetherby, 1990). Because they often display low rates of initiation and responsiveness (Rosenberg, 1982; Yoder, Davies, & Bishop, 1994), young children with developmental delays or sensory disorders also may experience input that differs substantially in quantity and quality from the input that high achieving, typically developing children receive despite the best intentions of their caregivers (e.g., Hart & Risley, 1995). The challenges faced by young children who initiate communication relatively infrequently may be further multiplied if their caregivers are relatively unresponsive.

Caregivers who are unresponsive to their young children's initiations and often display depressed or negative affect toward the child may represent a risk factor in terms of their children's emotional, social, and communicative development (Landry, Smith, Miller-Loncar, & Swank, 1997). Unresponsive caregivers often have children who are insecurely attached (Ainsworth, Blehar, Waters, & Wall, 1978), which is a major risk factor for poor social-emotional development (Bornstein, 1989). Furthermore, there is evidence that unresponsive caregivers can negate or minimize the positive transactional effects of early intervention efforts because they fail to respond to changes in their child's repertoire being generated by the intervention (Mahoney, Boyce, Fewell, Spiker, & Wheeden, 1998; Yoder & Warren, 1998). In short, the generation of transactional effects likely depends on sensitive, responsive caregivers who notice and nurture the child's growth.

By generating strong transactional effects in which caregivers scaffold development of emotional, social, and communicative skills, a multiplier effect may result whereby a relatively small dose of early intervention may lead to long-term effects (Yoder & Warren, 2001). These effects are necessary when considering that relatively "intensive" early intervention by a skilled practitioner may represent cumulatively only a few hours per week of a young child's potential learning time. For example, 5 hours per week of intensive interaction represents just 5% of the child's available social and communicative skill learning time, assuming the child is awake and learning 100 hours per week. Thus, unless direct intervention accounts for a large portion of a child's waking hours (an unlikely and possibly undesirable event), transactional effects may be mandatory for early intervention efforts to achieve their potential. This fact further implies that sensitive, responsive caregivers and teachers are a necessary, though not sufficient, component for early intervention to be optimally effective.

Defining Social Competence

There is no clear consensus on the definition of social competence (Saunders & Green, 1993). Schultz, Florio, and Erickson (1982) defined it as communicative knowledge that enables one to interact with others in socially appropriate and effective ways. Katz (1988) defined it as the capacity to initiate, develop, and maintain satisfying relationships with others, especially peers. Indeed, many researchers who study social competence in children place primary emphasis on peer interactions (e.g., Dodge, 1983; Howes, 1987, Wright, 1980).

It is necessary to consider what social competence may be during the infancy and toddler period. Even typically developing infants occasionally interact with peers; however, in part to avoid redundancy with Brown and Conroy (see Chapter 6), who primarily address peer interaction, this chapter emphasizes the aspects of social competence that precede peer interaction. With this in mind, this chapter has adapted the definition of social competence used by Bailey and Simeonsson (1985) because it is general enough to include adult–child interaction and the types of skills infants bring to social interaction. This definition of social competence is as follows: the infant's ability to engage with others in interactions that either 1) evoke nurturing environmental responses or achieve desired goals, 2) are mutually satisfying to both the child and the communicative partner, and 3) are consistent with the communicative partner's expectations for socially competent behavior.

This definition provides only a general conceptualization of social competence. Indeed, only general characteristics are likely to fit all cultures; however, to be useful for educational and assessment purposes, particular behaviors that are considered socially competent must be defined. These particular behaviors will vary across cultures (O'Reilly, Tokuno, & Ebata, 1986). Instead of vainly attempting to determine specific behaviors that would be considered socially competent in all cultures, this chapter includes a description of the socially competent toddler in Western industrialized culture.

Like Bailey and Simeonsson (1985), we acknowledge that the perceptions of the communicative partner are relevant to determining whether the partner considers the child with a disability socially competent; however, given that the perceptions of all potential communicative partners cannot be controlled and that the list of behaviors in the chapter may be used to guide goal selection, we have chosen to emphasize particular child behaviors that the dominant culture generally considers socially competent for a 24-month-old.

The following description is not complete. Instead, it is a sampling of the types of skills a socially competent 2-year-old in a Western culture would probably possess. The chapter describes *productive*, not *receptive*, behaviors because the former are more easily assessed and more is known about them (Bates, 1993). The various aspects of language are used to organize the description: pragmatics, phonology, prosody, semantics, and grammar. Logic and descriptions of typical development are used to infer possible precursors of the linguistic skills used for social purposes; however, little is known about whether there are causal links between early occurring and later occurring skills. Because available information on the achievement of developmental milestones is largely limited to research with small samples, only general age ranges are provided in Table 4.1.

Assessing Social Competence in Infants and Toddlers

There are four primary purposes of assessment: 1) screening for delays, 2) identification or classification for placement and funding purposes, 3) goal selection for intervention, and 4) program monitoring (Coggins, 1998). Screening instruments are normative instruments that are designed to be quick to administer. *Normative* or *norm-referenced* means that an individual's raw score is compared with those attained by many typically developing children at the same chronological age. Typically, if the child's score is below 90% of the children his or her chronological age, the target child is considered at risk for developmental delay. Screening instruments need to be quick to administer so that many children can be tested. The most promising screening instrument for children developmentally between 8 and 16 months is the Infant-Toddler Checklist, which is part of the Communication and Symbolic Behavior Scales Developmental Profile (Wetherby & Prizant, 1998). This parent report has good predictive validity for later language (A. Wetherby, personal communication, November 1998). The MacArthur Communicative Development Inventory, a parent report, is a popular and well-normed vocabulary-screening instrument (Fenson et al., 1993). In order to be used quickly, screening instruments cannot be very detailed in many areas of development. Therefore, those who "fail" a screening instrument are referred for more detailed evaluation.

Evaluations for identification and classification purposes are necessarily norm-referenced and are more comprehensive. Evaluations are used to determine the extent to which a delay occurs and to identify the broad areas of delay. After children begin to use intentional communication but before they begin to talk, the Communication and Symbolic Behavior Scales (CSBS) is a useful evaluation tool (Wetherby & Prizant, 1993). It measures the frequency of communication, the breadth of pragmatic functions, the extent to which communication repairs occur, the syllable and consonant structure of prelinguistic vocalizations, the broad types and frequency of gestures, and superficial information about vocabulary and length of utterance. It is among our best norm-referenced evaluation instruments during the prelinguistic and early linguistic period (McCathren, Yoder, & Warren, 1999). Once children begin to talk, normative language tests can be used to evaluate phonology, semantics, and grammar; however, there are no normative methods for evaluating the more detailed aspects of early discourse skills yet. Researchers usually compare performance with milestones expected at different ages for typical children, which are based on relatively small samples of conversational skills (e.g., Chapman & Miller, 1983).

Intervention planning does not need to rely on norm-referenced instruments because no detailed comparison to age-mates is necessary. If normative comparisons are made, they are made only to identify endpoint goals and mastery criteria. Again, there are no instruments to use for goal selection before the intentional communication stage (about 9 months of age in typically developing children). During the intentional communication to early linguistic stage, the CSBS and the Early Social-Communicative Scales (ESCS, Seibert, Hogan, & Mundy, 1982) can be used to select goals. The ESCS and CSBS both use semi-structured procedures to provoke children into communicating. The functions and forms used to communicate are the primary focus of both instruments. The CSBS has more information about the vocalizations and repair strategies than the ESCS does. Conversational language samples are necessary to assess the details of children's vocabulary, grammar, discourse, and intelligibility in conversation. Using norm-referenced tests for goal selection generally will not be sufficiently detailed and will not indicate how children behave under more natural conditions (Coggins, 1998).

High-quality progress monitoring requires the most detailed assessment and the most naturalistic measurement contexts possible. Social development should be assessed in the typical context of the child's important social interactions. Once a goal has been identified, it is broken into objectives that are better specified with regard to behavior, environment, and mastery criteria. Ideally, the objective identifies the environment in which the child's performance needs to be monitored. The mastery criteria should identify the degree of independence and the frequency or consistency with which the child is expected to perform

Table 4.1. Select characteristics of socially competent infants and toddlers by Western standards

Age	Area	Skill	Source
By 6 months	Prosody	Duration of cooing, 2–3 seconds	Chapman & Miller, 1983
		Variable intonation during cooing	Chapman & Miller, 1983
	Phonology	Mostly vowel-like sounds	Stoel-Gammon, 1998
6–12 months	Pragmatics	Vocal turn taking in communication games such as Pat-a-cake	Chapman & Miller, 1983
		Some response to partner's initiation between 12% and 67% of the time	Hays, Nash, & Pedersen, 1982
		Imitates other actions	Dunn & Kendrick, 1982
		Gestures and vocalizes to an adult while coordinating attention to an object or event	Adamson & Chance, 1998
		Prelinguistic forms of requesting, commenting, and protesting	Chapman, 1981
	Phonology	Multisyllabic vocalizations with consonants to communicate	Chapman & Miller, 1983
		Stops, nasals, and glides compose about 90% of the consonants used	Stoel-Gammon, 1998
		Vocal communication is about 20% of all vocalizations	Stoel-Gammon, 1998
	Prosody	Intonation varies by pragmatic function of the vocal communication	Stoel-Gammon, 1998
12–18 months	Pragmatics	Topic of conversations about routines or perceptually present objects, events, and people	Imbens-Bailey & Snow, 1996
		Approximately 38% of communications are immediately successful	Golinkoff, 1986
		Approximately 49% of communications are initially misunderstood by mother	Golinkoff, 1986
		Average of seven turns to repair a misunderstood message	Golinkoff, 1986
		Approximately 90% of requests for clarification are repaired	Wetherby, Alexander, & Prizant, 1998
		Approximately 64% of repairs modify the original message	Wetherby, et al., 1998
		Linguistic forms of requesting, commenting, and protest	Chapman, 1981

Table 4.1. *(continued)*

Age	Area	Skill	Source
	Phonology	Vocal or verbal communication is predominant type of vocalization	Stoel-Gammon, 1998
	Prosody	Longer bouts of jargoning or intonated babbling	Stoel-Gammon, 1998
	Semantics	50–100 spoken words—maternal report	Fenson et al., 1993
	Grammar	Mostly single word utterances	Miller, 1981
18–24 months	Pragmatics	Asks "what's that" and "where's that" questions	Chapman & Miller, 1983
		Initiates new topic following silence with less than a 2-second pause 13% of the time	Chapman, Miller, MacKenzie, & Bedrosian, 1981
		Continues the topic after mother's topic initiation 22% of the time	Chapman et al., 1981
		76% of repairs modify the original message; 17% modify the word; 39% modify the phrase	Wetherby et al., 1998
	Phonology	About 50% of spoken utterances understood by a stranger	Stoel-Gammon, 1998
	Semantics	100–350 spoken words—maternal report	Fenson et al., 1993
	Grammar	Early multiword utterances and early morphology	Miller, 1981

the behavior. Although normative information is unavailable to set frequency or consistency criteria for most behavioral components of social competency in infants and toddlers, the degree to which adults prompt or model the desired behavior in the natural interaction contexts can and should be indicated.

FACILITATING SOCIAL-COMMUNICATIVE DEVELOPMENT

At the most general level, only two basic strategies exist for facilitating social-communicative development in young children. One can directly teach (e.g., prompt, model, reinforce) communication and language skills. Alternatively, one can teach caregivers who interact frequently with the child to be highly responsive to the child's communication attempts whenever possible and to use relatively simple techniques such as linguistic mapping (e.g., labeling what the child prelinguistically requests or comments on). These strategies are not mutually exclusive. Furthermore, if caregivers are already highly responsive (as many clearly are), then the second tactic need not be specifically targeted, although even highly responsive parents may benefit from some fine tuning of their skills. In any case, the two tactics are complementary, and a comprehensive intervention program should attempt to use both strategies to the degree possible.

Indeed, it may be that neither strategy is sufficient with some young children in the absence of the other. Yoder and Warren (1998, 2001) reported that the effects of prelinguistic milieu teaching are substantially greater for children with mothers who are above average on a pretreatment measure of responsivity to their child's communication acts. Conversely, adult responsivity to children's communication attempts has been shown to have modest effects on language development for at least some children in the absence of specific elicitation techniques (Tannock & Girolametto, 1992; Wilcox & Shannon, 1998; Yoder, Warren, McCathren, & Leew, 1998). In short, optimal intervention outcomes may be achieved when high levels of adult responsivity in general are combined with specific intervention tactics aimed at evoking key aspects of communication in their children.

The following section first describes what is termed as *enabling contexts* (Warren & Yoder, 1998). This term refers to a small set of variables that support effective social communication and language learning irrespective of what specific approach or procedures are used. We describe several specific techniques collectively referred to as prelinguistic milieu teaching (PMT) and how these techniques can be used to establish an initial repertoire of proto-imperatives and proto-declaratives. We then present a brief overview of milieu language teaching techniques. These techniques are appropriate for use as children begin using words as a frequent mode of communication. Finally, we describe the use of responsive interaction techniques to enhance communicative development and to augment the use of PMT and milieu language teaching.

Enabling Contexts

Enabling contexts refer to the following set of procedures intended to provide an optimal environment for highly responsive caregiver–child interaction or the use of specific teaching techniques: 1) arranging the environment, 2) following the child's attentional lead, and 3) building social routines. They are to be used whenever possible to ensure a high degree of engagement by the child and support frequent teaching interactions between the child and adult. The basic formats for these procedures were developed for use in naturalistic early language intervention approaches such as milieu teaching (Warren, 1991) and responsive interaction teaching (Wilcox & Shannon, 1998).

Arranging the Environment

The value of attending to and specifying the arrangement of the child's immediate environment rests on the fact that children are most likely to initiate communication about things they need, want, or find interesting (Hart & Risley, 1968; Warren, 1991). This fact obviously implies that the child inhabits a stimulating, interesting, developmentally appropriate environment. More specifically, arranging the environment involves placing desired items (e.g., food, toys) either out of reach of the child or in a context in which adult assistance is necessary to gain access to them. This often happens quite naturally in homes and child care environments. In a classroom context, certain toys might be kept in clear plastic containers with lids on them that children cannot open without adult assistance. Crayons might be placed on the floor next to the adult where the child can see them but cannot easily reach them. Extra cupcakes might be placed in clear view but beyond the child's reach.

Communication opportunities also arise when the very predictability and order of an environment is violated. An adult can plan such events or they can capitalize on naturally occurring, unplanned events. In the course of daily life, events of this nature may occur frequently and can be used by observant caregivers as communication opportunities. The novelty of these events may create excellent opportunities for modeling and using declaratives.

Positioning refers to how adults place their bodies in relation to the child's body and a focal object. To the extent possible, the adult should directly face the child and place the focal object at the child's eye level (Musselwhite, 1986). With infants and toddlers, this may mean the adult will need to sit or even lay on the floor. This type of close, face-to-face contact facilitates coordinated joint attention between the adult and child (MacDonald, 1989). Sitting behind or above the child makes this type of interaction more difficult.

Following the Child's Attentional Lead

The quality of a young child's attention is substantially greater to objects or events of the child's choosing, rather than to objects or events of the adults choosing (Bruner, Roy, & Ratner, 1980). Furthermore, young children have difficulty deploying their attention on command for more than very short periods (Goldberg, 1977). Thus, following the child's attentional lead, a universal tenet of virtually all naturalistic early communication and language intervention approaches (Hepting & Goldstein, 1996), is employed to sustain the child's interest in activities and social interaction. In practice this tenet might mean that the adult plays with toys or engages in activities of interest to the child (typically selected by the child from an array of choices) in a manner similar to the child's play. Children who are passive and engage in low rates of action can make maintaining this procedure challenging. Adults can easily lapse into directive styles in which they dominate most interaction episodes with the child. Experience suggests that if the goal is to build initiations, then it is far better to simply adapt one's behavior to the child's initiation rate.

A technique that can be quite helpful with a young child who seldom initiates is contingent motor imitation (Gazdag & Warren, 2000). Contingent motor imitation is an exact, reduced, or slightly expanded imitation of the child's motor production that is performed by the adult immediately following the child's motor production. It represents a specific form of following the child's attentional lead. This simple technique may be used at the start of intervention to establish a basic form of turn taking between the child and adult that over time can be transformed into interaction and play routines. Contingent imitation may benefit children because it allows them to regulate the amount of social stimulation received, it increases the probability that adult input will be easily processed and understood (Dawson & Lewy, 1989), it may encourage children to imitate adult behavior (Snow, 1989), and it may result in more differentiated play schemes (Dawson & Adams, 1984).

Contingent vocal imitation offers many of the same advantages and benefits as contingent motor imitation. It occurs when adults follow children's vocalizations with a partial, exact, or modified vocal imitation. For example, a child might say "ba," which an adult might immediately imitate as "ba," or "ba ba." This type of vocal imitation (similar to motor imitation) allows children to regulate the amount of social stimulation they receive and may encourage children to increase their rate of vocalization and to spontaneously imitate adult vocalizations (Gazdag & Warren, 2000).

Building Social Routines

Arranging the environment and following the child's attentional lead support the development of social routines. Social routines, in turn, provide an excellent context for facilitating social-communicative development. Social routines are repetitive, predictable turn-taking games and rituals such as Peek-a-boo and Pat-a-cake. They can be established in the course of daily activities such as feeding, bathing, and dressing, as well as games and toy play. They also can be unconventional and unique to a given child. Social routines may last from a few seconds to a half-hour or more and may occur with a wide range of frequency. A child may engage in a specific routine for a few days or a few years. The predictable structure of social routines may help children learn and remember new skills. Once children learn predictable roles in a routine, they can devote greater attention to analyzing adult models of new ways to communicate (Conti-Ramsden & Friel-Patti, 1986; Nelson, 1989). In addition, the effectiveness of models may be enhanced because slight variations in the routine may create a "moderately novel" situation that is particularly salient to young children (Piaget & Inhelder, 1969).

Research with children who are typically developing and with children who have mental retardation has shown that social routines are particularly powerful stimuli for linguistic (Snow, Perlmann, & Nathan, 1987; Yoder & Davies, 1992) and prelinguistic communication (Bakeman & Adamson, 1986). Once a social routine is well established with a child, adults can often evoke a high rate of requests and comments by interrupting or modifying the routine. Social routines also provide a natural context for modeling these communication functions and related skills such as turn taking.

Prelinguistic Milieu Teaching Techniques

Social interaction routines set the stage for implementing specific techniques to prompt, model, and reinforce clear, frequent, intentional communication. These techniques also can be used in nonroutine interactions. Either way, occasions for the use of any specific technique is determined by the quality of children's engagement with objects of interest and their conversational partners. Prompts are used only when motivation to communicate is high (e.g., when the child is intently engaged in social interaction). Additional consequences can follow any intentional communication attempt. Specific teaching episodes should be brief, positive, and embedded in the ongoing stream of interaction. Our research suggests that PMT is most effective with children whose primary caregivers are at least moderately responsive to them (Yoder & Warren, 1998, 2001). Responsive interaction procedures (discussed later) may be more effective with children with low-responsive caregivers, at least initially.

Prompts

Prompts are used to evoke intentional communication attempts by the child or to evoke specific components of intentional communication. Two types of prompts, time delay and verbal prompts, can be used to facilitate communication attempts. A time delay for initiation is a nonverbal prompt that often functions as an interruption of an ongoing turn-taking routine. For example, if a child and adult were rolling a ball back and forth, the adult might interrupt this routine by withholding the ball and looking at the child expectantly until the child initiates a request to continue the routine. Verbal prompts for communication can be open-ended questions (e.g., "What?") intended to elicit communication responses. Verbal prompts for communication also can be used to elicit a specific component of communication. For example, when a young child requests without eye contact, the directive statement "Look at me" may be used to evoke eye contact. Intersection of gaze is a technique that allows the adult to establish eye contact, an essential component of coordinated joint attention. To intersect the child's gaze, a mom would move her eyes into the gaze of her child. This technique is then faded out as the child begins to regularly initiate and maintain eye contact.

Models

Models are used to support and enhance the vocal and gestural topography of the child's intentional communication attempts. Vocal models of sounds that the adult has heard the child produce (e.g., "ba") are used to emphasize the vocal component of communication and as contingent consequences to increase the rate of child vocalization. Likewise, gestural models are used to encourage the child to use and imitate gestures. For example, when an airplane passes overhead, the adult might point to it as a model for the child to use pointing as an element of commenting.

Additional Consequences

Child communication attempts such as requests and comments should be consequated in accordance with their intent: The child should receive whatever he or she requested, and comments should result in adult attention to the child's topic. Continued attention and interaction by the adult are assumed. These natural consequences may be supplemented with specific acknowledgement and/or linguistic mapping. Specific acknowledgement is provided by a smile and comment (that specifies the desired communication behavior that was used) after the child produces a targeted intentional communication component. For example, when a child makes eye contact with a caregiver in the course of initiating a request, the caregiver might break into a big smile and comment, "You looked at me!" while responding to the child's request. Frequent use of specific acknowledgement may disrupt the flow of interaction, and praise statements tend to lose their value for recipients if used too frequently. Therefore, these statements should be used primarily when a child is first acquiring a new behavior and thereafter only in response to some occurrences.

Linguistic mapping occurs when the adult verbally states the core meaning of the immediately preceding communication act. For example, a child might hold up a doll for the adult to see (a comment), and the adult might respond, "It's a baby." Research with both typically and atypically developing children has indicated that linguistic mapping can be a powerful contributor to vocabulary development (Nelson, 1989). Therefore, we encourage the frequent use of linguistic mapping as part of adult responses to intentional communication attempts.

Teaching Intentional Communication

The specific techniques described should be embedded into ongoing interactions and used as dictated by the context and the child's current communication goals. Some specific techniques may be used quite frequently (e.g., linguistic mapping), others only until the child begins to intentionally communicate (e.g., intersection of gaze). Yet, the enabling procedures of arranging the environment, following the child's attentional lead, and social routine building are to be used whenever possible.

Teaching Proto-Imperatives

It is helpful to first establish social routines that involve turn taking between the adult and child. How long this takes will depend on the child. Once an initial set of routines has been established and a particular routine has gone on for at least two turns, the adult may stop the routine by withholding a turn and look expectantly at the child (time delay for initiation). A verbal prompt also might be given, such as "What?" (to start the activity) or "Do you want this?" (while maintaining eye contact and holding up an object the child needs to resume the activity). If there is not an appropriate response to the interruption of the routine or if the child's response is incomplete (i.e., it is missing a component necessary to be considered intentional communication), then the adult may provide further assistance to the child. For example, if the child looks at a toy and displays a discrete action or provides a vocalization but does not make eye contact with the adult, then the adult might prompt "Look at me" and/or intersect the child's gaze. The adult also might provide a gestural model if needed to complete the communication act. Once the child begins to request across different routines intentionally, then prompts, models, and specific acknowledgements should be faded out. Linguistic mapping should continue as part of the adults' response to the requests, however.

Teaching Proto-Declaratives

Proto-declaratives are taught in a decidedly different manner from proto-imperatives (Yoder & Warren, 1999). The primary motivation for a proto-declarative is to recruit another's attention and to share affective states with him or her. It is often necessary for young children to first develop a positive relationship with adults before they will initiate proto-declaratives to them frequently. Thus, adults should wait until such a relationship has been established before attempting to facilitate the development of proto-declaratives directly. Of course, proto-declaratives may be modeled at any time.

Proto-declaratives are taught by modeling and by providing situations likely to stimulate their use. One such situation is the introduction of novel events or objects. This introduction can take many forms such as adding new toys or items within routines (which can be done frequently) or taking advantage of occasional occurrences (planned or unplanned) of silly or unusual events, a sabotaged routine, a walk, or a ride in the car. The adult should model proto-declaratives concurrent with or just after novel events. On occasion, when something novel occurs, the adult may pretend not to notice. The intent in this case is to set up a situation in which the child feels the need to direct the adult's attention to the object or event. Yet another approach is to let the child have the run of the room for a few minutes but with the adult clearly observing him from a short distance away. As the child "discovers" novel items in this manner, the child may then comment to the adult; however, our clinical observation has been that by far the majority of proto-declaratives occur about an object or event that the child has reason to believe the adult is already attending to. That is, they occur in a context in which both the child and adult are obviously engaged in joint attention (Carpenter et al., 1998).

Milieu Language Teaching Techniques

Milieu teaching procedures can be used to teach a wide range of early language skills (Warren & Kaiser, 1988). These procedures are particularly effective for teaching basic vocabulary and two- and three-term semantic relationships and teaching children to use language for social purposes (Kaiser, Yoder, & Keetz, 1992). Given the emphasis in this chapter on social competence, the effects of milieu teaching procedures on skills that directly influence social interaction are of the utmost relevance. For example, milieu approaches have been found to facilitate generalized intelligibility (Yoder, Kaiser, & Alpert, 1991), generalized talkativeness (Yoder, Kaiser, Goldstein, et al., 1995), and generalized child responsiveness in obligatory speech contexts (Warren, McQuarter, & Rogers-Warren, 1984). Finally, milieu procedures have been used in combination with responsive-interaction procedures to enhance both linguistic aspects of language development and social-communicative exchanges between parents and their young children with language delays (Kaiser, 1993).

Effective milieu language teaching requires the systematic use of the mand-model procedure and the incidental teaching procedure (e.g., Warren & Bambara, 1989). These procedures are complementary and follow the same basic steps in prompting and consequating a target response. They are designed to be embedded in conversational exchanges and are inherently social in nature. The distinction between the two procedures centers on who (the adult or the child) initiates the instructional episode within the social interaction. In the mand-model procedure, the adult initiates the teaching episode by "manding" a target response, typically by asking a question meant to evoke the target response. In the incidental teaching procedure, the child initiates the episode either verbally or nonverbally. The adult then prompts the target response by requesting a more elaborate response.

The main social-interaction effect of the mand-model procedure is to increase responsiveness and attentiveness to both environmental and verbal cues. As children's self-initiations and responsiveness to adult initiations increase, there should be a corresponding shift away from use of the mand-model procedure toward the use of the incidental teaching procedure. Because the incidental teaching procedure explicitly continues children's topic of conversation, it may be more likely to enhance social-conversation skills in general (Hart, 1985).

When using the incidental teaching procedure, the following basic steps are employed:

1. The child initiates an interaction. The adult establishes joint attention with the child.
2. The adult asks a question in response to the child's initiation. This is intended to prompt the target response. If the child responds with a partial target response, the adult may ask an elaborative question or in some cases immediately present a scaffolded model for the child to imitate.
3. If the child does not produce the target response and the child still appears receptive and interested, the adult may present another prompt. Otherwise, a model for the target response is presented.
4. An acceptable target response is reinforced functionally according to the child's apparent intent. Reinforcement might include access to a requested activity or material, provision of requested information, or continued participation in an activity or conversation. The adult may acknowledge a particularly noteworthy response by the child with praise and frequently will provide a further verbal expansion of the child's response to conclude the episode.

Responsive Interaction Approaches

There is considerable correlational evidence (Landrey et al., 1997; Murray & Hornbaker, 1997; Smith, Landry, Miller-Loncar, & Swank, 1997) and some experimental evidence (Yoder et al., 1998) suggesting that an optimal style for promoting social and cognitive competence fosters reciprocal interactions between parent and child that give the child some degree of control over the interaction. Responsive interaction techniques (Wilcox & Shannon, 1998) are intended to create just such an optimal style in caregivers. This approach is widely used in parent training (the Hanen Program [Manolson, 1985] is a good example of such an approach). Its major immediate goal is to increase the child's social-communicative skills by enhancing the quality of interaction between the adult and the child.

Responsive interaction techniques also have been referred to as focused stimulation (Leonard, 1981) and interactive modeling (Wilcox, Kouri, & Caswell, 1991). Like PMT and milieu teaching, these techniques require the provision of "enabling contexts" (e.g., following the child's attention lead) to maximize their effectiveness. Linguistic mapping is generally encouraged, too; however, responsive interaction approaches generally discourage the direct elicitation of specific child responses via requests to imitate, mands, or test questions because of the belief that child self-initiation is encouraged by responding to as opposed to prompting communication. Instead, focused input is provided based on the child's attentional lead. This input may include models (in the form of descriptive talk or linguistic mapping, not as elicited imitation prompts), expansions, and recasts to increase the saliency of the targeted language for the child.

A recast is a specific expansion or modification of a child's immediately preceding utterance in which new syntactic or semantic information is added (Nelson, 1989). For example, a child might say "throw ball" as a request to an adult. An adult may then recast this as "I'll throw the red ball to you." In theory, the temporal proximity and semantic overlap of the recast and the child's utterance aids the child in making comparisons between his or her utterance and the recast. Once an adult is skilled at creating "enabling contexts" for communication, the technique of recasting can be used virtually anytime and anywhere. In fact, recasts are a typical part of caregiver–child interaction (Nelson, 1989); however, recasts cannot be used until a child begins to communicate intentionally because they first require the child to produce an intentional communicative act at a minimum and are limited by the extent to which the child initiates. Thus, low initiation rates can stymie the effectiveness of this technique.

Several studies have found that responsive interaction approaches are more effective than milieu teaching approaches with children who have a mean length of utterance (MLU) above 2.5 but relatively less effective with children who have an MLU under 2.0 (e.g., Yoder et al., 1995; Wilcox et al. 1991). Their increased effectiveness as MLU increases is probably related to the development of children's short-term memory abilities. That is, as children are increasingly able to compare their own utterance with the adult utterance that immediately follows it, the effectiveness of the recasting aspect of the responsive interaction approach may increase (Camarata, 1995).

Our research (Yoder & Warren, 1998, 2001) has found that toddlers who have developmental delays as well as less responsive mothers demonstrated greater gains in intentional communication and vocabulary development as a result of a responsive small-group communication intervention (one that did not allow any direct elicitation prompts) than similar children with low responsive mothers who received PMT as an intervention. Anecdotal evidence suggested that some of these children focused their attention away from the referent of teaching when confronted with an explicit prompt to communicate in the PMT intervention sessions.

Why might young children with unresponsive mothers become passive or turn away from a prompt to communicate? Unresponsive mothers are likely to be both infrequent and directive interactants with their children (Hart & Risley, 1995; Landry et al., 1997). Directive means that a high proportion of the mother's interactions with her young child involve telling the child what to do. Children of infrequent interactants may expect to be left alone when adults are near. When faced with an adult who is undemanding, spatially close, attentive, and responsive (as in our responsive small-group intervention), children of infrequent interactants may become actively engaged more easily. In contrast, when faced with an adult who makes demands on them in the form of communication prompts (as in our PMT intervention), such children may withdraw or simply not respond. Children of directive, unresponsive mothers may learn early to expect adults to tell them how to behave, even in nonthreatening play situations (Hart & Risley, 1995). When faced with adults who give lots of prompts (again as in PMT intervention), these children may become passive communicators. For example, they may process the input from linguistic mapping of their prompted communications less effectively than that from responses to self-initiated communication. When faced with adults who do not give prompts but are unusually responsive (as in our responsive small group), children of directive mothers may use high rates of self-initiated, clear communication. Such communication may result in more easily processed adult responses, thereby increasing the efficacy of adult responses in facilitating future communications. Obviously, research is needed to test these hypotheses.

Global Interaction Approaches

An additional group of strategies might best be termed *global interaction approaches*. These strategies include approaches intended to specifically promote language development (e.g., MacDonald's [1985, 1989] conversational model), approaches intended to enhance attachment between young children and their primary caregivers (e.g., Lieberman, Weston, & Paul, 1991), and relatively comprehensive early intervention programs such as the Infant Health and Development Program

(1990). All of these programs aim to enhance caregiver responsiveness among other things. Although changes in caregiver–child interaction have been widely documented as a result of these types of efforts, specific changes in child language development have been more difficult to ascertain to date (e.g., Mahoney et al., 1998; McCollum & Hemmeter, 1997; Wilcox & Shannon, 1998).

Cross-Cultural Issues

The intervention approaches described previously reflect a set of biases about social-communicative development and the appropriate roles of caregivers and practitioners. The acceptability of these procedures, and hence their ultimate effectiveness, may vary in some cases because of differences in cultural values and beliefs (van Kleeck, 1994). Early social-communicative intervention is perhaps even more susceptible to problems associated with cultural differences than other forms of intervention for two reasons. First, it often takes place within the family context and carries an expectation that the caregivers will play an active role and even adopt a style of interaction with their child that directly violates some of their views of appropriate parent–child interaction (Bornstein, 1989). Second, the focus on communication and language development and differences is inherently one of the most sensitive areas for cross-cultural discourse. A range of basic class and ethnic differences are frequently manifested in language differences (Heath, 1989). Furthermore, even a basic goal such as "increase the child's rate of communicative initiations" can be problematic. For example, in her study of the Inuit people in northern Canada, Crago (1990) found that parents discouraged talkativeness in young children, considering it a sign of a learning problem.

Most potential sources of bias can be limited or at least identified through the careful collection and consideration of information on individual family values, beliefs, and desires. This information then can be used to modify intervention strategies to enhance their acceptability and thus their ultimate effectiveness. A thorough consideration of individual family differences should be a given with all families, irrespective of their cultural or ethnic background. Thus, embracing this perspective should place no additional burden on practitioners. It is in fact completely congruent with the notion of individualizing efforts to meet the unique concerns of the family and child, a widely held tenet of early intervention practices in many countries and cultures (Odom & McLean, 1996).

IMPLICATIONS FOR PRACTITIONERS AND PARENTS

The first 3 years of a child's life are a unique time during which the foundations of social, emotional, and communication skills are established. It is a time when parents may have the greatest effect on their children's development, positively or negatively. It is also a time when peer social interactions take a back seat to adult–child interaction. Yet, the social, emotional, and communicative foundations established during this period surely will have enormous implications for the later success of the child in peer interaction and other social contexts.

In the 1990s, knowledge of the myriad forces that shape child development exploded. Nevertheless, the ability to routinely profile early development, to determine an optimal intervention, and then to implement an optimal intervention in day to day practice will continue to be challenged. Still, a sufficient knowledge base is available to offer a modest set of clinical implications for practitioners and parents.

First, social and linguistic responsivity by caregivers is an important ingredient in promoting optimal child development and ensuring that specific targeted interventions have maximal effects; however, responsivity by itself is probably not sufficient to promote optimal development in young children with serious developmental delays and disorders. Some combination of highly responsive caregiving and specific intervention strategies may turn out to be the most efficacious approach with many of these children. Further research is needed to determine which comprehensive strategy is most effective. The authors' prediction is that ultimately researchers will determine that somewhat different strategies are optimally effective with children who have substantially different histories and current profiles of development. For example, a child with a history of exposure to an unresponsive environment will necessitate a somewhat different approach than a child with a history of exposure to a highly responsive environment even if the two children are similar in other important ways (e.g., both have Down syndrome).

Second, young children benefit from enabling contexts such as following their attentional lead and establishing playful social routines irrespective of which specific intervention technique may be used. These "enabling contexts," whether established in homes or in child care centers, are manifestations of highly responsive environments specifically attuned to the interests and concerns of the child.

Third, when supported by a responsive environment, specific procedures such as prelinguistic milieu teaching can be used to effectively establish and enhance social-communicative development. In the absence of such a responsive environment at home, then responsive interaction approaches may be relatively more effective, at least during the course of prelinguistic communication development.

Fourth, because social-communicative skills are learned hour by hour, day by day, specific interventions must take advantage of the ripple effects associated with the transactional model of social-communicative development in order to achieve meaningful changes. As the chapter has noted several times, the fuel that drives the transactional model is sensitive, highly responsive parenting.

CONCLUSION

All children increase in their social skills to the extent that they interact with others. This fact is as true for infants and toddlers who may primarily interact with caregivers as it is for older children whose social world increasingly revolves around peer interactions. During the first 24 months of developmental life, the foundational skills of social competence are established in the context of caregiver–child interactions. Hart and Risley (1995) described a style of everyday parenting of typically developing toddlers (all their child participants were younger than 3 years of age) that seemed to ensure not only socially competent children but also children who eventually demonstrated larger vocabularies, greater success in school, and even higher IQ scores than children who received less of this style of parenting. These parents talked a lot to their children, they listened attentively to their children, they treated them kindly, they gave them choices, and they told them about things in the parents' world. In short, they were highly responsive to their children. This style certainly reflects a cultural bias; however, in Western information-age societies, this style in combination with specific targeted interventions as dictated by individual child concerns, is likely to be as appropriate for enhancing the social competence of young children with developmental delays and disorders as it appears to be for typically developing children.

REFERENCES

Adamson, L., & Bakeman, R. (1991). The development of shared attention in infancy. *Annals of Child Development, 8,* 1–41.

Adamson, L.B., & Chance, S.E. (1998). Coordinating attention to people, objects, and language. In S.F. Warren & J. Reichle (Series Eds.) & A.M. Wetherby, S.F. Warren, & J. Reichle (Vol. Eds.), *Communication and language intervention series: Vol. 7. Transitions in prelinguistic communication* (pp. 15–38). Baltimore: Paul H. Brookes Publishing Co.

Ainsworth, M.D., Blehar, M.C., Waters, E., & Wall, S. (1978). *Patterns of attachment: A psychological study of the strange situations.* Mahwah, NJ: Lawrence Erlbaum Associates.

Bailey, D., & Simeonsson, R. (1985). A functional model of social competence. *Topics in Early Childhood Special Education, 4,* 20–31.

Bakeman, R., & Adamson, L.B. (1986). Infants' conventionalized acts: Gestures and words with mothers and peers. *Infant Behavior and Development, 9,* 215–230.

Bates, E. (1993). Comprehension and production in early language development. In S. Savage-Rumbaugh, J. Murphy, R. Sevcik, K. Brakke, S. Williams, & D. Rumbaugh (Eds.), *Language comprehension in ape and child* (pp. 222–242). Chicago: University of Chicago Press.

Bornstein, M.H. (Ed.). (1989). *Maternal responsiveness: Characteristics and consequences.* San Francisco: Jossey-Bass.

Bruner, J.S. (1976). From communication to language: A psychological perspective. *Cognition, 3,* 155–187.

Bruner, J., Roy, C., & Ratner, R. (1980). The beginnings of request. In K.E. Nelson (Ed.), *Children's language* (Vol. 3, pp. 91–138). New York: Gardner Press.

Camarata, S.C. (1995). A rationale for naturalistic speech intelligibility intervention. In S.F. Warren & J. Reichle (Series Eds.) & M. Fey, J. Windsor, & S.F. Warren (Vol. Eds.), *Communication and language intervention series: Vol. 5. Language intervention: Preschool through the elementary years* (pp. 63–84). Baltimore: Paul H. Brookes Publishing Co.

Carpenter, M., Nagell, K., & Tomasello, M. (1998). Social cognition, joint attention, and communicative competence from 9 to 15 months of age. *Monographs of the Society for Research in Child Development, 63*(Serial No. 4).

Chapman, R. (1981). Exploring children's communicative intent. In J. Miller (Ed.), *Assessing language production in children: Experimental procedures* (pp. 111–138). Baltimore: University Park Press.

Chapman, R., & Miller, J. (1983). Early stages of discourse comprehension and production: Implications for assessment and intervention. In R.M. Golinkoff (Ed.), *The transition from prelinguistic to linguistic communication* (pp. 219–233). Mahwah, NJ: Lawrence Erlbaum Associates.

Chapman, R., Miller, J., MacKenzie, H., & Bedrosian, J. (1981, August). *The development of discourse skills in the second year of life.* Paper presented at the Second International Congress for the Study of Child Language, University of British Columbia, Vancouver, Canada.

Coggins, T. (1998). Clinical assessment of emerging language: How to gather evidence and make informed decisions. In S.F. Warren & J. Reichle (Series Eds.) & A.M. Wetherby, S.F. Warren, & J. Reichle (Vol. Eds.), *Communication and language intervention series: Vol. 7. Transitions in prelinguistic communication* (pp. 233–259). Baltimore: Paul H. Brookes Publishing Co.

Conti-Ramsden, G., & Friel-Patti, S. (1986). Mother–child dialogues: Considerations of cognitive complexity for young language learning children. *British Journal of Disorders of Communication, 21,* 245–255.

Crago, M. (1990). Development of communicative competence in Inuit children: Implications for speech-language pathology. *Journal of Childhood Communication Disorders, 13,* 73–83.

Dawson, G., & Adams, A. (1984). Imitation and social responsiveness in autistic children. *Journal of Abnormal Child Psychology, 12,* 209–226.

Dawson, G., & Lewy, A. (1989). Reciprocal subcortical-cortical influences in autism: The role of attentional mechanisms. In G. Dawson (Ed.), *Autism: Nature, diagnosis, and treatment* (pp. 144–173). New York: Guilford Press.

DeCasper, A.J., & Fifer, W.P. (1980). Of human bonding: Newborns prefer their mothers' voices. *Science, 208,* 1174–1176.

Dodge, K. (1983). Behavioral antecedents of peer social status. *Child Development, 54,* 1386–1399.

Dunn, J., & Kendrick, C. (1982). *Siblings: Love, envy, and understanding.* Cambridge, MA: Harvard University Press.

Feagans, L., & Farran, D.C. (1982). *The language of children reared in poverty: Implications for evaluation and intervention.* San Diego: Academic Press.

Fenson, L., Dale, P., Reznick, J.S., Thal, D., Bates, E., Hartung, J., Pethick, S., & Reilly, J. (1993). *MacArthur Communicative Development Inventories (CDI).* San Diego: Singular Publishing Group.

Gazdag, G.E., & Warren, S.F. (2000). The effects of adult contingent imitation on the development of young children's vocal imitations. *Journal of Early Intervention, 23,* 24–35.

Goldberg, S. (1977). Social competence in infancy: A model of parent–infant interaction. *Merrill-Palmer Quarterly, 23,* 163–177.

Golinkoff, R.M. (1986). "I beg your pardon?": The preverbal negotiation of failed messages. *Journal of Child Language, 13,* 455–476.

Gottfried, A.W. (Ed.). (1984). *Home environment and early cognitive development: Longitudinal research.* San Diego: Academic Press.

Hart, B. (1985). Naturalistic language training techniques. In S.F. Warren & A. Rogers-Warren (Eds.), *Teaching functional language* (pp. 63–88). Baltimore: University Park Press.

Hart, B., & Risley, T.R. (1968). Establishing the use of descriptive adjectives in the spontaneous speech of disadvantaged preschool children. *Journal of Applied Behavior Analysis, 1,* 109–120.

Hart, B., & Risley, T.R. (1992). American parenting of language-learning children: Persisting differences in family–child interactions observed in natural home environments. *Developmental Psychology, 28(6),* 1096–1105.

Hart, B., & Risley, T.R. (1995). *Meaningful differences in the everyday experience of young American children.* Baltimore: Paul H. Brookes Publishing Co.

Hays, D., Nash, A., & Pedersen, J. (1982). Dyadic interaction in the first year of life. In K. Rubin & H. Ross (Eds.), *Peer relationships and social skills in childhood* (pp. 11–40). New York: Springer-Verlag.

Heath, S.B. (1989). The learner as cultural member. In M.L. Rice & R.L. Schiefelbusch (Eds.), *The teachability of language* (pp. 333–350). Baltimore: Paul H. Brookes Publishing Co.

Hepting, N.H., & Goldstein, H. (1996). What's natural about naturalistic language intervention? *Journal of Early Intervention, 20,* 250–278.

Howes, C. (1987). Social competency with peers: Contributions from child care. *Early Childhood Research Quarterly, 2,* 155–167.

Imbens-Bailey, A., & Snow, C. (1997). Making meaning in parent–child interaction: A pragmatic approach. In C. Mandell & A. McCabe (Eds.), *The problem of meaning: Behavioral and cognitive perspectives* (pp. 261–296). Amsterdam: North-Holland.

Infant Health and Development Program. (1990). Enhancing the outcomes of low birth-weight, premature infants: A multi-site randomized trial. *Journal of the American Medical Association, 263,* 3035–3042.

Kaiser, A.P. (1993). Parent-implemented language intervention. In S.F. Warren & J. Reichle (Series Eds.) & A.P. Kaiser & D.B. Gray (Vol. Eds.), *Communication and language intervention series: Vol. 2. Enhancing children's communication: Research foundations for intervention* (pp. 63–84). Baltimore: Paul H. Brookes Publishing Co.

Kaiser, A.P., Yoder, P.J., & Keetz, A. (1992). Evaluating milieu teaching. In S.F. Warren & J. Reichle (Series & Vol. Eds.), *Communication and language intervention series: Vol. 1. Causes and effects in communication and language intervention* (pp. 9–48). Baltimore: Paul H. Brookes Publishing Co.

Katz, L. (1988). What should young children be learning. *ERIC Digest* (pp. 47–48). Urbana, IL: Clearinghouse on Elementary and Early Childhood Education.

Landry, S.H., Smith, K.E., Miller-Loncar, C.L., & Swank, P.R. (1997). The relation of change in maternal interactive styles to the developing social competence of full-term and preterm children. *Child Development, 69,* 105–123.

Leonard, L. (1981). Facilitating linguistic skills in children with specific language impairment. *Applied Psycholinguistic, 2,* 89–118.

Lieberman, A.F., Weston, D.R., & Paul, J.H. (1991). Preventive intervention and outcome with anxiously attached dyads. *Child Development, 62,* 199–209.

Locke, J.L. (1993). *The child's path to spoken language.* Cambridge, MA: Harvard University Press.

MacDonald, J. (1985). Language through conversation: A model for intervention with language delayed persons. In S. Warren & A. Rogers-Warren (Eds.), *Teaching functional language* (pp. 89–122). Baltimore: University Park Press.

MacDonald, J. (1989). *Becoming partners with children: From play to conversation.* San Antonio, TX: Special Press.

Mahoney, G., Boyce, G., Fewell, R.R., Spiker, D., & Wheeden, C.A. (1998). The relationship of parent–child interaction to the effectiveness of early intervention services for at-risk children and children with disabilities. *Topics in Early Childhood Special Education, 18,* 5–17.

Manolson, H.A. (1985). *It takes two to talk: A Hanen early language parent guidebook.* (Available from Hanen Early Language Resource Center, 152 Bloor Street West, Toronto, Canada 40126)

McCathren, R., Yoder, P.J., & Warren, S.F. (1999). The relationship between prelinguistic vocalization and later expressive vocabulary in young children with developmental delay. *Journal of Speech, Language, and Hearing Research, 42,* 915–924.

McCollum, J.A., & Hemmeter, M.L. (1997). Parent-child interaction intervention when children have disabilities. In M.J. Guralnick (Ed.), *The effectiveness of early intervention* (pp. 549–576). Baltimore: Paul H. Brookes Publishing Co.

McLean, J., & Snyder-McLean, L. (1978). *A transactional approach to early language training.* Columbus, OH: Charles E. Merrill.

Miller, J. (1981). *Assessing language production in children.* Needham Heights, MA: Allyn & Bacon.

Murray, A.D., & Hornbaker, A.V. (1997). Maternal direction and facilitative interaction styles: Associations with language and cognitive development of low risk and high risk toddlers. *Development and Psychopathology, 9,* 507–516.

Musselwhite, C.R. (1986). *Adaptive play for special needs children.* San Diego: College-Hill Press.

Nelson, K.E. (1989). Strategies for first language learning. In M.L. Rice & R.L. Schiefebusch (Eds.), *The teachabilitiy of language* (pp. 263–310). Baltimore: Paul H. Brookes Publishing Co.

Odom, S.L., & McLean, M.E. (1996). *Early intervention/Early childhood special education recommended practices.* Austin, TX: PRO-ED.

O'Reilly, J.P., Tokuno, K.A., & Ebata, A.T. (1986). Cultural differences between Americans of Japanese and European ancestry in parental valuing of social competence. *Journal of Comparative Family Studies, 17,* 87–97.

Piaget, J., & Inhelder, B. (1969). *The psychology of the child.* New York: Basic Books.

Prizant, B., & Wetherby, A. (1990). Toward an integrated view of early language and communication development and socioemotional development. *Topics in Language Disorders, 10,* 1–16.

Rosenberg, S. (1982). The language of the mentally retarded: Development, progress, and intervention. In S. Rosenberg (Ed.), *Handbook of applied psycholingusitics* (pp. 329–392). Mahwah, NJ: Lawrence Erlbaum Associates.

Sachs, J. (1997). Communication development in infancy. In J.L. Gleason (Ed.), *The development of language* (pp. 40–68). Needham Heights, MA: Allyn & Bacon.

Sameroff, A.J. (1983). Developmental systems: Contexts and evolution. In P.H. Mussen (Ed.), *Handbook of Child Psychology* (Vol. 1, pp. 237–294). New York: John Wiley & Sons.

Sameroff, A.J., & Chandler, M.J. (1975). Reproductive risk and the continuum of caretaking casualty. In F.D. Horowitz, M. Hetherington, S. Scarr-Salapatek, & G. Siegel (Eds.), *Review of child development research* (Vol. 4, pp. 187–244). Chicago: University of Chicago Press.

Saunders, S.D., & Green, V. (1993). Evaluating the social competence of young children: A review of the literature. *Early Child Development and Care, 87,* 39–46.

Scheffelin, B., & Ochs, E. (1986). *Language socialization across cultures.* New York: Cambridge University Press.

Schultz, J.J., Florio, S., & Erickson, F. (1982). Where's the floor? Aspects of the cultural organization of social relationships in communication at home and in school. In P. Gilmore & A.A. Glatthorn (Eds.), *Children in and out of school: Ethnography and education.* Washington, DC: Center for Applied Linguistics.

Seibert, J., Hogan, A., & Mundy, P. (1982). Assessing interactional competencies: The Early Social-Communicative Scales. *Infant Mental Health Journal, 3,* 244–259.

Shore, R. (1997). *Rethinking the brain. New insights into early development.* New York: Families and Work Institute.

Smith, K.E., Landry, S.H., Miller-Loncar, C.L., & Swank, P.R. (1997). Characteristics that help mothers maintain their infants' focus of attention. *Journal of Applied Developmental Psychology, 18,* 587–601.

Snow, C.E. (1989). Imitativeness: A trait or a skill? In G.E. Speidel & K.E. Nelson (Eds.), *The many faces of imitation in language learning* (pp. 73–90). New York: Springer-Verlag.

Snow, C.E., Perlmann, R., & Nathan, D. (1987). What routines are different: Toward a multiple factors model of the relation between input and language acquisition. In K.E. Nelson & A. Van Kleeck (Eds.), *Child language* (Vol. 6, pp. 65–97). Mahwah, NJ: Lawrence Erlbaum Associates.

Stoel-Gammon, C. (1998). Role of babbling and phonology in early linguistic development. In S.F. Warren & J. Reichle (Series Eds.) & A.M. Wetherby, S.F. Warren, & J. Reichle (Vol. Eds.), *Communication and language intervention series: Vol. 7. Transitions in prelinguistic communication* (pp. 87–110). Baltimore: Paul H. Brookes Publishing Co.

Tannock, R., & Girolametto, L. (1992). Reassessing parent-focused language intervention programs. In S.F. Warren & J. Reichle (Series & Vol. Eds.) *Communication and language intervention series: Vol. 1. Causes and effects in communication and language intervention.* (pp. 49–79). Baltimore: Paul H. Brookes Publishing Co.

van Kleeck, A. (1994). Potential cultural bias in training parents as conversational partners with their children who have delays in language development. *American Journal of Speech-Language Pathology, 31,* 67–78.

Warren, S.F. (1991). Enhancing communication and language development with milieu teaching procedures. In E. Cipani (Ed.), *A guide for developing language competence in preschool children with severe and moderate handicaps* (pp. 68–93). Springfield, IL: Charles C Thomas.

Warren, S.F., & Bambara, L.M. (1989). An experimental analysis of milieu language intervention: Teaching the action-object form. *Journal of Speech and Hearing Disorders, 54,* 448–461.

Warren, S.F., & Kaiser, A.P. (1988). Research in early language intervention. In S.L. Odom & M.B. Karnes (Eds.), *Early intervention in infants and children with handicaps: An empirical base* (pp. 89–108). Baltimore: Paul H. Brookes Publishing Co.

Warren, S.F., McQuarter, R.J., & Rogers-Warren, A. (1984). The effects of mands and models on the speech of unresponsive language delayed preschool children. *Journal of Speech and Hearing Disorders, 49,* 42–52.

Warren, S.F., & Yoder, P.J. (1998). Facilitating the transition from preintentional to intentional communication. In S.F. Warren & J. Reichle (Series Eds.) & A.M. Wetherby, S.F. Warren, & J. Reichle (Vol. Eds.), *Communication and language intervention series: Vol. 7. Transitions in prelinguistic communication* (pp. 365–384). Baltimore: Paul H. Brookes Publishing Co.

Wetherby, A.M., Alexander, D.G., & Prizant, B.M. (1998). The ontogeny and role of repair strategies. In S.F. Warren & J. Reichle (Series Eds.) & A.M. Wetherby, S.F. Warren, & J. Reichle (Vol. Eds.), *Communication and language intervention series: Vol. 7. Transitions in prelinguistic communication* (pp. 135–159). Baltimore: Paul H. Brookes Publishing Co.

Wetherby, A., & Prizant, B. (1993). *Communication and Symbolic Behavior Scales manual: Normed edition.* Itasca, IL: The Riverside Publishing Co.

Wetherby, A., & Prizant, B. (1998). *Communication and Symbolic Behavior Scales Developmental Profile, Research edition.* Chicago: Applied Symbolix.

Wilcox, M.J., Kouri, T., & Caswell, S. (1991). Early language intervention: A comparison of classroom and individual treatment. *American Journal of Speech-Language Pathology, 1,* 49–62.

Wilcox, M.J., & Shannon, M.S. (1998). Facilitating the transition from prelinguistic to linguistic communication. In S.F. Warren & J. Reichle (Series Eds.) & A.M. Wetherby, S.F. Warren, & J. Reichle (Vol. Eds.), *Communication and language intervention series: Vol. 7. Transitions in prelinguistic communication* (pp. 385–416). Baltimore: Paul H. Brookes Publishing Co.

Wright, M.J. (1980). Measuring the social competence of preschool children. *Canadian Journal of Behavioural Sciences, 12,* 17–32.

Yoder, P.J., & Davies, B. (1992). Do children with developmental delays use more frequent and diverse language in verbal routines? *American Journal on Mental Retardation, 97,* 197–208.

Yoder, P.J., Davies, B., & Bishop, K. (1994). Adult interaction style effects on the language sampling and transcription process with children who have developmental disabilities. *American Journal on Mental Retardation, 99,* 270–282.

Yoder, P.J., Kaiser, A.P., & Alpert, C. (1991). An exploratory study of the inter-action between language teaching methods and child characteristics. *Journal of Speech and Hearing Research, 34,* 155–167.

Yoder, P.J., Kaiser, A.P., Goldstein, H., Alpert, C., Mousetis, L., Kaczmarek, L., & Fischer, R. (1995). An exploratory comparison of milieu teaching and responsive interaction in the classroom. *Journal of Early Intervention, 19,* 218–242.

Yoder, P.J., & Warren, S.F. (1998). Maternal responsivity predicts the prelinguis-tic communication intervention that facilitates generalized intentional com-munication. *Journal of Speech, Language, and Hearing Research, 41,* 1207–1219.

Yoder, P.J., & Warren, S.F. (1999). Self-initiated proto-declaratives and proto-imperatives can be facilitated in prelingusitic children with developmental disabilities. *Journal of Early Intervention, 22,* 337–354.

Yoder, P.J., & Warren, S.F. (2001). Relative treatment effects of two prelinguis-tic communication interventions on language development in toddlers with developmental delays vary by maternal characteristics. *Journal of Speech, Lan-guage, and Hearing Research, 44,* 224–237.

Yoder, P.J., Warren, S.F., McCathren, R., & Leew, S.V. (1998). Does adult re-sponsivity to child behavior facilitate communication development? In S.F. Warren & J. Reichle (Series Eds.) & A.M. Wetherby, S.F. Warren, & J. Reichle (Vol. Eds.), *Communication and language intervention series: Vol. 7. Tran-sitions in prelingusitic communication* (pp. 39–58). Baltimore: Paul H. Brookes Publishing Co.

5

Infants and Toddlers

Putting Research into Practice

Shirley V. Leew, Steven F. Warren, and Paul J. Yoder

Young children who exhibit social impairments vary tremendously. A minor cognitive or learning disability can create severe social problems for one child, whereas a more severe cognitive limitation might cause relatively minor social impairments for another. Social difficulties can be situation specific, exacerbated by special circumstances, or elicited by unexpected changes in the environment.

The following case studies are hypothetical composites based on many children encountered during years of practice in the field. The idealized intervention approaches are based on this extensive personal experience as well as the practices and research discussed in Chapter 4. They represent a family-focused approach in which the family's needs, capabilities, and involvement are primary considerations. The interventions focus on the social needs of two young children and demonstrate how the whole child should be considered in targeting social-communicative development. These hypothetical children have multiple needs; however, only those aspects of a comprehensive intervention approach directly relevant to social-communicative development are discussed here. These case descriptions are intended to demonstrate how the skilled integration and coordination of knowledge, treatments, and approaches can culminate in the achievement of social-communicative goals for children at a developmental age of 24 months or younger.

DAVID

David is 36 months old. His birth was unremarkable. The second child in a family of three children, David appeared to be developing typically until his second birthday. At this point, his parents became concerned with his lack of speech in comparison with other children; when David was 24 months old, they requested a speech-language assessment. The assessment process began 2 months later, and an intervention program was in place by the time he was 30 months old. His parents had no concerns about his cognitive abilities. The speech-language pathologist who provided the initial assessment suspected more global delays because of his lack of imaginative play skills and his resistance to social involvement. David was very difficult to engage in simple play activities, and he showed signs of rigidity with simple objects such as blocks. The assessment revealed that his receptive and expressive communication skills were at a developmental level below 12 months, though he would perseverate complex phrases from television programs and videotapes. Based on the speech-language pathologist's observations and results on The Rossetti Infant-Toddler Scale (Rossetti, 1990) that suggested delays in play and interaction, David was referred to an assessment team for a comprehensive diagnostic evaluation.

The Diagnostic Evaluation

The assessment team included a psychologist, a pediatrician, a physiotherapist, a speech-language pathologist, an audiologist, and an occupational therapist. The assessment was carried out at home and in a specialized play school and involved substantial parent participation. Both dynamic assessment methods (Kublin, Wetherby, Crais, & Prizant, 1998) and standardized assessments were carried out over an 8-week period in both environments (i.e., when David was 26–28 months of age).

Medical Assessment

The developmental psychologist and the pediatrician diagnosed David with autism spectrum disorder based on the Childhood Autism Ratings Scale (CARS; Schopler, Reichler, & Renner, 1986). The diagnosis was made because of his language impairment, his inability to respond to social cues, and his lack of play skills. David obtained a score of 34.5, which is above the cutoff score of 30 for a diagnosis of autism. He displayed many of the behavior characteristics consistent with the *Diagnostic and Statistical Manual of Mental Disorders, Fourth Edition* (DSM-IV; American Psychiatric Association, 1994), description of autism. These included 1) a qualitative impairment in reciprocal interaction; 2) a qualitative impairment in communication; and 3) restricted, repetitive, and stereotyped patterns of behaviors, interests, and activities. A comprehensive audiological examination, including auditory brainstem responses, indicated that David's hearing was normal.

Dynamic Assessment and Observations

A dynamic assessment approach was used to observe David (Kublin et al., 1998). In addition to taking a nonintrusive inventory of David's social functioning through observation, the dynamic assessment involved having team members interact with David at different times to determine the effectiveness and acceptability of different kinds and levels of support. Thus, the dynamic assessment approach yielded information about which strategies might be successful in enhancing David's social behavior.

These structured observations of David across environments indicated that in his family environment, his asocial behaviors were less pronounced than in the clinic or at the child development center. During dynamic assessment, different strategies to use with David were suggested to the family. Clinicians observed that with prompting from adults he could be encouraged to expand his communicative function repertoire beyond behavioral regulation, and he would engage in structured play interactions involving turn taking when using preferred objects. These trial interventions and observations provided the team with knowledge about how the family felt about David and his social-communicative impairments. The family provided helpful information during the assessment process and was receptive to advice about how to assist David in becoming more social at home. Because the parents were actively involved in the assessment, they became more aware of how David's social impairments affected the family's functioning. His parents also were better prepared to participate in designing David's intervention program and to be effective advocates for their son.

Observations at home yielded a number of conclusions. David demonstrated acceptable approach behavior and affect sharing with familiar people. He had limited spontaneous imitation skills for sounds, single words, gestures, or games, and he demonstrated rigid, limited, and nonsymbolic play skills. He rarely initiated communication except for regulating other people in the pursuit of getting food or particular videotapes that were out of reach, and he never initiated playful interactions, daily routine activities, or comments.

Observations made at the development center yielded the following conclusions: David avoided interaction bids from his peers by flopping to the floor. He avoided eye gaze, and when confronted with social bids, he often emitted high-pitched vocalizations. David exhibited rigid play behaviors such as putting objects in containers or holes and lining up cars and blocks. He became very upset when these routines were disrupted or if therapists tried to play reciprocally. Attention to any activity other than those just mentioned was limited. Communication was largely absent except for expressions of distress and anxiety through negative affect.

Standardized Assessment

On the Vineland Adaptive Behavior Scales (Sparrow, Balla, & Cicchetti, 1984), an index of overall adaptive functioning, David obtained an age equivalent score of 1 year, 10 months. This score indicated a mild impairment for a child of 30 months. On the Mental Scale of the Bayley Scales of Infant Development, Second Edition (Bayley, 1993), David obtained an approximate age equivalent score of 29 months. He was able to attend to a story, complete a nine-piece puzzle in a timely fashion, match disks on the basis of color, discriminate among pictures, and build with and stack blocks. These results suggested good visual cognition. Based on the Communication and Symbolic Behavior Scales (CSBS; Wetherby & Prizant, 1993), David demonstrated mild to moderate social-communicative impairments.

Assessment Interpretations

As is common with children with autism, David demonstrated an uneven pattern of development. His visual skills and some of his daily living skills were areas of relative strength. His play, social, communicative, and language skills were delayed or impaired. In terms of his social-communicative functioning, David demonstrated significant impairments in reciprocity, vocal-verbal tasks, and communicative functions. Reciprocity is the ability to stay actively in interactions, take appropriate turns, persist in communicating for the desired response, and in general, keep an interaction going. David did little of this during the administration of the CSBS. He inconsistently paid attention to objects and to books. His typical response was to take his mother's hand and guide it to a desired object. Then, he would wait for her to act.

Vocal-verbal behaviors were present in the form of "chunks" and included real words, but their communicative intent was unclear in most instances because of a lack of eye gaze. David would not imitate nonverbal vocalizations (e.g., car sounds, animal sounds). He did not use communicative gestures at all (i.e., giving, showing, pushing away, reaching, pointing, waving, nodding, shaking head).

During testing, the only communicative functions David demonstrated were to protest and to regulate the behavior of the adult (protoimperative). David did not attempt to attract adults' attention or to direct adults' attention to an object (proto-declarative). There was no attempt to repair a communicative behavior if the adult did not respond correctly. Instead, David would avoid further contact or would scream and cry. David also demonstrated a low rate of communicative acts (i.e., less than one per minute) during the administration of the CSBS.

Intervention Goals

The rich information gathered during 8 weeks of observation and through the variety of assessment methods was used to establish a comprehensive intervention plan. The intervention team consisted of the parents and select professionals, including the early childhood special education teacher in David's inclusive play school, the speech-language pathologist, the psychologist, and two trained rehabilitation aides. The team met to prepare an individualized family service plan (IFSP). The special education teacher was chosen to serve as service coordinator and to document goals and strategies. The family decided at the outset that they wanted monthly meetings with all service providers to ensure the communication necessary for a transdisciplinary approach (Raver, 1991). By consistently sharing observations and experiences with each other, all of the adults could incorporate methods and strategies that were most successful for David while accomplishing all goals of the intervention. For example, the speech-language pathologist suggested targeting the expansion of communicative functions to include prelinguistic commenting or proto-declaratives. By explaining the expectations that she had for David for this communicative function, the special educator, the parents, and the other therapists began to expect them, too. They became increasingly proficient at expecting and prompting communicative behavior. Similarly, when a rehabilitation aide discovered that puzzles were a preferred activity, the speech-language pathologist began to develop routines using puzzles and to set the stage for communication. This transdisciplinary approach ensured that David was treated holistically in every intervention interaction and all of his strengths and needs were well known to whomever was with him. Biannual social goals were selected as follows:

1. David's family will develop social responsiveness skills in order to help David become a social participant in his family. The service coordinator will apply an ecological partnership model and monitor social-communicative development at the 6-month review using the ECO Adult Communication Evaluation checklist (MacDonald, 1989).

2. David will develop meaningful and reciprocal social communication, including nonverbal and verbal behaviors. The speech-language pathologist will monitor this development at the 6-month review using the CSBS.
3. David will initiate social interactions. Qualitative information will be reviewed at the 6-month review to determine if he is accomplishing this and in what contexts.

Short-term social objectives were to be evaluated at monthly meetings. In keeping with the transactional theory of development and its implied importance to social communication, the team established goals for both the caregivers and David. By increasing the frequency and clarity of David's communicative behaviors (prelinguistic and verbal), the adults around him would be more likely to provide appropriate linguistic input. Evaluation of progress was based on qualitative reports regarding the frequency and generalization of targeted behavior. When all team members reported increased frequency of a particular behavior, progress was judged to be good. If only one person observed a change, progress was judged to be minimal. Caregiver transactional objectives included

1. Adults will improve their responsiveness to David by enhancing their skill at attributing communicative value to David's behavior and by providing appropriate language stimulation. To this end, caregivers will observe videotapes of David and will count and analyze behaviors as they relate to social functioning.
2. Adults will develop their ability to interpret David's behavior (protests, requests, bids for interaction, affective attunement, persistence) to facilitate interactions and to provide appropriate linguistic mapping.
3. Adults will develop their turn-taking strategies to develop reciprocal interactions with David. These strategies include following David's lead, waiting and time delay, prompts, and contingent imitation.
4. Adults will arrange David's environment at home and at play school to provide inviting and predictable social and play experiences. Adults will provide opportunities to develop play routines around preferred objects within these environments. The special education teacher will teach the others environmental arrangement strategies.
5. Adults will learn to use visual supports in conjunction with their verbal communication to aid David's comprehension of different situations. They will model the use of gestures to clarify David's requests. Adults will use environmental arrangement within the

play routines to facilitate intentional requesting and commenting. For example, clear containers with preferred objects in them and toys out of reach in the room will be used as communication temptations.

6. Adults will provide specific acknowledgment ("you showed me") and natural consequences for emerging social-communicative behaviors such as gesturing, vocalizing, and coordinating attention.

David's objectives in the transactional process included

1. David will develop turn-taking routines in play with adults and peers in which the attention focus is clearly shared. Initially, these routines will be established around preferred objects and with responsive adults. Peers will be engaged once the routines have become established.

2. David will increase his rate of verbal and nonverbal communication supported by models, prompts, and natural consequences so that he will become an active social partner.

3. David will learn to imitate communicative gestures (pointing, showing, and reaching) and vocalizations within his established play routines.

4. David will develop intentional use of single words. Adults will acknowledge his meaningful use of proto-words and words and provide appropriate verbal models consistently based on David's repertoire of vocalizations and verbalizations.

5. David will develop and expand his repertoire of intentional pre-linguistic and verbal communication functions of behavioral regulation (proto-imperatives), commenting (proto-declaratives), invitations to play, protests, and repairs.

6. David will imitate vocalizations in play, such as car noises, animal sounds, and songs. These vocalizations will be prompted within routines with a responsive adult who uses time delay and specific acknowledgment for desired communication.

7. David will develop constructive and symbolic play schemes. The rehabilitation aides will expand David's object repertoire by modeling play at appropriate levels when David is engaged in preferred play routines.

8. David will learn to coordinate his attention (e.g., from object to person, person to person, person to object) exhibited by eye gaze shifts to enhance his communication clarity.

Table 5.1 summarizes the findings of the assessment.

Table 5.1. David's social assessment summary

Social strengths	Social needs
Typical cognitive functioning	Responsive adults
Self-help and daily living skills	Reciprocity
Family support	Expanded conventional communicative functions
Sustained attention	
Affect sharing	Verbal/expressive language development
Development of imitation	
Attention shifts (coordinated and joint attention)	Development of play schemes

The qualitative changes observed in individual sessions were re-corded in a journal. Often, there were subtle changes in David's behavior that would not be reflected in a formal assessment but nevertheless marked achievement and progress. For example, when David began spontaneously shifting his eyes from his activity to a person in play routines, the rehabilitation aide noted it, realizing its importance for social communication. The daily recording of similar qualitative observations provided important feedback to the team. Thus, observations revealed behavior changes by tracking typical development in David's areas of strength and by monitoring the gradual achievement of social goals relating to the IFSP.

Intervention

In this section, the environments, personnel, and process for achieving the IFSP goals are described. David attended an inclusive child development center located near his home, and he received intensive home-based programming that stressed education of the family. The major focus of the program was the development of social communication. In addition to acting as the service coordinator of the program for David, the early childhood special education teacher was responsible for ensuring that David participated in developmentally appropriate activities at the child development center and that he had opportunities for social interactions with his peer group. She supervised the rehabilitation aides and taught them how to provide nonintrusive assistance for David.

The speech-language pathologist saw David for 45 minutes each week at the child development center for individual language therapy and was available to consult in the home as needed. She conducted biweekly sessions to teach the parents and aides to enhance their facilitative interaction styles with David. David's development was monitored using analyses of prelinguistic pragmatic skills and verbal language gathered through communication samples. She used videotapes of David with various caregivers to illustrate the consequences of communication and to highlight David's social-communicative behaviors. She monitored language development by collecting and counting qualitative observations, by recording monthly audiotape samples during her therapy sessions for language analysis, and by observing David at the child development center to assess generalization. These analyses were used to ascertain whether targeted communicative behaviors were established, emerging, or not occurring.

The family provided the team with ongoing information about how David's behavior affected their daily lives and what particular challenges existed for them. The family was taught to follow David's lead and to exhibit affective attunement (Kublin et al., 1998). They were taught how to use contingent responding and to imitate David's behavior to establish social contact and rudimentary turn taking. They also were shown how to create communication opportunities for David by arranging his environment so communication was necessary and how to use gestures and pictures to support their verbal communication, thereby increasing his ability to interpret and symbolize his home routines.

One rehabilitation aide accompanied David to school each morning to provide assistance to the special education teacher and to scaffold social interactions for David. The aides provided a crucial consistent link between the home and the school on a daily basis and were most responsible for implementing an integrated or transactional approach to David's treatment.

David attended his inclusive child development center (where learning was play based) four mornings per week for 2½ hours. David had a personal rehabilitation aide assist him in the school. In order to achieve the goal of independence, the aides withdrew support as soon as possible and only intervened when breakdowns in social interactions were apparent. The aides also facilitated home–school communication on a daily basis. At home, David's afternoons and sometimes evenings were spent in specified social intervention program activities with the rehabilitation aide and engaged in activities and outings with his parents and siblings.

Outcomes

Outcome measures were gathered using daily qualitative observations documented in a communal journal and formal reevaluations at 3 and

6 months (chronological age = 33 and 36 months) through behavior checklists (e.g., The Rossetti Infant-Toddler Scale; Rossetti, 1990) and standardized assessment measures (e.g., CSBS).

Observed Outcomes

Qualitative observations provided insights as to how David began to stay in interactions and develop small turn-taking routines with a supportive adult. As the adult adopted the facilitating strategies outlined in the IFSP, David began to attend longer to objects and to his partner. These essential changes were noted in the journal within the first 2 weeks of program implementation at home. Because of these observations, the team began to expect the same results at the child development center.

In circle and large-group activities, the special education teacher attempted to assist David in waiting his turn, staying for the whole time, and attending to her from increasing distances. After 2 months of gradually increasing expectations and gradually decreasing support from his aide, David was staying for music and story time about 80% of the time. The expectation was that within the next 4 weeks, he would stay 100% of the time. If David would not stay in large-group activities, he was removed to a nonpreferred area of the room and interactive adult attention was withdrawn until either the group time was over or he indicated that he would like to rejoin the group. The expectations placed on David for participating were the same for all of the children. His disruptive behavior was interpreted and verbally described for him as such, but the consequences of his behavior were the same as they would be for any of the children who disrupted the larger group.

David's social language was increasing in rate and diversity of pragmatic function. He used words to protest ("no," "stop"), to request objects ("want milk"), to request comfort from an adult ("hug," "sleep"), to greet ("Derek"), and to comment ("plane"). David's expressive vocabulary increased rapidly suggesting that the responsive changes made to his social environment were effective. The adults made social language more salient through their contingent responding to his behavior, enabling David to identify and imitate appropriate language more easily. Although David was encouraged to use communicative gestures for commenting, protesting, and requesting, at the 6-month review there was little progress in terms of spontaneous use.

By the 6-month review, David was showing increased social competence at home and at school. His affect overall had become more positive, and he anticipated his daily routines with animation. The rehabilitation aides at the school were able to sit apart from David in large-group activities. He was imitating actions on objects, as well as expanding schemes associated with those objects. The family also was more positive about David's role within the family.

Formal Assessment Outcomes

A formal reassessment of language, cognitive, and social skills was carried out after 6 months of his program when David was 36 months old. Because David's social behavior had improved and his use of verbal language had increased, more language measures were used than at the initial assessment phase. He now was able to participate in vocabulary tests that used pictures and a phonology inventory based on object identification because of the development of his expressive vocabulary. The psychologist also was able to use more verbal measures that were not possible at the outset. The early childhood special education teacher assessed social skills at the child development center using the CSBS (Wetherby & Prizant, 1993).

David demonstrated significant development in language comprehension and expression. The Preschool Language Scale–3 (Zimmerman, Steiner, & Pond, 1992) was used, as well as the CSBS. He was demonstrating knowledge of position words such as *in, on,* and *off.* David also understood some early pronouns, such as *me* and *him,* and could follow simple verbal instructions that involved the number concept of one. In addition, he could point to action pictures (e.g., point to run*).* Expressively, David was beginning to answer simple questions that required labels ("What's that?"). He was beginning to combine two or three words spontaneously and to answer yes/no questions but with an overgeneralized "yes" response. Expressive and receptive single word vocabulary measures indicated significant development.

Table 5.2 summarizes the formal test results at the 6-month review. These new results suggest a mild social-communicative impairment. The teacher reported that because of his increasing verbal skills, David was beginning to participate in classroom activities with his peers with minimal adult assistance. This participation had the result of increasing the incidence of positive peer interactions. His cooperative play remained limited, but the school staff reported increased time spent in parallel play at various centers in the school. His functional level was now at about 30 months.

David's Future

At 36 months of age, David has made significant gains in his social development in the areas of language, play, and social interaction. He continues to be challenged when transitions are required and when changes

Table 5.2. Formal posttest results for David (chronological age = 36 months)

Measure	Standard score	Standard deviation	Pre-intervention
Peabody Picture Vocabulary Test	90	−.75	unable to administer
Expressive One Word Picture Vocabulary Test	85	−1	unable to administer
Preschool Language Scale–3	85	−1	unable to administer
Communication and Symbolic Behavior Scales			
Communicative Functions	−.5	>1	
Communicative Means Gestural	>−1	>−1	
Communication Means Vocal	−1	−2	
Communication Means Verbal	−1	>−2	
Reciprocity	−1	−2	
Social-Affective Signaling	−.5	−1	
Symbolic	−1	>−1	

occur in his regular routines. Continued support is necessary to assist the family in determining strategies and appropriate environments for maintaining progress and continued social involvement. Speech and language intervention should continue. As David acquires more language, his phonological development will require formal analysis. In the immediate future, his expressive language development continues to be delayed, and he requires support for using language in social situations. Therapy should continue to be play based with an emphasis on expanding his repertoire of action schemes on familiar objects. David will most likely require occasional scaffolding in even the most familiar and supportive social environments. A focus on deliberate peer involvement in the home, school, and community will be needed as his other abilities develop. He remains socially indifferent with peers. His parents should attempt to provide him with developmentally appropriate participation in community activities, such as swimming lessons. Although David's cognitive development and behavior may not be major concerns, the psychologist should provide consultation to the caregivers in David's various environments to monitor progress.

Given the level of support for David and his family at his young age, David's prognosis for future inclusion into regular educational environments is favorable. Because David is now 3 years old and soon will enter the early childhood education system in his city, a transition IFSP meeting is scheduled. David's family feels confident in their ability to advocate for appropriate services for David.

KRISTIN

Kristin is 12 months old (adjusted age = 10 months) and has cerebral palsy and a bilateral hearing impairment. She was born at 28 weeks' gestation weighing 915 grams (about 2 pounds) to a single, 16-year-old mother (Tracey), by emergency cesarean section because of fetal distress. Kristin had breathing difficulties and upon delivery was immediately intubated and placed on a ventilator. The ventilator was removed after 10 days. Kristin was then in an incubator for 4 weeks and fed through a nasogastric tube during that time. The pediatrician recommended nonnutritive sucking (using a pacifier) to improve oxygenation and to provide Kristin a method for self-quieting (Als, 1986). Her bio-states were erratic, with no well-defined alertness or sleep cycle. The nurses and the family complied with a policy of careful handling and long resting periods. The neonatal intensive care unit (NICU) environment was controlled so that light and noise were muted to encourage rest and relaxation for the infants.

Under the guidance of the medical team in the NICU, Kristin was exposed to waterbed flotation. This exposure had the effect of modulating her movement and tone patterns and reducing her irritability. She began to appear more alert by 4 weeks, which greatly enhanced early interactions with her caregivers (Als, 1986). Unfortunately, Tracey visited irregularly and was unresponsive to Kristin's bids for changes in state, levels of alertness, or physical discomfort. Tracey became irritable and distressed if Kristin fussed or cried and usually insisted on having a nurse take over.

Although Kristin left the NICU after 4 weeks, she remained in the hospital until her weight increased and her development was stable. This period of time allowed for an interdisciplinary assessment through observation and comprehensive program planning. Improved stability was reflected in well-defined sleep and alert states, respiratory control, temperature regulation, and digestive functioning. With assistance, Kristin's movements and postures were regulated to some extent. Kristin went home after 10 weeks weighing 1,900 grams (about 4 pounds). By that time, she was following objects visually, could maintain an alert state for up to 1 hour, and appeared to be healthy.

Much had been learned during these 4 weeks about how to regulate Kristin's physical states and to stimulate her during her alert, attentive state; however, convincing Tracey to practice in the hospital was extremely difficult. Kristin would obviously benefit from a supportive and responsive social environment and could learn to induce social behavior from responsive, sensitive caregivers.

Tracey was poorly equipped to care for her infant daughter who had such complicated special needs. Although this young mother was often very loving and gentle, she was inconsistent in her general child care practices and proved incapable of independently applying the recommendations of the hospital staff. Soon after Kristin went home, Tracey went back to high school full time. At that time, Tracey's mother began to provide child care for Kristin, with the expectation that Tracey would take over when she got home from school.

Discharge Assessments at Ten Weeks of Age

The pediatrician found impairments in muscle tone and deep tendon reflexes. She also observed tremors (clonus) in the arms and legs. Kristin subsequently was diagnosed with spastic quadriplegia cerebral palsy (increased muscle tone in the arms and legs). Ongoing monitoring while Kristin was in the nursery revealed persistence of primitive reflexes preventing attainment of motor milestones at expected ages.

The compulsory hearing screening in the NICU revealed a lack of response to noises and depressed reactions to even intense auditory stimuli. She would not waken from sleep to loud noises at her cribside. An auditory brain stem response assessment conducted when Kristin was 2 months old (chronological age) revealed severe bilateral sensorineural abnormalities. This assessment did not require Kristin to be awake or to make behavior responses. The conclusion based on observation and formal assessment was a severe to profound bilateral hearing impairment.

Because Kristin was fed through a nasogastric tube for the first 4 weeks of her life and she experienced difficulties with oral motor movements secondary to cerebral palsy, the social environment of feeding was addressed by the occupational therapist, the physiotherapist, and the speech-language pathologist. Kristin needed to be positioned for efficient sucking and swallowing and to allow for visual interaction with her caregiver. The slightest distraction could cause Kristin to experience increased tone that would interrupt feeding and interaction and cause Kristin and her mother distress.

Kristin's ability to engage in age-appropriate play activities was severely limited by her physical disabilities. Her ability to observe her environment and to experience her own body was diminished because of her physical limitations. When appropriately positioned and supported, however, Kristin showed interest in watching others. She showed increased attention to interesting objects but had extreme difficulty turning her head if they were out of her immediate visual range.

Assessment of Kristin's language development was ongoing. As is common among infants with hearing impairments, the monotonous vowel babbling that begins at about 6 months of age was at risk of not growing in complexity later on without amplification and auditory training. Kristin's hearing loss, her poor oral motor control, and her difficulties engaging in interactions because of physical discomfort were immediate concerns.

The physical and occupational therapy assessments provided information about how to position, hold, and handle Kristin. In order to stimulate Kristen within natural social interactions, she needed to be free of discomfort. The physical therapist was able to identify ways to hold Kristin so that feeding was pleasurable. The physical assessment also identified ways to ensure Kristin was physically included so she could see people and events during social activities in the home. Table 5.3 presents a summary of the initial assessment findings regarding Kristin's social development.

Home Intervention

Extensive counseling during the postnatal period was available to Tracey to help avert her feelings of low self-esteem, self-blame, depression, and anger that had the potential to affect Kristin's social development as well (Als, 1986). Tracey felt guilty and sad about her infant and the circumstances of her birth. Without professional assistance, there was a risk of Tracey's completely rejecting her daughter. Tracey was strongly encouraged to attend a weekly support group for a year following Kristin's discharge to help her deal with the emotions and challenges facing her. Tracey needed to learn how to take pride in Kristin as a unique person who would develop, given competent care.

Table 5.3.   Kristin's discharge assessment summary

Social strengths	Social needs
Visual attention	Consistent positive stimulation by caregivers
Responsive with appropriate handling	Responsiveness by caregivers
	Auditory training
	Augmented communication
	Augmented play
	Positioning and movement
	Intentional expressive visual communication

A home-based intervention program was planned prior to Kristin's leaving the hospital. Much of the intervention focus would be teaching the caregivers about how to facilitate interactions with the infant, given the extent of Kristin's disabilities. The importance of the primary mother–daughter relationship to Kristin's current and lifelong social development necessitated teaching Tracey and the grandparents how to interact responsively with and stimulate Kristin. She required multisensory stimulation to ensure the initiation and development of transactional learning. The early childhood special educator coordinated training for primary caregivers in the NICU. Once Kristin was discharged, responsibility for the intervention program was transferred to the outreach services of a child development facility in the community. Because of the very early identification of developmental risk factors (by 10 weeks of age), this intervention could be preventive and prescriptive but also could be responsive to problems.

Once Kristin was home, the special education teacher from the child development center visited the family on a weekly basis and was available by telephone for queries or emergencies. The program became an integrated team effort involving the family, the early childhood special education teacher, the psychologist, the speech-language pathologist, the occupational therapist, and the physical therapist. The designated service coordinator of the IFSP, the early childhood special educator, was responsible for coordination and integration within the program.

The IFSP meeting took place within 2 weeks of Kristin arriving home (chronological age = 12 weeks) from the hospital. The following social goals were established at that time with the intent of the team being to monitor Kristin's development regularly and to make revisions as necessary. This provision was included because the prognosis for Kristen's rate of development was unpredictable due to the severity of her disabilities and the complexity of her needs, not the least of which was acceptance by her family members.

Annual social goals were established with a plan for review in 7 months when Kristen was 12 months of age. These goals were as follows:

1. Kristin's mother and grandparents will develop responsive, facilitative, interactive styles with the infant to ensure adequate attachment and social learning.
2. Kristin will develop precursor behaviors to social communication, including reciprocity in interactions with caregivers, eye contact and eye gaze behaviors, facial and gestural imitation of caregivers, and positive affect sharing in interactions.

3. Kristin will use a conventional, augmentative communication system, the specifics of which will be determined as progress is made through ongoing dynamic assessment.
4. Kristin will develop object play, including mouthing, handling, and cause and effect. Suitable objects will be presented to her throughout the day and will be readily available in her crib.
5. Kristin will develop her ability to respond to auditory information by learning to use residual hearing through amplification and auditory training.
6. Kristin will develop intentional prelinguistic communication, including behavioral regulation, protesting, and commenting.

Short-term program objectives were established with an agreement to review them at monthly meetings, as follows:

1. Adults will position Kristin (i.e., handling and seating) for interactions so that discomfort and physical effort are minimized and controlled movement is maximized.
2. Adults will develop facilitative interaction styles that will include environmental arrangement, social routine building, following Kristin's lead, and time delay prompts.
3. Adults will provide "enabling contexts" using stimulating physical-social environments for Kristin and ensuring multisensory input (i.e., visual, tactile, kinesthetic, olfactory) to maximize interest and involvement.
4. Kristin will receive hearing aids and auditory training, and auditory information will be augmented with additional sensory information, especially visual input.
5. Kristin will develop oral motor skills and vocalizing behavior to promote communication development.
6. Tracey will enroll in a weekly support group at the child development center where she will learn about special needs and will network with mothers like herself.

Kristin's social behavior depended on all aspects of her development. Physical stability was needed to decrease irritability. Contingent responsiveness to emerging communicative behavior on the part of caregivers was encouraged to elicit imitation behavior and communication clarity (Warren & Yoder, 1998). Hearing aids were fitted and auditory training began to help Kristin make use of her residual hearing. Oral motor development proceeded to facilitate the development of positive affect expression and perhaps speech. Kristin required consistent positive and responsive interactions with an adult in order to learn about social relatedness. The primary adult in her life became her grandmother, who felt reluctant to usurp her own daughter's role of mother, and therefore family counseling and support became a primary concern.

Goals, Methods, and Progress

Tracey needed to learn how to interpret Kristin's expressions of internal state and to regulate interactions for both of them. In this way, she would be able to teach Kristin about effective social communication (Stern, 1977). Tracey was with Kristin in the late afternoons and evenings but was unable to be present for many of the day sessions with the special educator. This absence presented a major obstacle to Kristin's social development with her mother, jeopardizing the development of attachment behaviors. The long-term goal for Kristin and her mother primarily, and the other caregivers secondarily, was to develop social relationships through enjoyable interactions. To achieve that goal, all partners needed to feel competent in their interaction styles (MacDonald, 1989; Stern, 1977). The special education teacher showed the family that interactions with Kristin could be enjoyable once Kristin was comfortable and able to attend. She also taught them how to interpret Kristin's behavior as preintentional and prelinguistic communication and how to appreciate it as development on the way to competence. They learned how to follow Kristin's lead by watching her face and eyes, how to respond contingently to Kristin's behaviors to promote the development of intentional communication, and how to specifically acknowledge any attempts by Kristin to communicate. They also learned to gain Kristin's attention before attempting interactions, to provide her with objects that were interesting, and to rely on visual, tactile, and olfactory stimulation while not overwhelming Kristin. They learned about Kristin's levels of functioning and how to avoid overstimulation and were encouraged to note small developments and to celebrate her progress, however incremental.

Kristin's grandmother reluctantly became the primary caregiver during the day once Tracey went back to school and was present for most of the home-based sessions with the early childhood special educator. Her opinions and observations were integral to the development of the program and her ability to interact competently with Kristin served as a model for Tracey.

The measures of the success of the program were typical social milestones, such as the development of stranger anxiety (i.e., a common measure of emotional attachment between an infant and her primary

caregiver), a purposeful smile, Kristin's willingness to interact with positive affect with adults, her maintenance of visual contact with her partners, her increasing interest in objects, her imitation of gestures and
facial expressions, and the emerging intentional use of body movement
and gestures for communication. The early childhood specialist assisted
the caregivers and monitored to ensure they were developing enjoy-
ment in their interactions with Kristin. They were shown how Kristin
responded positively to environmental and social enhancements and
how social supports increased the time and effort Kristin would give to
interactions. Viewing videotaped interactions occasionally provided the
adults with concrete information about these processes. The family's reports of positive exchanges indicated how well things were going.

The special educator coordinated consultation visits in the home
by an audiologist, a pediatric physiotherapist, a pediatric occupational
therapist, a speech-language pathologist, and a developmental psychologist. Following monthly consultation visits with the family and the service coordinator, team meetings were held to discuss progress, to ensure
the appropriateness of objectives, and to continually monitor the program. The regular team meetings enabled a holistic intervention approach. This consistent sharing of information resulted in the intensive
theoretical and practical education of the family that augmented their
feelings of increasing competence and their understanding of Kristin as
a person. They were able to identify subtle development and to understand the plan for the future. They also were constantly reinforced by
the support of the team.

Outcomes at Twelve Months of Age

Kristin benefited from the early diagnoses and dynamic intervention
planning that occurred in this first year. Initially, her physical care and
development was of foremost concern and was crucial to building a
foundation for a supportive social environment. She responded well to
physical training by learning to attend visually while in supported positioning. The increasing ability of her family to modify Kristin's positions
to ensure social participation was essential for her social development.

Intensive parental support and training was fundamental to the
establishment of mutually reciprocal relationships based on feelings of
competence. The physical, sensory, and social-emotional deficits that
Kristin faced were compounded by the fact that her mother was extremely young and emotionally unprepared to raise a child. Because of
intensive and inclusive intervention planning that included specific social responsiveness training to her caregivers, and emotional support

for her mother, Kristin's development was probably maximized. Kristin and her caregivers were able to begin to form strong positive interpersonal relationships.

Kristin learned to use hearing amplification to localize loud sounds and to identify certain objects. The severity of her hearing impairment greatly restricted her ability to develop verbal communication, but the identification of her strong visual orientation during her NICU stay helped identify a mode for augmenting communication from the start.

Kristin was beginning to attend to pictures and photographs and to attempt imitation of gestures, such as showing and pushing away when she was stabilized in an appropriate sitting position. Intentional pointing still was extremely difficult for Kristin, even with her trunk and head stabilized. Because of the nature of her cerebral palsy, it became obvious that a gestural system of communication would not be an immediate option for her. Intentional vocalizations and articulation were major challenges for Kristin because of motor control problems of her vocal tract and mouth. Kristin's eyes were her best communication mode, and distinct facial expressions were beginning to be discernible. Kristin's grandmother and mother were learning to interpret Kristin's emotional and physical state by observing her eyes and face and to respond to these expressions with confidence. As a result of her mother's new responsiveness, Kristin had developed intentional proto-imperatives and protests using her eyes, facial expressions, and gross head movements and was functioning at the 6- to 9-month age level for social communication with familiar caregivers (based on The Rossetti Infant-Toddler Scale).

Kristin's Future

As Kristin entered her second year of life, many challenges still faced her. Her IFSP meeting addressed the following:

1. The development of play skills, including augmented reciprocal games with adults and augmented toy manipulation
2. The dynamic assessment and development of an intentional technology-assisted augmentative communication system
3. The assessment of physical independence training that would eventually affect her mobility for social approach
4. The development of upper body strength for gaining access to assistive technology to be used in communication training
5. Continued parental support to address needs, such as inclusion into activities in the community and an inclusive child development center in their area

6. Voice assessment and subsequent training to assist in the development of intentional use of vocalizations for communicative functions
7. Appropriate cognitive skills assessment
8. Continued prelinguistic training to include the expansion of communicative functions (i.e., proto-declaratives) and other social interaction skills

CONCLUSION

The preceding case studies demonstrate how early intensive intervention that complements caregiver training and involvement can facilitate the social-communicative development of infants and toddlers with disabilities. Both case studies adhere to the transactional model of development and intervention in the targeting of parent and caregiver training as well as the specific social-behavioral goals for the children. The assessments of both David and Kristin involved distinct methods for initial screening, program planning, and monitoring of progress. The adult targeted skills included becoming optimally sensitive and responsive to the communication of the children and learning global interaction approaches as well as specific prelinguistic mileu teaching and milieu language teaching techniques (see Chapter 4) to develop the frequency and the quality of children's nonverbal and verbal communication. The adult objectives were intended to create an enabling and responsive environment for the infant or toddler with disabilities. Child goals included emotional, behavioral, prelinguistic, and linguistic objectives that were theoretically correlated with optimal social, language, and cognitive development. Goals for the individual programs were established in a family-centered environment that included an inclusive team approach. Communication among all caregivers and professionals was well coordinated and maximized using the IFSP format. Because these idealized interventions were swift and intense, optimum social-communicative development was enhanced.

REFERENCES

Als, H. (1986). *A synactive model of neonatal behavioral organization: Framework for the assessment of neurobehavioral development in the premature infant and for support of infants and parents in the neonatal intensive care environment*. Binghamton, NY: The Haworth Press.
American Psychiatric Association. (1994). *Diagnostic and statistical manual of mental disorders* (4th ed.). Washington, DC: Author.
Bayley, N. (1993). *Bayley Scales of Infant Development*. San Antonio, TX: Psychological Corporation & Harcourt Educational Measurement.

Kublin, K.S., Wetherby, A.M., Crais, E.R., & Prizant B.M. (1998). Prelinguistic dynamic assessment: A transactional perspective. In S.F. Warren & J. Reichle (Series Eds.) & A.M. Wetherby, S.F. Warren, & J. Reichle (Vol. Eds.), *Communication and language intervention series: Vol. 7. Transitions in prelinguistic communication* (pp. 285–312). Baltimore: Paul H. Brookes Publishing Co.

MacDonald, J.D. (1989). *On becoming partners with children.* Chicago: The Riverside Publishing Co.

Raver, S.A. (1991). *Strategies for teaching at-risk and handicapped infants and toddlers: A transdisciplinary approach.* New York: Macmillan.

Rossetti, L. (1990). *The Rossetti Infant–Toddler Scale.* East Moline, IL: LinguiSystems.

Schopler, E., Reichler, R.J., & Renner, B.R. (1986). *The Childhood Autism Ratings Scale (CARS) for diagnostic screening and classification of autism.* New York: Irvington.

Sparrow, S., Balla, D., & Cicchetti, D. (1984). *Vineland Adaptive Behavior Scales (VABS).* Circle Pines, MN: American Guidance Service.

Stern, D. (1977). *The first relationship: Infant and mother.* Cambridge, MA: Harvard University Press.

Warren, S.F., & Yoder, P.J. (1998). Facilitating the transition from preintentional to intentional communication. In S.F. Warren & J. Reichle (Series Eds.) & A.M. Wetherby, S.F. Warren, & J. Reichle (Vol. Eds.), *Communication and language intervention series: Vol. 7. Transitions in prelinguistic communication* (pp. 365–384). Baltimore: Paul H. Brookes Publishing Co.

Wetherby A.M., & Prizant, B.M. (1993). *Communication and symbolic behavior scales.* Itasca, IL: The Riverside Publishing Co.

Zimmerman, I., Steiner, V., & Pond, R. (1992). *Preschool Language Scale–3 (PLS–3).* San Antonio, TX: The Psychological Corporation.

6

Promoting Peer-Related Social-Communicative Competence in Preschool Children

William H. Brown and Maureen A. Conroy

Child development theorists with diverse perspectives suggest that successful adult–child and child–child transactions provide both a context and a mechanism for the emergence of children's developmental abilities such as social, language, and cognitive competencies (see Bijou, 1993; Flavel, 1977; Piaget, 1926; Vygotsky, 1978). Since the 1970s, communicative competence in young children has been recognized as an important feature of child development (e.g., Baudonniere, Garcia-Werebe, Michel, & Liegois, 1989; Dyson & Genishi, 1993) and a critical component of early intervention efforts with young children with developmental delays (e.g., Bricker, 1993; McLean & Cripe, 1997; Notari & Cole, 1993). Similarly, social competence has been recognized as a fundamental facet of the development of young children with (e.g., Gresham & MacMillan, 1997; Guralnick, 1994; Odom, McConnell, & McEvoy, 1992) and without developmental delays (e.g., Hartup, 1992; Ladd & Coleman, 1993; Newcomb & Bagwell, 1995).

Separating communicative competence from social competence would be difficult at best. Indeed, many researchers have argued that social competence is influenced by and influences the continued emergence of important developmental abilities throughout early childhood (Guralnick, 1992; Hartup & Moore, 1990; Odom, McConnell, et al., 1992). Hence, interventions that focus on improving both social and communicative competence (hereafter called social-communicative competence) of children with developmental delays have been, and will continue to be, a critical component of early intervention efforts with young children with disabilities and their families (Bricker, 1992, 1993).

In spite of the frequent recognition of the interrelatedness of social and communicative competence (e.g., Baudonniere et al., 1989; Guralnick, 1992), traditionally these two dimensions of child development have been studied separately, particularly with respect to intervention research. The purpose of this chapter is to integrate research findings that are relevant to practitioners and researchers who are interested in both social competence and communication intervention for preschool-age children. First, an ecological perspective is proposed to provide a conceptual framework for understanding young children's social-communicative competence. Next, we review intervention strategies that have been designed to promote peer-related social-communicative competencies of preschool children with developmental delays. Then, we discuss four critical challenges in promoting young children's social-communicative competence. Finally, we offer recommendations for future research on promoting peer-related social-communicative competence of preschool children with developmental delays.

AN ECOLOGICAL PERSPECTIVE

Since the mid-1960s, ecological perspectives on human development (Bronfenbrenner, 1979; Hobbs, 1966) have provided an influential conceptual framework for practitioners and researchers who are interested in addressing child development from a strength-based perspective. The fundamental assumptions of ecological perspectives are that 1) children's behavior and development are multiply determined by both internal and external factors, 2) potent developmental variables are transactional in nature, and 3) influential developmental factors may operate at various levels of analysis. Researchers have investigated a range of potential influences from moment-to-moment transactions (e.g., parent–child interactions, child–child interactions) to more distal factors (e.g., social policies that support inclusion of children with developmental delays in early childhood environments, cultural factors that affect parent–child interactions) (Odom et al., 1996). An ecological approach guides practitioners and researchers to investigate factors within individuals (e.g., temperament, developmental status) *and* their social and physical environments (e.g., behavioral environments, cultural factors) for explanations of behavior and development.

Investigators have argued for employing ecological approaches to enhance future intervention efforts (Goldstein & Kaczmarek, 1992; Odom & Brown, 1993; Odom et al., 1996; Peck, 1989, 1993; Vincent, Salisbury, Strain, McCormick, & Tessier, 1990). Specifically, because peers constitute a significant aspect of young children's ecology, Goldstein and Kaczmarek (1992) recommended peer-mediated interaction interventions to promote preschool children's social-communicative interactions. They proposed individualized analyses of communicative strategies that enhance young children's peer interactions and social-communicative development. For example, instead of global analyses of social initiations, responses, and interactions, they advised detailed analyses of children's comments on activities, their requests for information, and any acknowledgments of their communicative attempts (Ferrell, 1990, as cited in Goldstein & Kaczmarek, 1992). Similarly, Peck (1989) recommended that interventionists carefully assess and intervene with young children who have communicative competence difficulties in real-world environments (i.e., with peers in common classroom contexts).

The adoption of an ecological perspective for social-communicative competence for young children with developmental delays has several important implications for promoting young children's social-communicative behavior and development. First, measurement of social-communicative abilities should be conducted within typical contexts (e.g., preschools, homes) and familiar social circumstances (e.g., with teachers, parents, peers). Naturalistic assessment procedures are warranted to determine preschool children's present social-communicative competencies within authentic circumstances in which they have learned and developed. Second, social environments must be assessed carefully and, if necessary, altered to provide young children with developmental delays optimal environmental circumstances for promoting social-communicative interactions. For example, a range of interesting and meaningful activities that facilitate children's active engagement *and* responsive social partners should be made available to children with social-communicative delays (Bricker, 1998; Odom & Brown, 1993). Third, social-communicative behaviors that are chosen for assessment and intervention should be social-communicative behavioral strategies that have a high likelihood of evoking and maintaining positive child–child interactions (Brown, Odom, & Holcombe, 1996; Goldstein & Kaczmarek, 1992). Fourth, initial social-communicative assessment and subsequent intervention should be directly linked to ensure that practitioners achieve meaningful developmental outcomes (see Bagnato, Neisworth, & Munson, 1997; Bricker & Pretti-Frontczak, 1996). Fifth, to promote generalization and maintenance of critical social-communicative abilities in important behavioral environments with significant participants in those environments, interventionists should be prepared to monitor and intervene with empirically valid strategies to foster the continued emergence of young children's social-communicative competence (Brown & Odom, 1994; Ostrosky, Kaiser, & Odom, 1993).

INTERVENTIONS TO PROMOTE
SOCIAL-COMMUNICATIVE COMPETENCE

During the 1920s and 1930s, psychologists and educators studied young children's development in a network of child welfare stations across the nation (e.g., University of Iowa, University of Minnesota). In the area of children's social development, a number of influential descriptive studies (e.g., Parten, 1932) and arguably the first intervention study (Jack, 1934) were conducted during the "heyday" of child development research (Renshaw, 1981). Interventions to improve young children's social interactions with peers began in earnest in the 1960s and for young children with identified disabilities in the 1970s (see Odom, McConnell, & McEvoy, 1992, and Shores, 1987, for reviews). Most social interaction interventions either changed environmental arrangements, altered social contingencies (i.e., teacher- and peer-mediated interventions), or combined these strategies to promote peer interactions.

The rationale for social interaction interventions has been straightforward. Essentially, young children without a rich history of peer interactions miss a primary route for acquiring not only social interaction skills but other important developmental abilities that might be learned, practiced, and elaborated while interacting with peers (Guralnick, 1992; Hartup, 1992; Ladd & Coleman, 1993). A primary assumption is that active social participation will become reinforcing and result in additional social interactions (i.e., "social entrapment;" Baer & Wolf, 1970; McConnell, 1987) resulting in learning in other environments and with other people in the future (i.e., generalization and maintenance of newly acquired social interaction and related skills).

As mentioned in the introduction to this chapter, intervention research on social and communicative competence has developed separately. Thus, we will selectively review examples of child–child social interaction interventions (see Brown & Conroy, 1997; McEvoy, Odom, & McConnell, 1992, and Odom & Brown, 1993, for reviews) and then a smaller number of studies that have focused on young children's social-communicative competence (see Goldstein & Kaczmarek, 1992, and Ostrosky et al., 1993, for reviews).

Environmental Arrangements

One intervention strategy for promoting young children's peer interactions has been systematic arrangement of preschool environments (Odom & Brown, 1993; Sainato & Carta, 1992). Environmental arrangements refer to purposeful changes in the physical and social context of environments and not direct alterations in contingency relationships among participants (e.g., teacher prompting of social interaction, praise for social initiations to peers) (Brown, Bryson-Brockmann, & Fox, 1986).

Several arrangements of the physical environment have been demonstrated to influence young children's social behavior. For example, Quilitch and Risley (1973) found that the availability of some types of materials influenced young children's peer interactions. Specifically, they noted that some toys were "social toys" (e.g., board games, balls) whereas other toys were "isolate toys" (e.g., puzzles, crayons). Quilitch and Risley's (1973) systematic analysis of toys showed that careful selection of materials may increase the likelihood of peer interactions. The seminal work of Quilitch and Risley has been replicated with young children with developmental delays (e.g., Beckman & Kohl, 1984; Lieber & Beckman, 1991; Martin, Brady, & Williams, 1989). Brown, Fox, and Brady (1987) found that limiting the amount of space made available to young children (i.e., 19 versus 58 square feet per child) promoted their social behavior when controlling for the type of available toys, teacher interactions with children, and familiarity of children. The Brown and colleagues (1987) spatial analysis showed that careful consideration of room arrangements that support children's proximity may increase young children's social responding with peers.

In another intervention study, DeKlyen and Odom (1989) found that peer interactions among young children with and without developmental delays increased as a function of the activity structure employed by teachers. When teachers structured play activities (e.g., assigned roles, discussed expectations for the activity), children interacted more frequently. Guralnick, Connor, Hammond, Gottman, and Kinnish (1995) demonstrated that the presence of children without developmental delays (i.e., heterogenous versus homogeneous groups) increased the likelihood of peer interaction for young children with developmental delays. Similarly, Strain (1983) showed that inclusion of children without disabilities in heterogeneous playgroups produced better generalization than homogeneous playgroups with only young children with autism. When planning for and promoting peer interactions among preschool children, environmental arrangement studies have indicated the potential importance of several ecological factors within preschool environments including 1) toys and materials, 2) physical room arrangements, 3) teacher implemented structure for activities, and 4) the presence of socially sophisticated and responsive peers.

Although several investigators have shown that environmental arrangements are effective in improving preschool children's social interactions, results of many environmental arrangements have been modest and sometimes have not produced the hoped-for effects on young children's social behavior (Brown et al., 1987; Odom & Brown, 1993). For example, McEvoy, McConnell, Odom, and Skellenger (1991) failed to improve peer interactions for children with developmental delays when implementing an environmental arrangement intervention package (i.e., limited space assignment, structured play activities, mixed grouping of children with and without disabilities) in four classrooms. Similarly, Hecimovic, Fox, Shores, and Strain (1985) failed to obtain generalized social responding with heterogeneous playgroups. In spite of these failures to replicate previous findings, environmental arrangements continue to have appeal for practitioners for several reasons. First, environmental arrangements have been relatively easy to implement and have not had deleterious effects on the children involved in the interventions (Brown et al., 1987). Second, surveys (Odom, McConnell, & Chandler, 1994) and direct observations (McConnell, McEvoy, & Odom, 1992) indicate that teachers both prefer and implement environmental arrangement interventions more often than interventions that alter the social contingencies in their classrooms. Finally, and perhaps most important, environmental manipulations may interact with the alteration of more powerful social contingencies (i.e., teacher- and peer-mediated interventions) to improve peer interactions. In spite of the modest effects associated with environmental alterations, careful use of ecological factors may provide teachers with important environment events that enhance preschool children's peer interactions (Brown et al., 1986; Sainato & Carta, 1992).

Alterations in Social Contingencies: Teacher- and Peer-Mediated Interventions

Since the 1960s, many investigators have demonstrated that systematic alterations of social contingencies within preschool environments can improve children's social interactions with peers (Goldstein & Kaczmarek, 1992; McEvoy et al., 1992; Ostrosky et al., 1993; Odom & Brown, 1993; Shores, 1987). Most social interaction interventions for preschoolers have been based on either an applied behavior analysis (see Odom & McConnell, 1992) or a cognitive-social learning (see Mize, 1995) conceptual framework. Moreover, most of the intervention strategies entail adults systematically encouraging (e.g., verbal prompts, visual cues) and acknowledging (e.g., verbal praise, tangible rewards) social behavior that results in peer interactions. Alteration of social contingencies may be divided into teacher- and peer-mediated intervention strategies (McEvoy et al., 1992; Odom & Brown, 1993; Strain & Fox, 1981).

Interventionists who have used teacher-mediated strategies have employed adults to 1) provide putative reinforcement for positive social responding (Allen, Hart, Buell, Harris, & Wolf, 1964; Strain, Shores, & Kerr, 1976; Wahler, 1967), 2) issue prompts for engagement in social interaction (Antia & Kreimeyer, 1988; Odom & Strain, 1986), 3) lead social interaction training groups in which they teach or provide practice for specific social behavior (Goldstein, Wickstrom, Hoyson, Jamieson, & Odom, 1988; Mize & Ladd, 1990), or use some combination of the three intervention strategies (McConnell, Sisson, Cort, & Strain, 1991; Odom, Hoyson, Jamieson, & Strain, 1985). For example, Allen and colleagues (1964) demonstrated that systematically modifying teachers' attention to an "isolate child" (child with minimal peer interaction) was sufficient to alter her social interactions with adults and peers in her nursery school. Specifically, teachers ignored initiations to adults while socially attending to the girl's social interactions with peers. The new social contingency increased positive social responding with peers whereas initiations to adults decreased. Reversals in the social contingencies (i.e., adult attention made contingent on interactions with adult) clearly showed that teacher attention was a powerful influence on the young girl's social behavior. Since the Allen and colleagues (1964) study, the use of adult praise and attention (or other putative reinforcers) to improve young children's social interactions with peers has been replicated often with young children with developmental difficulties (Goldstein & Kaczmarek, 1992; McEvoy et al., 1992; Odom & Brown, 1993; Shores, 1987; Strain & Fox, 1981).

Interventionists also employ teacher prompts to promote young children's social interactions with peers. For example, Odom and Strain (1986) systematically used prompting procedures to increase the social initiations of young children with autism. Although adult cues for children to socially interact with one another have been employed often, prompting procedures usually have been used in combination with other tactics such as teacher reinforcement and social skills training groups (e.g., Odom, Chandler, Ostrosky, McConnell, & Reaney, 1992; Odom et al., 1985).

In spite of the repeated demonstrations of the effectiveness of teacher-mediated intervention strategies in the 1960s and 1970s, several significant problems have been evident. First, many of the intervention strategies were implemented in relatively controlled circumstances by either researchers or well-trained practitioners who were supported by research personnel. Hence, the generality of the intervention procedures for many teachers in typical preschool environments is suspect. Second, participating children often become overly dependent on teacher prompts or reinforcement when interventions relied extensively on manipulating antecedent and consequent events (Odom & Strain, 1986). Although some investigators use systematic fading and thinning procedures as a method to overcome children's overreliance on teacher prompts and reinforcements (Odom, Chandler, et al., 1992; Timm, Strain, & Eller, 1979), researchers have noted that those procedures were time consuming and required relatively sophisticated personnel to implement appropriately (Brown & Odom, 1994; Strain & Fox, 1981). Finally, Strain and Fox (1981) discussed the distinct possibility that ill-timed teacher prompts and reinforcement may actually disrupt young children's ongoing peer interaction.

To address the potential problems associated with teacher-mediated intervention strategies, researchers have investigated peer-mediated strategies to improve young children's social interactions with peers. Similar to teacher-mediated intervention strategies, investigators who used peer-mediated strategies had teachers manipulate antecedent and consequent conditions (e.g., teacher prompts, teacher praise, small-group lessons) to promote children's peer interactions. Also, similar to teacher-mediated strategies, the ultimate goal of the intervention has been to increase and improve the social interactions of young children with social competence difficulties (Shores, 1987; Strain & Fox, 1981).

Unlike teacher-mediated interventions, researchers who used peer-mediated strategies first intervened with socially sophisticated peers to increase their social initiations to children with developmental delays. Frequently, after initial peer training, researchers have prompted and reinforced the trained peers' social initiations to children with developmental delays for some period. Typically, increased peer initiations resulted in increased child–child social interactions and in some cases "spillover" effects to children who were not targeted for intervention (Strain, Shores, & Timm, 1977).

Combined Social Interaction Interventions

The work of interventionists in the 1960s and 1970s has been important to the development and refinement of social interaction intervention strategies into relatively comprehensive intervention packages. By the 1980s and 1990s, researchers had begun to employ intervention packages to improve young children's social interactions with peers (Brown, Ragland, & Bishop, 1989; English, Goldstein, Shafer, & Kaczmarek, 1997; Goldstein et al., 1988; McConnell et al., 1991; Odom & McConnell, 1993). Most often, these intervention packages included teaching specific social behaviors or roles to children with and without developmental delays and using teacher praise and prompts for children to participate in peer interactions during common preschool activities.

One line of social interaction research implemented friendship activities within the context of common preschool activities such as simple songs and games (Brown, Ragland, & Fox, 1988; McEvoy et al., 1988; Twardosz, Nordquist, Simon, & Botkin, 1983). Similar to other social interaction interventions, the primary goal of friendship activities is to increase the number of opportunities for peer interaction and hence improve the social interactions of children with and without developmental delays. When implementing friendship activities, interventionists restructure the preschool environment to support children's interactions by systematically integrating teacher praise and prompts for social behaviors that have a high probability of evoking peer social responses (e.g., affection, compliments) with supplementary discussions of the importance of friendships. For example, while playing Musical Chairs teachers might encourage children to give one another hugs or compliments after the music stops and for children to rush for their chairs. Teachers' prompts and praise statements for peer interaction can be employed with individual dyads of children as well as with the entire group of participants. Twardosz and colleagues (1983) demonstrated that friendship activities improved the social interactions of preschool children who were socially withdrawn. Replications by Brown and colleagues (1988) and McEvoy and colleagues (1988) have shown that friendship activities can be effective with young children with more significant developmental difficulties, including autism, mental retardation, and behavior disorders.

Unlike many of the social interaction intervention studies that have been characterized by restricting and structuring training in separate training environments with specific prompts and praise statements for social interaction (e.g., McConnell et al., 1991; Odom et al., 1985), friendship activities have been implemented within the relatively chaotic conditions of naturally occurring preschool routines and activities. Hence, the procedures have been characterized as "naturalistic peer interventions" (Brown & Conroy, 1997; Brown & Odom, 1995). Teachers' use of friendship activities may be more teacher friendly than interventions that require a thorough understanding of behavior analysis principles or other intensive intervention strategies that require separate training sessions outside of the context of everyday classroom activities. Nevertheless, comparisons of the effectiveness of friendship activities and more intensive and structured social interaction interventions have not been reported.

For children with severe disabilities, a direct instruction approach with teaching of specific social-communicative behavior may be indicated (e.g., Dragsow, Halle, & Ostrosky, 1998; Dragsow, Halle, Ostrosky,

& Harbers, 1996). For example, Drasgow and his colleagues (1998) demonstrated that systematic prompting procedures and well-specified alterations of social contingencies (i.e., differential reinforcement of alternative forms of communicative behavior) may be required to establish an initial repertoire of social-communicative behavior that is more conventional than primitive repertoires (e.g., reaching, grabbing, screaming). Moreover, their work has suggested that with some children, alterations of the social contingencies may have to be performed in all the environments in which generalization and maintenance of newly acquired social-communicative behavior are planned.

McConnell and his colleagues (1991) provided another example of a combined social interaction intervention. They demonstrated that intensive social skills training within a structured instructional environment (i.e., teacher-directed instruction outside of children's classrooms) was effective in teaching preschool children with behavior disorders specific social behaviors that they could then perform during role-play assessment; however, only modest changes in peer interactions during free play resulted from isolated social skills training alone. Subsequent interventions within free play produced significant improvements in the social behavior of participating children. Specifically, individual coaching (i.e., teacher prompts and praise statements for target children's social behavior) increased the overall rates of target children's social initiations, and about half of those initiations received peer responses. The positive effects of the individual coaching strategy, however, were primarily seen on target children's social behavior (i.e., increased social initiations and improved responsiveness to peer initiations). With group coaching (i.e., systematically rotated teachers' prompts and praise statements for social interaction for both target children and peers and a group contingency for increased social interaction) the investigators achieved improvements in both peer social initiations to target children and peer responsiveness to target children's social initiations. Thus, the effects of group coaching were seen primarily on peers' social behavior.

In discussing these differential effects of individual and group coaching strategies, McConnell and his colleagues noted that rates of social behavior for target children and their peers varied independently of one another. They further argued that the independence of the target child and peer effects may be a critical factor for planning generalization and maintenance of social interactions. They noted that generalized effects for two of the four target children seemed to result from a "behavioral entrapment process" evidenced by social reciprocity with an equitable balance of social roles for young children with and without developmental delays. It is likely that greater generalization and maintenance of young children's social behavior will result if individual and group coaching strategies are combined.

Social-Communicative Interventions

Most of the social interaction intervention investigations cited previously are characterized by the use of global measures of children's social behavior such as 1) sharing, 2) share requests, 3) play organizers, 4) assistance, 5) affection, and 6) compliments. The investigators recorded the effects of these measures on children's social initiations, social responses, and social interactions (i.e., defined by a social response to a social initiation) (Brown et al., 1996; Odom & Ogawa, 1992). Although these behavioral codes may be further categorized as verbal or nonverbal (e.g., vocal/verbal initiation, motor/gestural response), they are often aggregated to report session-by-session composite rates of children's social behavior. In spite of their global nature, these types of measures have been useful in demonstrating the efficacy of intervention procedures for improving preschool children's overall rates of peer interactions (Brown et al., 1996; Odom, McConnell, et al., 1992; Shores, 1987).

Unfortunately, this approach has only allowed the analysis of changes in overall social interaction (or initiations) and has not permitted careful analysis of children's communicative behavior per se. For example, unless investigators have monitored and recorded well-specified categories of child behavior (e.g., verbal requests for information), they might miss or overlook changes in critical types of communicative behavior. Therefore, the changes in social interaction reported in previous studies may represent increases in simple motor/gestural social behavior as opposed to sophisticated vocal/verbal social behavior. Without better specification of behavioral categories, reviewers of research will not know which precise types of social-communicative behavior changed.

Relative to a significant number of social interaction studies in the extant literature, investigations of interventions to promote young children's peer interactions and peer communications have been limited in number. During the 1990s, however, Goldstein and his colleagues carefully examined interventions that focus on both peer interactions and peer social-communicative behavior (English et al., 1997; Goldstein & Cisar, 1992; Goldstein, English, Shafer, & Kaczmarek, 1997; Goldstein & Ferrell, 1987; Goldstein, Kaczmarek, Pennington, & Shafer, 1992; Goldstein & Wickstrom, 1986; Goldstein et al., 1988). Although similar to previous peer-mediated social interaction interventions, Goldstein and his colleagues have systematically extended that line of inquiry to refine the social strategies taught to children and to better specify the verbal categories used to assess peer interactions. Goldstein and colleagues have taught preschool children to 1) establish eye contact; 2) establish joint attention; 3) verbally describe their play; 4) prompt requests with a sequence; 5) respond to children's verbal initiations by repeating, expanding, or requesting clarification; and 6) redirect social play activity while carefully assessing both verbal (i.e., comments, verbal requests, action requests, on-topic responses, imitative responses, nonsocial utterances) and nonverbal child behavior (i.e., nonverbal responses, no response).

In an early study, Goldstein and Wickstrom (1986) taught peers without developmental delays important behavioral strategies that promoted peer interactions of children with developmental difficulties. Specifically, Goldstein and Wickstrom (1986) provided peers without disabilities with direct instruction on six behavioral strategies: establishing eye contact; establishing joint attention; descriptive talking; prompting requests; responding to peers by repeating, elaborating, or requesting clarification; and redirecting play activities. Following peer training, children were prompted during free play to implement the behavioral strategies with target children with developmental delays. Increased rates of social-communicative interaction were achieved with immediate effects on communicative responding of target children and their peers. Although peer interaction rates were variable, following the termination of teacher prompting of peers to use the six strategies, all three children with developmental delays maintained their increased frequency of peer initiations and responses. Following intervention, the interaction changes noted by Goldstein and Wickstrom (1986) were clearly communicative in nature. Indeed, on-topic responses, an important indicator of conversation and social reciprocity, primarily accounted for increases in communicative interactions of two of the three children.

In another investigation, Goldstein and Cisar (1992) demonstrated that young children with and without developmental delays can learn social scripts (e.g., a booth attendant at a carnival game, an assistant at the carnival game, a customer participating in a carnival game for the carnival social script) during small-group lessons and that when prompted by teachers, preschool children will employ newly acquired sociodramatic behavior during classroom activities. Initially, Goldstein and Cisar (1992) showed that teachers' overviews of sociodramatic scripts and their general prompting for children to interact with one another failed to produce improvements in peer interactions of three children with autistic behaviors. Nevertheless, systematic training with triads composed of two children without disabilities and one child with autism across three sociodramatic scripts (i.e., pet shop, carnival, magic show) increased participating children's overall social behavior during play activities. Children's increased social responding included both targeted verbal and nonverbal social behavior and theme-related verbal and nonverbal social behavior.

Although most of the children's improvements in social-communicative interactions were attributable to increases in their targeted script behavior, Goldstein and Cisar (1992) noted that other theme-related behavior that was performed less often may have represented an important form of response generalization. In addition, children generalized their newly acquired social behavior to a different environment (i.e., free play activities in their classroom) and with different albeit similarly trained peers in the free play environment. Hence, Goldstein and Cisar (1992) have demonstrated that careful instruction in sociodramatic scripts, which provides children with common behavioral repertoires, can result in improved social and communicative interactions among peers with and without developmental delays.

In a series of similar studies, Goldstein and his colleagues systematically replicated their social-communicative intervention procedures by refining a peer intervention training package, called Buddy Skills-Training Program, for promoting children's peer interactions and social-communicative behavior (English et al., 1997; Goldstein et al., 1997). For example, English and colleagues (1997) assessed target children and trained peers' (i.e., buddies) verbal and nonverbal communicative acts including 1) verbal requests for attention, 2) verbal requests, 3) comments, 4) verbal responses, 5) nonverbal requests for attention, 6) nonverbal requests, and 7) nonverbal responses.

Following buddy skills-training, peer interactions between children with and without developmental delays increased significantly and social validity measures of children's social behavior before and after intervention indicated qualitative improvements in children's peer interactions. English and colleagues' (1997) observational system allowed careful analysis of changes in children's social and communicative interactions during nonintervention and intervention conditions. Specifically, all four target children with disabilities had low rates of social interaction and few communicative acts prior to peer buddy skills-training intervention. During two intervention phases (i.e., peer and dyadic strategy-use conditions), peer "buddies" had many more communicative acts with target children.

During the peer buddy skills-training, peers without developmental delays were taught three "buddy skills": 1) to maintain proximity with the assigned partner, 2) to say the partner's name to establish joint attention and to suggest playing together or talking about their play, and 3) to maintain proximity while continuing to play and talk with their assigned partner. These behavioral strategies were described in a specific instruction, "Stay with your friend, play with your friend, and talk with your friend," which was later condensed into a verbal mnemonic of "STAY-PLAY-TALK" (English et al., 1997). A subsequent dyadic training phase, in which target children were taught a modified version of the "STAY-PLAY-TALK with your buddy" strategy, was used to assess the additive effects of training target children in the buddy skills-training behavioral strategy.

The overall results of the English and colleagues (1997) buddy skills-training included immediate improvements in the frequency of peers and target children's social-communicative acts and subsequent peer interactions during 10-minute observations across the day (i.e., 4 minutes during free play, 3 minutes during snack, and 3 minutes during large-group activities). Specifically, following an initial peer strategy use phase, both trained peers and target children had many more social-communicative acts and subsequent peer interactions. In addition, both trained peers and target children continued their increased communicative acts and peer interactions with only slight improvements in the probability of social interactions during a subsequent dyadic strategy-use condition. English and her colleagues (1997) noted that the second intervention phase in which target children were taught the buddy strategies had only a minimal effect on the social responsiveness of children with developmental delays. Nevertheless, it appears appropriate to provide young children with developmental delays with similar successful behavioral strategies to improve the likelihood of social reciprocity. Again, the careful investigation of the nature of social reciprocity awaits further empirical verification.

CONTINUING CHALLENGES IN PROMOTING SOCIAL-COMMUNICATIVE COMPETENCE

Since the 1970s, significant improvements have been made in intervention strategies to improve young children's social interactions with peers. Environmental arrangements and teacher- and peer-mediated strategies have been systematically developed, refined, and evaluated. Investigators have developed an effective technology for improving young children's social interactions with peers. Nevertheless, several significant challenges continue to exist for researchers and practitioners who are interested in having a positive influence on young children's peer-related social-communicative competence. These critical challenges include 1) promoting generalization and maintenance of important social behavior, 2) identifying and validating effective social behavior, 3) supporting children's peer relations and friendships, and 4) translating research into practice.

Generalization and Maintenance of Young Children's Social Behavior

Historically, generalization and maintenance of newly acquired behavior have been considered critical and necessary dimensions of any effective intervention technology (Baer, Wolf, & Risley, 1968, 1987; Stokes & Baer, 1977). Generalization and maintenance have been defined as "the occurrence of relevant behavior under different nontraining conditions (i.e., across subjects, environments, people, behaviors, and/or time) without the scheduling of the same events in those conditions as had been scheduled in the training conditions" (Stokes & Baer, 1977, p. 350). Although intervention strategies have been effective in promoting children's acquisition and use of social behavior, most often interventions have not been as efficacious in producing well-generalized social responding without the employment of additional procedures (e.g., response-dependent fading, sequential modification of environments, retraining strategies) (Brown & Odom, 1994; Chandler, Lubeck, & Fowler, 1992; McEvoy et al., 1992; Odom & Brown, 1993; Odom & McConnell, 1992; Stokes & Osnes, 1986; Strain & Fox, 1981). Chandler and her colleagues' (1992) review of the preschool social interaction intervention literature illustrated the state of affairs. Of 45 investigations analyzed by Chandler and her colleagues, only 14 studies with successful generalization and another 8 studies with partial generalization were noted. Stokes and Osnes (1986) and Brown and Odom (1994) proposed employing a conceptual framework that includes three fundamental strategies for planning for generalization and maintenance of young children's social interactions with peers: 1) taking advantage of natural communities of reinforcement, 2) training diversely, and 3) incorporating functional mediators.

Taking Advantage of Natural Communities of Reinforcement

Baer and Wolf (1970) asserted that preschool children's social behavior was well suited for gaining access to "natural communities of reinforcement." They reasoned that children's social participation within preschools can function to improve and maintain their peer interactions. For children who rarely interact with peers, preschool teachers can use prompts and praise statements (or other antecedent and consequent events) to systematically "introduce" children to the existing social contingencies and the potential social rewards of peer interactions. This process has generated positive learning histories, and across time, interventionists have been able to fade their level of assistance with children targeted for intervention. The fundamental assumption of the process has been that existing social contingencies within preschool environments will become effective in maintaining children's social behavior. Hence, newly acquired or elaborated social responding will be "entrapped" by the social interactions of peers in important environments. Most of the social interaction intervention strategies employed to date have been based, at least partially, on the notion of social entrapment. Indeed, the opportunity to respond socially is at the heart of both teacher- and peer-mediated intervention strategies; however, entrapment typically has been discussed in post hoc analyses of generalization and maintenance of children's social behavior (Brown & Odom, 1994).

The concept of entry into natural communities of reinforcement has intuitive appeal and some empirical support. Nevertheless, Stokes and Osnes (1986) cautioned that literature about the entry into natural communities of reinforcement has been limited empirically and is speculative in nature. At least three critical assumptions have been inherent in approaches that rely on an entrapment process: 1) acquisition of a fluent repertoire of social behavior (see Brown & Odom, 1994), 2) the presence of socially sophisticated and responsive peers (see Strain, 1983), and 3) the absence of significant maladaptive behavior (see Stokes & Osnes, 1986). These assumptions have not invalidated the utility of employing natural communities of reinforcement to improve young children's social behavior. Rather, they identify potential difficulties and remind us that interventionists should be judicious in their use of tactics to promote access to existing social contingencies in preschools.

The tactic of teaching children to recruit social reinforcement (i.e., initiate and respond in social situations with peers) has been effective in improving social responding in the short term and has produced generalization and maintenance for at least some children on some occasions (Chandler et al., 1992). For example, a number of studies have shown that young children with social interaction difficulties respond well to social initiations by peers (e.g., Goldstein et al., 1997; McConnell et al., 1991; Strain et al., 1977), and McConnell (1987) employed an entrapment process to promote generalization and maintenance of preschool children's social behavior. These types of studies have indicated that both the acquisition and fluent use of functional social initiation skills (e.g., sharing, descriptive talking, verbal requests), as well as learning to be responsive to initiations by peers, may promote entry into natural communities of reinforcement. Hence, the opportunity to respond socially may have been (and will continue to be) a critical element in producing generalization and maintenance of young children's social behavior.

Moreover, review of studies that have reported generalization and maintenance has shown that the length of intervention may be related to entry into natural communities of reinforcement. Specifically, Chandler and colleagues (1992) noted that the most effective intervention strategies in terms of producing generalization had many more training sessions than less successful interventions (i.e., mean of 36 training sessions for successful generalization versus mean of 16 training sessions for unsuccessful generalization). Therefore, young children's frequent opportunities to respond socially have been linked to generalization and maintenance of social behavior. This fact makes careful monitoring of children's peer interactions following intervention in nonintervention environments a critical assessment component of any comprehensive social skills intervention strategy.

Training Diversely

Another basic strategy for promoting generalization and maintenance of young children's social interactions with peers has been training diversely (Brown & Odom, 1994; Stokes & Osnes, 1986). When using this strategy, investigators have employed several tactics including training across multiple exemplars, training loosely, and using indiscriminable contingencies. For example, Brady and colleagues (1984) used a multiple peer exemplar tactic to facilitate generalization of social interaction to peers without disabilities. Sequential training across three peers promoted generalized social responding with peers without disabilities who were not involved in social skills interaction training. Similar positive intervention outcomes might be predicted from concurrent training of peer interaction across peers and environments. Most social interaction interventions have used either sequential or concurrent training of peers and to date it has remained unclear which strategy has been most effective.

Training loosely is another tactic that has been employed by interventionists, and this approach is basically a variant of training multiple peer and social response exemplars. Instead of conducting training sessions outside of classroom contexts (e.g., McConnell et al., 1991), some investigators have embedded interventions within the relatively chaotic conditions of routine preschool activities and have provided opportunities to train loosely. For example, the friendship activities discussed previously produced cross-environment generalization to nonintervention free play environments, which were conducted at least 23 hours after the implementation of intervention (Brown et al., 1988; McEvoy et al., 1988; Twardosz et al., 1983). Generalization to peers who are not involved in friendship activities and short-term maintenance of social behavior following the termination of intervention also have been reported (McEvoy et al., 1988). Training loosely is an intervention tactic that has been teacher friendly and beneficial to preschool children as a less intrusive means of providing additional opportunities and practice to respond socially to peers (see Brown & Conroy, 1997).

Using indiscriminable contingencies is another tactic for training diversely. Several methods for making contingencies indiscriminable have been used with preschool children. For example, following initial intervention, Timm and colleagues (1979) systematically faded teachers' prompts and attention based on continued social responding by target children and their peers. Another method of making contingencies indiscriminable has been the employment of delayed reinforcement. Fowler and Baer (1981) showed that withholding teacher feedback and delaying reinforcement of children's social responding were sufficient to promote generalization of peer interaction during free play periods.

A final method of making contingencies less discriminable has been the sequential modification of environments or conditions. Odom and colleagues (1985) employed sequential modification of environments by monitoring young children's social behavior in three preschool environments (i.e., structured play, table activities, and learning centers) and using a peer-mediated intervention in the structured play environment. When target children's social interactions with peers failed to change in nonintervention situations, Odom and colleagues (1985) sequentially employed the peer-mediated intervention across the remaining two environments to promote improved peer interactions.

Although *retraining* techniques have not satisfied the strict definition of generalization and maintenance offered by Stokes and Baer (1977), they have been a pragmatic response to increasing the number of teaching and learning opportunities in important social environments, particularly with children with significant developmental difficulties who may require more intensive and sustained social interaction intervention. Indeed, the careful work of Drasgow and colleagues (1998) reminds us that for children with severe disabilities, retraining strategies may be critical for improving social-communicative behavior.

Incorporating Functional Mediators

A final strategy for programming generalization and maintenance of children's social interactions with peers is the integration of functional mediators into social interaction interventions. Functional mediators have been common stimuli or verbal behavior that are presented in nontraining contexts. For example, in an early example of using common stimuli to promote generalization, Redd (1970) showed that the presence of an adult who was associated with a previous history of reinforcement was sufficient to evoke children's cooperative play in nontraining environments. Another variant of using common social stimuli has been to employ children's language and cognitive abilities to promote generalized social responding. Sainato, Goldstein, and Strain (1992) demonstrated that self-monitoring procedures that included forecasting how to get peers to play, reviewing four procedures for promoting peer interaction, and self-evaluating the effectiveness of those procedures promoted trained peers' continued social interaction with children with autism. Hence, verbal mediation procedures were used to facilitate peers' social initiations without having to rely on more intrusive teacher praising and prompting strategies during children's play activities.

In summary, three basic strategies and a number of accompanying tactics for promoting generalization and maintenance of young children's social behavior have been investigated and recommended to improve peer-related social competence interventions since the 1970s. Nevertheless, following initial social interaction interventions, generalization and maintenance of young children's peer interactions has continued to be elusive and frequently nonexistent (Brown & Odom, 1994; Chandler et al., 1992; Stokes & Osnes, 1986; Strain & Fox, 1981). As Brown and Odom (1994) argued, to view a lack of generalization and maintenance of young children's social behavior pessimistically is counterproductive at best. A more productive approach is to systematically plan for generalization and maintenance across significant social responses, people, environments, and time by using those strategies and tactics known to promote generality of social behavior. Direct assessment of generalization and maintenance with time sampling techniques or periodic social probes should allow interventionists to carefully monitor and analyze generalization and maintenance. Moreover, pragmatically, if generalization and maintenance are not forthcoming, additional supplemental strategies should be employed to facilitate generalized social responding.

Many of the current social interaction intervention packages available for use by practitioners have incorporated many of the strategies and tactics known to promote generalization and maintenance (e.g., Brown et al., 1989; English et al., 1997; Goldstein et al., 1988; McConnell et al., 1991; Odom & McConnell, 1993). As a general principle, social interaction interventions should focus on teaching and providing practice for critical social behavior (Goldstein & Ferrell, 1987; Tremblay,

Strain, Hendrickson, & Shores, 1981) and should be conducted with several familiar peers (Brown et al., 1988) in multiple preschool environments and situations (English et al., 1997) and across sustained periods of time (Chandler et al., 1992; McConnell et al., 1991). Generalization and maintenance to important circumstances should be monitored carefully, and when necessary, retraining and sequential modification procedures should be employed to ensure that young children have multiple opportunities to participate in many positive social interactions with peers in important social environments and across prolonged periods of time.

Identification and Validation of Effective Social Behavior

A second critical challenge for interventionists interested in promoting young children's socially competent behavior is identification and empirical validation of effective social behaviors that promote and support frequent social initiations, social responses, and sustained and meaningful peer interactions. Effective social-communicative behavior might be viewed as social responses that are exhibited often by young children during peer interactions, can be taught effectively and efficiently, and evoke social reciprocity resulting in sustained and meaningful social participation. Although researchers have begun to discuss the importance of the relationship between peer interactions and social-communicative competence, few investigators have identified and examined effective peer-related, social-communication competencies. Therefore, we examine the social behaviors employed in several peer interaction and social-communicative competencies intervention studies.

Social Behaviors Employed in Peer Interaction Intervention Studies

Numerous peer interaction researchers have investigated social behavior that promotes social interactions between children with and without developmental delays. For the most part, behavioral categories identified by investigators have been global in nature (Brown et al., 1996; McEvoy et al., 1992; Shores, 1987). For example, many researchers have defined social behavior as motor/gestural behavior, vocal/verbal behavior, or a combination of those two forms (e.g., Fox, Shores, Lindeman, & Strain, 1986; Shores, 1987; Strain & Shores, 1977; Strain et al., 1976; Strain et al., 1977). In addition, investigators have delineated the reciprocal nature of vocal/verbal and motor/gestural social behavior by further cataloging those behaviors as positive or negative ongoing social interactions.

In an attempt to refine behavioral categories for young children's social interaction interventions, Tremblay and her colleagues (1981) studied a small sample of preschool children without disabilities. They identified and descriptively validated specific social initiations that were effective (i.e., resulted in positive peer responses at least 50% of the time) in evoking social responses from peers. The specific social initiations that were effective included play organizing, affection, assistance, sharing, and rough-and-tumble play. Since the initial descriptive work of Tremblay and her colleagues, play organizing, affection, assistance, and sharing have been empirically validated frequently as social initiations that can be taught to children with and without developmental delays and that the acquisition of those social behaviors can promote peer interactions (McEvoy et al., 1992; Odom & Brown, 1993; Shores, 1987). Other peer interaction researchers have suggested additional social behaviors that have included conversing, dispensing information, responding (Odom & Ogawa, 1992); initiating, complimenting, and requesting (Odom, McEvoy, Ostrosky, & Bishop, 1987); and commenting, questioning, requesting, and information-seeking (Guralnick & Paul-Brown, 1980).

In summary, peer interaction intervention researchers have identified global social behaviors that promote peer interactions among children with and without developmental delays. Although peer interaction researchers have neither defined explicitly nor described their behavior measures in terms of social-communicative abilities, many of the social behaviors they have employed are clearly related to young children's social-communicative competence (i.e., they represent a combination of social and communicative abilities and may well promote communicative competence). Peer interaction intervention investigators have provided an initial foundation for identifying the social-communicative competencies that relate to promoting and supporting young children's peer interactions and communicative competence.

Social Behaviors Employed in Peer Intervention Studies

Researchers have begun to explicitly examine peer-related, social-communicative competence in preschool children with and without developmental delays. Goldstein and colleagues have identified several social-communicative competencies that promote peer interactions (Goldstein & Ferrell, 1987; Goldstein & Kaczmarek, 1992; Goldstein & Wickstrom, 1986; Goldstein et al., 1988). Similar to the behavior measures used in peer interaction intervention research, the identified competencies have represented relatively global behavioral categories; however, the social competencies employed by Goldstein and colleagues have included critical social behaviors discussed in the pragmatics literature (Guralnick & Paul-Brown, 1980; Wetherby & Prizant, 1992). These social competencies are more clearly related to communication and language development than the measures typically used by peer interaction investigators. The social-communication behaviors investigated have been establishing eye contact, establishing a joint focus of attention, using descriptive talk, responding appropriately to an initiation by repeating, expanding, or clarifying a peer's comments, suggesting joint play, prompting requests, and redirecting play activities. Goldstein and his colleagues have empirically validated these social competencies in a series of intervention studies.

Ostrosky and colleagues (1993) also suggested that social competencies such as turn taking, topic maintenance, and responsiveness are critical social behaviors that characterize peer-related, social-communicative competence. They argued for the examination of the social purpose or social goals of children's behavior, and they suggested four specific peer-related, social-communicative goals: 1) expressing a need or a want, 2) transferring information, 3) obtaining social closeness, and 4) using social etiquette that might be important during peer interactions. Investigators who are interested in peer-related, social-communicative competence have begun to investigate social behaviors that are directly related to both improved peer interactions and enhanced communication among young children. Hence, they have begun to address the important issue of which social behaviors are critical for promoting and supporting young children's peer-related social competence.

Validation of Effective Social Behavior

Although researchers have identified some peer-related, social-communicative competencies for young children, a clear and concise subset of those competencies that are effective in promoting peer interactions has not been established. Future validation of effective social behavior is needed to further refine behavioral categories for assessment purposes. Normative standards for young children's peer interactions, particularly children with developmental delays, do not exist as of 2001, and the influences of physical and social contextual factors are not well delineated. Consequently, careful analyses of children within common preschool environments should yield important information about which behaviors might influence young children's social interactions.

For example, Ferrell (1990) employed an ecobehavioral approach to study young children's peer interactions by observing the social interactions of children without disabilities in dyads with peers with moderate and severe disabilities. Careful descriptive and comparative analyses, which included the frequency and proportion of global and specific social behaviors, sequential analyses to identify social behaviors that evoked reciprocal responding, and qualitative analyses of resultant peer interactions, were used to better determine the behavioral targets for future peer-mediated interventions. The ecological analyses revealed that 1) joint attention to objects or activities was directly related to communicative behavior that evoked social responses; 2) descriptive comments on current activities occurred frequently, and both comments and requests for information were likely to result in peer interaction; and 3) social responding that acknowledged the communicative attempt of a peer promoted continued peer interaction more often than other types of social responses. Careful ecological analysis of factors related to young children's social behavior during high-quality peer interactions is a useful approach to identifying and validating which interactive behaviors might be important behavioral targets for future peer-related, social competence interventions.

Brown and colleagues (1996) reviewed the literature on observational assessment of preschool children's peer interactions. Based on the previous work of a number of researchers in the fields of applied behavior analysis, pragmatics, and social problem solving, they delineated a relatively comprehensive taxonomy of young children's social behavior with peers. Specifically, they argued for further refinement of behavior measures and an expanded conceptual framework that focused on children's social goals and behavioral strategies used to achieve those goals (Ostrosky et al., 1993). Brown and his colleagues defined social goals as "the intended outcomes or purposes of children's social interactions (i.e., outcomes if the interaction had been successful)," and they also described behavioral strategies as "the social behaviors that children use in attempts to achieve their social goals" (1996, p. 28). The specific social goals delineated by Brown and colleagues included aggression, assistance, attention, comfort-support, information seeking, information providing, object-related play, pretend play, self-action, and stop-action. The specific behavioral strategies they discussed were sharing, physical assistance, affection, commenting, calling, complimentary statements, gestural communication, need statements, object aggression, play noises, personal aggression, questions, requests/commands, role assignment, and suggestions.

Careful descriptive analyses of young children's social goals and the behavioral strategies they use to achieve their goals (e.g., frequency, conditional probabilities of evoking positive peer interactions) should result in a better understanding of young children's peer interactions and their social competence. Normative analyses of social behavior will allow researchers to better understand which social goals are typical for young children and which behavioral strategies are used during positive peer interactions. Moreover, once important social goals and behavioral strategies are identified, those goals and strategies can be further validated by determining if young children can be taught to employ the identified behavioral strategies to improve peer interactions.

Both normative and ecobehavioral approaches for analyzing young children's social behavior with peers represent two much needed areas of research to further develop a new generation of behavioral strategies for improving young children's peer-related, social competence. First, social behaviors that have a high probability of success in producing meaningful and sustained social interactions for children without disabilities must be identified. Second, those behaviors will need to be further validated in intervention studies to determine if young children with peer-related, social competence problems can acquire and fluently use those behavioral strategies to improve their peer interactions. For example, for young children who are disruptive during play, acquisition of effective social behavior for soliciting play partners has clear clinical significance (Kopp, Baker, & Brown, 1992; Putallaz & Wasserman, 1990). A better understanding of effective social behaviors may allow teachers to better promote and support a particular child's emerging social competence in common preschool activities (Brown et al., 1996). Finally, the fine-grained analyses of social behavior recommended by Goldstein and Kaczmarek (1992) and Brown and colleagues (1996) might assist interventionists in developing and implementing highly individualized interventions that are linked directly to children's peer-related difficulties (Kazdin, 1985).

Peer Relationships and Friendship Formation

A third critical challenge for researchers and practitioners who are interested in improving young children's social competence is the implementation of a more comprehensive intervention perspective that includes promoting better peer relations and the meaningful establishment of peer relationships and friendships. Whereas a number of intervention strategies that produce short-term improvements in peer interactions have been developed and evaluated, few interventionists have adequately addressed the development of young children's peer relationships and friendships (Brown & Odom, 1994; Favazza & Odom, 1997; Haring, 1992; Newcomb & Bagwell, 1995; Richardson & Schwartz, 1998). Although better peer relationships and friendships are implicit goals of most interventionists, to date, most researchers have failed to focus directly on peer relationships or use sufficient measures to clearly indicate whether the social status and social networks of children who have been targeted for social competence intervention have changed meaningfully. To their credit, several researchers have included socio-metric assessment as one of their outcome measures. Nevertheless, following intervention, clear changes in peer status have been obtained inconsistently. For example, using very similar intervention procedures, Goldstein and colleagues (1997) achieved changes in peer status, whereas English and colleagues (1997) failed to obtain improvements in peer preference. Moreover, alterations in peer status may have represented ephemeral changes during intervention and not the development of friendships across time.

If better peer relationships and friendships are to be an explicit goal of social competence interventions, then interventionists will need to adopt a broader perspective (Haring, 1992). For example, with older children with moderate and severe disabilities, Haring and Breen (1992) demonstrated that a peer-mediated social network intervention strategy was effective in increasing both the quantity and quality of peer interaction while supporting the development of friendships among children with and without disabilities. Specifically, Haring and Breen established peer networks through regular meetings with the purpose of systematically planning and implementing a peer group intervention for adolescents with severe disabilities. Several peers without disabilities, students with severe disabilities, and an adult facilitator met weekly to discuss the social interactions of students with and without disabilities, to plan strategies to promote positive peer interactions, to provide positive peer support for peer group participation, to role play specific interaction strategies for students with and without disabilities, to plan additional social competence interventions identified by members of the peer network, and to assess satisfaction with the intervention strategies as well as the peer network. The peer group intervention was successful in increasing the frequency of peer interactions, increasing the number of opportunities for peer interactions, and improving the appropriateness of peer interactions. In addition, the peer network strategy promoted and supported better peer relationships and the development of friendship among the participants.

With appropriate modifications for preschool children, similar peer group interventions that focus on both improved peer interactions and enhanced peer relationships might be planned, implemented, and evaluated. Indeed, recent work by Goldstein and his colleagues on "peer buddy skills-training strategies" (English et al., 1997; Goldstein et al., 1997) has incorporated intervention components (or might easily incorporate additional components) that are complementary to the formation of social networks (e.g., assigning peer buddies, matching peer buddies' schedules, social skills training to promote peer interactions, discussions and feedback for positive peer interactions, explicit discussions of friendships). It appears, however, that this approach may need further enhancement to achieve meaningful social relationships and friendships.

Another contextual component that might be used to enhance contemporary peer interaction strategies has been the systematic use of affective-based intervention strategies (e.g., positive and realistic stories about children with disabilities). These interventions might promote children's understanding of and sensitivity to other children's disabilities as well as their social interactions with peers with developmental delays. For example, with kindergarten children, Favazza and Odom (1997) showed that a "high-contact" intervention package consisting of indirect experiences (i.e., 15-minute stories and discussions about children with disabilities), direct experiences (i.e., structured play with children with disabilities), and home reading (i.e., parent reading one of the stories from a previous classroom discussion group) enhanced children's attitudes about and acceptance of people with disabilities. Specifically, Favazza and Odom (1997) demonstrated that a "high-contact" group demonstrated significantly greater social acceptance relative to a "low-contact" group (i.e., mainstreaming of children with and without disabilities during recess, lunch, music, or library without systematic intervention) and a "no-contact" group at another school.

Although several social competence intervention packages have included components that discussed children's differential abilities (English et al., 1997) and friendship with young children with developmental delays (Brown et al., 1988), those intervention packages focused primarily on increasing the number of opportunities to interact rather than enhancing children's understanding of and sensitivity to children with disabilities. Affective interventions may be important for improving peer interaction in the short-run and, more importantly, peer relationships and friendships in the long-term (see Favazza & Odom, 1997; Haring, 1992). It should be noted that peer interaction and peer acceptance intervention strategies can be complementary to one another. Indeed, the combination of the intervention strategies should enhance the comprehensive nature of contemporary social competence interventions and one would hope increase the power of those interventions. Nevertheless, the use of these two intervention strategies in combination awaits empirical validation to determine which components are necessary for both the short-term improvement of peer interactions and the long-term development of friendships.

In addition to broadening the focus of interventions, researchers and practitioners will need to employ assessment procedures that evaluate multiple dimensions of intervention strategies (e.g., child–child interaction, peer attitudes, children's social status) across much longer periods of time to demonstrate the effectiveness and efficiency of combined interventions. For example, if interventionists are interested in improved peer interactions, enhanced attitudes about children with disabilities, and peer relations and friendships, they might use a multi-method assessment approach by employing direct observation methods to assess child–child social interaction, modified attitude scales to address young children's perspectives of peers with disabilities (e.g., Acceptance Scale for Kindergartens [ASK; Favazza & Odom, 1997]), sociometrics to evaluate peer acceptance (e.g., Goldstein et al., 1997), and social network or clique analyses to assess peer relations and friendships (e.g., Yan et al., 1990).

Translating Research into Practice

A final critical challenge for researchers and practitioners is translating social competence interventions into practice in preschools. Many researchers and practitioners have lamented a long-standing problem with the widespread adoption of effective intervention strategies in educational environments (Brady, Gunter, & Langford, 1985; Brown & Odom, 1995; McConnell et al., 1992; Odom, 1988; Odom, McLean, Johnson, & LaMontagne, 1995; Schwartz, Carta, & Grant, 1996; Witt & Elliot, 1985). A fundamental fact has been that even the most robust intervention strategy, if not used by practitioners, will be impotent in promoting and supporting young children's development. Indeed, McConnell and colleagues (1992) argued that the impact of any intervention has been an interaction between its effectiveness and the likelihood of practitioners implementing it.

Several reasons exist for a failure to translate research findings into everyday practice. First, researchers have not necessarily disseminated their findings in a manner that is "user friendly" for many important consumers (i.e., practitioner- and parent-oriented publications) (Schwartz et al., 1996). Many of the most effective intervention strategies have never been translated in sufficient detail to allow practitioners to implement them within their preschools. Second, many powerful intervention strategies have not been ecologically valid (Brooks & Baumeister, 1977). Specifically, many interventions have lacked ecological validity because they require additional or specially trained personnel, modified materials, and technical assistance that are not readily available to most preschool practitioners. Finally, most empirically validated interventions have not included practitioners on the research teams that developed, implemented, and evaluated those intervention strategies. Hence, empirically validated interventions may fulfill rigorous experimental criteria for scientific believability but fail to achieve a critical social criterion of teacher acceptability and subsequent use.

Even when recommended intervention practices were developed through consensus-based approaches and a majority of practitioners and researchers surveyed responded to those "best practices" as acceptable, few respondents indicated that they implemented the intervention strategies frequently (Odom et al., 1995). In recent studies examining the use of recommended language intervention practices, Schwartz and her colleagues (1996) showed that preschool children who were exposed to higher levels of "best practice" had 1) higher rates of engagement, 2) higher rates of verbalizations, and 3) greater communication improvements as indicated by standardized tests as well as parental and teacher reports. The findings of Schwartz and colleagues (1996) have been similar to other convergent descriptive (e.g., Carta, Sainato, & Greenwood, 1988; Hart & Risley, 1992) and experimental (e.g., Greenwood, Delquadri, & Hall, 1984) evidence in which children's opportunities to respond have been associated with significant developmental and behavioral gains.

With respect to translating research concerning effective social interaction interventions for young children into everyday practice, only limited information regarding the extent to which intervention strategies have been used is available. For example, with a national survey of 131 practitioners, Odom and colleagues (1994) found that teachers reported a significant need for effective social interaction interventions and a need for technical assistance in implementing social interaction interventions. Results of the survey indicated that teachers were concerned about having effective social competence interventions for young children, that teachers believed that a variety of intervention strategies are acceptable and feasible, and that teachers reported using, at least to some extent, several contemporary intervention strategies in their preschools. However, in another study, which employed direct observation methods for a sample of 22 preschools, McConnell and his colleagues (1992) found that classroom teachers were employing empirically validated social interaction interventions at a moderate to low level of implementation and were much more likely to use structural and indirect intervention methods with groups of young children (e.g., environmental arrangements, discussions of friendships) than to implement intensive, individualized intervention strategies with young children (e.g., teacher prompting, praising of target child's peer interaction).

Current evidence suggests that although preschool teachers value social competence interventions, they are reluctant to employ many of those intervention strategies in their programs, particularly the interventions that appear to be the most effective albeit most labor intensive for practitioners. With respect to translating research into practice, it appears that a significant gap between "what we know" and "what we do" continues to exist (Brown & Odom, 1995; McConnell et al., 1992; Odom, 1988).

To improve the translation of social competence intervention strategies into practice, researchers and practitioners must assess more than the efficacy of particular intervention strategies. Researchers must be willing to assess acceptability and feasibility of social competence interventions and the individual components of those interventions (McConnell et al., 1992). Effective intervention strategies must be evaluated under circumstances that exist in most early childhood and early childhood special education programs. For example, for social competence interventions to be both acceptable and feasible, interventions will need to be easily implemented by preschool teachers (both professionals and paraprofessionals), the primary intervention agents, within the context of common preschool activities. In addition, teachers who implement intervention strategies should be involved directly in assessing both acceptability and feasibility of potential intervention strategies. The nature of any technical assistance required to initiate interventions and sustain them also will need to be evaluated. Finally, the broader effect of the implementation of social competence interventions must be evaluated under naturalistic conditions within community-based preschools.

When an array of social interaction intervention strategies that are effective, acceptable, and feasible for teachers have been developed, refined, and carefully evaluated, only then will practitioners have the practical tools needed to translate well-researched interventions into pervasive preschool practices that influence young children's social competence. Moreover, to achieve acceptability and feasibility, parents and practitioners (e.g., teachers, administrators) should participate in the research and development of social competence interventions (McConnell et al., 1992; Schwartz et al., 1996).

CONCLUSION AND RECOMMENDATIONS

Since the 1970s, researchers and practitioners have begun acquiring a solid knowledge base concerning the social-communicative competence of young children with developmental delays. Nevertheless, a number of critical questions need to be addressed. Brown and Odom delineated several fundamental questions that continue to outline an important research agenda for researchers and practitioners who are interested in improving the social-communicative competence of young children with and without disabilities:

1. Which social responses are most likely to produce young children's social interactions?
2. Which social situations and settings are most likely to facilitate and support young children's social interactions?
3. What learning history is necessary and sufficient to produce sustained social interactions?
4. What constitutes an adequate social repertoire for young children to participate effectively in their communities, homes, and schools?
5. What environmental supports will be needed to facilitate generalization and maintenance of newly acquired social behavior to children's communities, homes, and schools, particularly for children with significant developmental difficulties (e.g., severe autism, significant mental retardation, multiple disabilities)?
6. What social skills interventions will be perceived as useful and hence more likely to be used by interventionists (e.g., teachers) in children's communities, homes, and schools?
7. What learning history and environmental supports are necessary and sufficient to produce children's meaningful social relationships and friendships? (1994, p. 114)

When these fundamental questions are adequately addressed, there will be a functional knowledge base for young children's social competence and for promoting and supporting the peer-related social-communicative competence of young children with and without developmental delays.

REFERENCES

Allen, K.E., Hart, B., Buell, J.S., Harris, F.R., & Wolf, M.M. (1964). Effects of social reinforcement on isolate behavior of a nursery school child. *Child Development, 35,* 511–518.

Antia, S.D., & Kreimeyer, K.H. (1988). Maintenance of positive peer interaction in preschool hearing-impaired children. *Volta Review, 90,* 206–216.

Baer, D.M., & Wolf, M.M. (1970). The entry into natural communities of reinforcement. In R. Ulrich, H.H. Sachnick, & J. Mabry (Eds.), *Control of human behavior* (pp. 319–324). Glenview, IL: Scott Foresman.

Baer, D.M., Wolf, M.M., & Risley, T.R. (1968). Some current dimensions of applied behavior analysis. *Journal of Applied Behavior Analysis, 1,* 91–97.

Baer, D.M., Wolf, M.M., & Risley, T.R. (1987). Some still-current dimensions of applied behavior analysis. *Journal of Applied Behavior Analysis, 20,* 313–327.

Bagnato, S.J., Neisworth, J.T., & Munson, S.M. (1997). *LINKing assessment and early intervention: An authentic curriculum-based approach.* Baltimore: Paul H. Brookes Publishing Co.

Baudonniere, P.M., Garcia-Werebe, M.J., Michel, J., & Liegois, J. (1989). Development of communicative competencies in early childhood. A model and results. In B. Schneider, G. Attili, J. Nadel, & R. Wessberg (Eds.), *Social competence in developmental perspective* (pp. 175–195). Norwell, MA: Kluwer Academic/Plenum Publishers.

Beckman, P.J., & Kohl, F.L. (1984). The effects of social and isolate toys on the interactions and play of integrated and nonintegrated groups of preschoolers. *Education and Training of the Mentally Retarded, 19,* 169–174.

Bijou, S.W. (1993). *Behavior analysis of child development* (2nd ed.). New York: Context Books.

Brady, M.P., Gunter, P., & Langford, C.A. (1985). Why aren't research results in practice? In M.P. Brady & P. Gunter (Eds.), *Integrating moderately and severely handicapped learners: Strategies that work* (pp. 282–294). Springfield, IL: Charles C Thomas.

Brady, M.P., Shores, R.E., Gunter, P., McEvoy, M.A., Fox, J.J., & White, C. (1984). Generalization of a severely handicapped adolescent's social interaction behavior via multiple peers in a classroom setting. *Journal of The Association for Persons with Severe Handicaps, 9,* 278–286.

Bricker, D. (1992). The changing nature of communication and language intervention. In S.F. Warren & J. Reichle (Series & Vol. Eds.), *Communication and language intervention series: Vol. 1. Causes and effects in communication and language intervention* (pp. 361–375). Baltimore: Paul H. Brookes Publishing Co.

Bricker, D. (1993). Then, now, and the path between: A brief history of language intervention. In S.F. Warren & J. Reichle (Series Eds.) & A.P. Kaiser & D.B. Gray (Vol. Eds.), *Communication and language intervention series: Vol. 2. Enhancing children's communication: Research foundations for intervention* (pp. 11–34). Baltimore: Paul H. Brookes Publishing Co.

Bricker, D., & Pretti-Frontczak, K. (Eds.). (1996). *Assessment, evaluation, and programming system for infants and children: Vol. 3. AEPS measurement for three to six years.* Baltimore: Paul H. Brookes Publishing Co.

Bricker, D., (with Pretti-Frontczak, K, & McComas, N.). (1998). *An activity-based approach to early intervention* (2nd ed.). Baltimore: Paul H. Brookes Publishing Co.

Bronfenbrenner, U. (1979). *The ecology of human development: Experiments by nature and design.* Cambridge, MA: Harvard University Press.

Brooks, P.H., & Baumeister, A.A. (1977). A plea for consideration of ecological validity in the experimental psychology of mental retardation. *American Journal of Mental Deficiency, 81,* 407–416.

Brown, W.H., Bryson-Brockmann, W.A., & Fox, J.J. (1986). The usefulness of J.R. Kantor's setting event concept for research on children's social behavior. *Child and Family Behavior Therapy, 8,* 15–25.

Brown, W.H., & Conroy, M.A. (1997). Promoting and supporting peer interactions in inclusive classrooms: Effective strategies for early childhood educators. In W.H. Brown & M.A. Conroy (Eds.), *Inclusion of preschool children with developmental delays in early childhood programs* (pp. 79–108). Little Rock, AR: Southern Early Childhood Association.

Brown, W.H., Fox, J.J., & Brady, M.P. (1987). Effects of spatial density on 3- and 4-year-old children's socially directed behavior during freeplay: An investigation of a setting factor. *Education and Treatment of Children, 10,* 247–258.

Brown, W.H., & Odom, S.L. (1994). Strategies and tactics for promoting generalization and maintenance of young children's social behavior. *Research in Developmental Disabilities, 15,* 99–118.

Brown, W.H., & Odom, S.L. (1995). Naturalistic peer interventions for promoting preschool children's social interactions. *Preventing School Failure, 39,* 38–43.

Brown, W.H., Odom, S.L., & Holcombe, A. (1996). Observational assessment of young children's social behavior with peers. *Early Childhood Research Quarterly, 11,* 19–40.

Brown, W.H., Ragland, E.U., & Bishop, N. (1989). *A socialization curriculum for preschool programs that integrate children with handicaps.* Nashville: John F. Kennedy Center for Research on Education and Human Development, Peabody College of Vanderbilt University.

Brown, W.H., Ragland, E.U., & Fox, J.J. (1988). Effects of group socialization procedures on the social interactions of preschool children. *Research in Developmental Disabilities, 9,* 359–376.

Carta, J.J., Sainato, D.M., & Greenwood, C.R. (1988). Advances in the ecological assessment of classroom instruction for young children with handicaps. In S.L. Odom & M.B. Karnes (Eds.), *Early intervention for infants and children with handicaps: An empirical base* (pp. 217–239). Baltimore: Paul H. Brookes Publishing Co.

Chandler, L.K., Lubeck, R.C., & Fowler, S.A. (1992). Generalization and maintenance of preschool children's social skills: A critical review and analysis. *Journal of Applied Behavior Analysis, 25,* 415–428.

DeKlyen, M., & Odom, S.L. (1989). Activity structure and social interactions with peers in developmentally integrated play groups. *Journal of Early Intervention, 13,* 342–352.

Drasgow, E., Halle, J.W., & Ostrosky, M.M. (1998). Effects of differential reinforcement on the generalization of a replacement mand in three children with severe language delays. *Journal of Applied Behavior Analysis, 31,* 357–374.

Drasgow, E., Halle, J.W., Ostrosky, M.M., & Harbers, H.M. (1996). Using behavioral indication and functional communication training to establish an initial sign repertoire with a young child with severe disabilities. *Topics in Early Childhood Special Education, 16,* 500–521.

Dyson, A., & Genishi, C. (1993). Visions of children as language users: Language and language education in early childhood. In B. Spodeck (Ed.), *Handbook of research on the education of young children* (pp. 122–136). New York: Macmillan.

English, K., Goldstein, H., Shafer, K., & Kaczmarek, L. (1997). Promoting interactions among preschoolers with and without disabilities: Effects of a buddy system skills-training program. *Exceptional Children, 63,* 229–243.

Favazza, P.C., & Odom, S.L. (1997). Promoting positive attitudes of kindergarten-age children toward people with disabilities. *Exceptional Children, 63,* 405–418.

Ferrell, D.R. (1990). *Communicative interaction between handicapped and nonhandicapped preschool children: Identifying facilitative strategies.* Unpublished doctoral dissertation, University of Pittsburgh.

Flavel, J.H. (1977). *Cognitive development.* Upper Saddle River, NJ: Prentice-Hall.

Fowler, S.A., & Baer, D.M. (1981). "Do I have to be good all day?" The timing of delayed reinforcement as a factor in generalization. *Journal of Applied Behavior Analysis, 14,* 13–24.

Fox, J., Shores, R., Lindeman, D., & Strain, P. (1986). Maintaining social initiations with withdrawn handicapped and nonhandicapped preschoolers through a response-dependent fading tactic. *Journal of Abnormal Child Psychology, 14,* 387–396.

Goldstein, H., & Cisar, C.L. (1992). Promoting interaction during sociodramatic play: Teaching scripts to typical preschoolers and classmates with disabilities. *Journal of Applied Behavior Analysis, 25,* 265–280.

Goldstein, H., English, K., Shafer, K., & Kaczmarek, L. (1997). Interaction among preschoolers with and without disabilities: Effects of across-the-day peer intervention. *Journal of Speech, Language, and Hearing Research, 40,* 33–48.

Goldstein, H., & Ferrell, D. (1987). Augmenting communicative interaction between handicapped and nonhandicapped preschool children. *Journal of Speech and Hearing Disorders, 52,* 200–211.

Goldstein, H., & Kaczmarek, L. (1992). Promoting communicative interaction among children in integrated intervention settings. In S.F. Warren & J. Reichle (Series & Vol. Eds.), *Communication and language intervention series: Vol. 1. Causes and effects in communication and language intervention* (pp. 81–112). Baltimore: Paul H. Brookes Publishing Co.

Goldstein, H., Kaczmarek, L., Pennington, R., & Shafer, K. (1992). Peer-mediated intervention: Attending to, commenting on, and acknowledging the behavior of preschoolers with autism. *Journal of Applied Behavior Analysis, 25,* 289–305.

Goldstein, H., & Wickstrom, S. (1986). Peer intervention effects on communicative interaction among handicapped and nonhandicapped preschoolers. *Journal of Applied Behavior Analysis, 19,* 209–214.

Goldstein, H., Wickstrom, S., Hoyson, M., Jamieson, B., & Odom, S. (1988). Effects of sociodramatic play training on social and communicative interaction. *Education and Treatment of Children, 11,* 97–117.

Greenwood, C.R., Delquadri, J.C., & Hall, R.V. (1984). Opportunity to respond and student academic performance. In W.L. Heward, T.E. Heron, D.F. Hill, & J. Trap-Porter (Eds.), *Focus on behavior analysis in education* (pp. 58–88). New York: Merrill.

Gresham, F.M., & MacMillan, D.L. (1997). Social competence and affective characteristics of students with mild disabilities. *Review of Educational Research, 67*(4), 377–415.

Guralnick, M.J. (1992). A hierarchical model for understanding children's peer-related social competence. In S.L. Odom, S.R. McConnell, & M.A. McEvoy (Eds.), *Social competence of young children with disabilities: Issues and strategies for intervention* (pp. 37–64). Baltimore: Paul H. Brookes Publishing Co.

Guralnick, M.J. (1994). Social competence with peers: Outcome and process in early childhood special education. In P.L. Safford (Ed.), *Yearbook in early childhood education: Vol. 5. Early childhood special education* (pp. 45–71). New York: Teachers College Press.

Guralnick, M.J., Connor, R.T., Hammond, M., Gottman, J.M., & Kinnish, K. (1995). Immediate effects of mainstreamed settings on the social interactions and social integration of preschool children. *American Journal on Mental Retardation, 100,* 359–377.

Guralnick, M.J., & Paul-Brown, D.P. (1980). Communicative adjustments during behavior request episodes among children at different developmental levels. *Child Development, 55,* 911–919.

Haring, T.G. (1992). The context of social competence: Relations, relationships, and generalization. In S.L. Odom, S.R. McConnell, & M.A. McEvoy (Eds.), *Social competence of young children with disabilities: Issues and strategies for intervention* (pp. 307–320). Baltimore: Paul H. Brookes Publishing Co.

Haring, T.G., & Breen, C.G. (1992). A peer-mediated social network intervention to enhance the social integration of persons with moderate and severe disabilities. *Journal of Applied Behavior Analysis, 25,* 319–333.

Hart, B., & Risley, T.R. (1992). American parenting of language-learning children: Persisting differences in family–child interactions observed in natural home environments. *Developmental Psychology, 28,* 1096–1105.

Hartup, W.W. (1992). Peer relations in early and middle childhood. In V. Van-Hasselt & M. Hersen (Eds.), *Handbook of social development* (pp. 257–281). New York: Kluwer Academic/Plenum Publishers.

Hartup, W.W., & Moore, S.G. (1990). Early peer relations: Developmental significance and prognostic implications. *Early Childhood Research Quarterly, 5,* 1–17.

Hecimovic, A., Fox, J.J., Shores, R.E., & Strain, P.S. (1985). An analysis of developmentally integrated and segregated free play setting and the generalization of newly-acquired social behaviors of socially withdrawn preschoolers. *Behavioral Assessment, 7,* 367–388.

Hobbs, N. (1966). Helping disturbed children: Psychological and ecological strategies. *American Psychologist, 21,* 1105–1115.

Jack, L.M. (1934). An experimental study of ascendent behavior in preschool children. *University of Iowa Studies in Child Welfare, 9*(3), 9–65.

Kazdin, A.E. (1985). Selection of target behaviors: The relationship of the treatment focus to clinical dysfunction. *Behavioral Assessment, 7,* 33–47.

Kopp, C.B., Baker, B.L., & Brown, K.W. (1992). Social skills and their correlates: Preschoolers with developmental delays. *American Journal on Mental Retardation, 96,* 357–366.

Ladd, G.W., & Coleman, C.C. (1993). Young children's peer relationships: Forms, features, and functions. In B. Spodeck (Ed.), *Handbook of research on the education of young children* (pp. 57–76). New York: Macmillan.

Lieber, J., & Beckman, P.J. (1991). The role of toys in individual and dyadic play among young children with handicaps. *Journal of Applied Developmental Psychology, 12,* 189–203.

Martin, S.S., Brady, M.P., & Williams, R.E. (1989). Effects of toys on the social behavior of preschool children in integrated and nonintegrated groups: Investigation of a setting event. *Journal of Early Intervention, 13,* 153–161.

McConnell, S.R. (1987). Entrapment effects and the generalization and maintenance of social skills training for elementary school students with behavior disorders. *Behavioral Disorders, 12,* 252–263.

McConnell, S.R., McEvoy, M.A., & Odom, S.L. (1992). Implementation of social competence interventions in early childhood special education classes: Current practices and future directions. In S.L. Odom, S.R. McConnell, & M.A. McEvoy (Eds.), *Social competence of young children with disabilities: Issues and strategies for intervention* (pp. 277–306). Baltimore: Paul H. Brookes Publishing Co.

McConnell, S.R., Sisson, L.A., Cort, C.A., & Strain, P.S. (1991). Effects of social skills training and contingency management on reciprocal interaction of preschool children with behavioral handicaps. *Journal of Special Education, 24,* 473–495.

McEvoy, M.A., McConnell, S.R., Odom, S.L., & Skellenger, A. (1991). *Analysis of an environmental arrangements intervention for young children with disabilities.* Unpublished paper from the Vanderbilt-Minnesota Social Interaction Project, Vanderbilt University, John F. Kennedy Center, Nashville.

McEvoy, M.A., Nordquist, V.M., Twardosz, S. Heckaman, K., Wehby, J.H., & Denny, R.K. (1988). Promoting autistic children's peer interaction in an integrated early childhood setting using affection activities. *Journal of Applied Behavior Analysis, 21,* 193–200.

McEvoy, M.A., Odom, S.L., & McConnell, S.R. (1992). Peer social competence intervention for young children with disabilities. In S.L. Odom, S.R. McConnell, & M.A. McEvoy (Eds.), *Social competence of young children with disabilities: Issues and strategies for intervention* (pp. 113–134). Baltimore: Paul H. Brookes Publishing Co.

McLean, L.K., & Cripe, J.W. (1997). The effectiveness of early intervention for children with communication disorders. In M.J. Guralnick (Ed.), *The effectiveness of early intervention* (pp. 349–428). Baltimore: Paul H. Brookes Publishing Co.

Mize, J. (1995). Coaching preschool children in social skills: A cognitive-social learning curriculum. In G. Cartledge & J.F. Milburn (Eds.), *Teaching social skills to children and youth: Innovative approaches* (3rd ed., pp. 237–261). Needham Heights, MA: Allyn & Bacon.

Mize, J., & Ladd, G.W. (1990). A cognitive-social learning approach to social skills training with low-status preschool children. *Developmental Psychology, 26,* 388–397.

Newcomb, A.F., & Bagwell, C.L. (1995). Children's friendship relations: A meta-analytic review. *Psychological Bulletin, 117,* 306–347.

Notari, A., & Cole, K. (1993). Language intervention: Research implications for service delivery. In C.A. Peck, S.L. Odom, & D.D. Bricker (Eds.), *Integrating young children with disabilities into community programs: Ecological perspectives on research and implementation* (pp. 17–38). Baltimore: Paul H. Brookes Publishing Co.

Odom, S.L. (1988). Research in early childhood special education. In S.L. Odom & M.B. Karnes (Eds.), *Early intervention for infants and children with handicaps: An empirical base* (pp. 1–21). Baltimore: Paul H. Brookes Publishing Co.

Odom, S.L., & Brown, W.H. (1993). Social interaction skills interventions for young children with disabilities in integrated settings. In C.A. Peck, S.L. Odom, & D. Bricker (Eds.), *Integrating young children with disabilities into community programs: Ecological perspectives on research and implementation* (pp. 39–64). Baltimore: Paul H. Brookes Publishing Co.

Odom, S.L., Chandler, L.K., Ostrosky, M., McConnell, S.R., & Reaney, S. (1992). Fading teacher prompts from peer-initiation interventions for young children with disabilities. *Journal of Applied Behavior Analysis, 25,* 307–317.

Odom, S.L., Hoyson, M., Jamieson, B., & Strain, P.S. (1985). Increasing handicapped preschoolers' peer social interactions: Cross-setting and component analysis. *Journal of Applied Behavior Analysis, 18,* 3–16.

Odom, S.L., & McConnell, S.R. (1992). Improving social competence: An applied behavior analysis perspective. *Journal of Applied Behavior Analysis, 25,* 239–244.

Odom, S.L., & McConnell, S.R. (1993). *Play time/social time: Organizing your classroom to build interaction skills.* San Antonio, TX: Communication Skill Builders.

Odom, S.L., McConnell, S.R., & Chandler, L.K. (1994). Acceptability and feasibility of classroom-based social interaction interventions for young children with disabilities. *Exceptional Children, 60,* 226–236.

Odom, S.L., McConnell, S.R., & McEvoy, M.A. (1992). Peer-related social competence and its significance for young children with disabilities. In S.L. Odom, S.R. McConnell, & M.A. McEvoy (Eds.), *Social competence of young children with disabilities: Issues and strategies for intervention* (pp. 3–36). Baltimore: Paul H. Brookes Publishing Co.

Odom, S.L., McEvoy, M.A., Ostrosky, M., & Bishop, L. (1987, May). *Observing the functional classes of social interactions of preschool children.* Paper presented at the annual convention of the Association for Behavior Analysis, Nashville.

Odom, S.L., McLean, M.E., Johnson, L.J., & LaMontagne, M.J. (1995). Recommended practice in early childhood special education: Validation and current use. *Journal of Early Intervention, 19,* 1–17.

Odom, S.L., & Ogawa, I. (1992). Direct observation of young children's social interaction with peers: A review of methodology. *Behavioral Assessment, 14,* 407–441.

Odom, S.L., Peck, C.A., Hanson, M., Beckman, P.J., Kaiser, A.P., Lieber, J., Brown, W.H., Horn, E.M., & Schwartz, I.S. (1996). Inclusion of young children with disabilities: An ecological analysis. *Social Policy Report of the Society for Research in Child Development, 10,* 18–30.

Odom, S.L., & Strain, P.S. (1986). A comparison of peer initiation and teacher-antecedent interventions for promoting reciprocal social interaction of autistic preschoolers. *Journal of Applied Behavior Analysis, 19,* 59–72.

Ostrosky, M.M., Kaiser, A.P., & Odom, S.L. (1993). Facilitating children's social communicative interactions through the use of peer-mediated interventions. In S.F. Warren & J. Reichle (Series Eds.) & A.P. Kaiser & D.B. Gray (Vol. Eds.), *Communication and language intervention series: Vol. 2. Enhancing children's communication: Research foundations for intervention* (pp. 159–187). Baltimore: Paul H. Brookes Publishing Co.

Parten, M.B. (1932). Social participation among preschool children. *Journal of Abnormal and Social Psychology, 27,* 243–269.

Peck, C.A. (1989). Assessment of social communicative competence: Evaluating environments. *Seminars in Speech and Language, 10,* 1–15.

Peck, C.A. (1993). Ecological perspectives on the implementation of integrated early childhood programs. In C.A. Peck, S.L. Odom, & D.D. Bricker (Eds.), *Integrating young children with disabilities into community programs: Ecological perspectives on research and implementation* (pp. 3-15). Baltimore: Paul H. Brookes Publishing Co.

Piaget, J. (1926). *Language and thought in the child.* London: Kegan & Paul.

Putallaz, M., & Wasserman, A. (1990). Children's entry behavior. In S.R. Asher & J. Gottman (Eds.), *Peer rejection in childhood* (pp. 60–89). New York: Cambridge University Press.

Quilitch, H.R., & Risley, T.R. (1973). The effects of play materials on social play. *Journal of Applied Behavior Analysis, 6,* 575–578.

Redd, W.H. (1970). Generalization of adult's stimulus control of children's behavior. *Journal of Experimental Child Psychology, 9,* 286–296.

Renshaw, P.D. (1981). The roots of peer interaction research: A historical analysis of the 1930s. In S.R. Asher & J.M. Gottman (Eds.), *The development of children's friendships* (pp. 29–52). New York: Cambridge University Press.

Richardson, P., & Schwartz, I.S. (1998). Making friends in preschool: Friendship patterns of young children with disabilities. In L.H. Meyer, H.-S. Park, M. Grenot-Scheyer, I.S. Schwartz, & B. Harry (Eds.), *Making friends: The influences of culture and development* (pp. 65-80). Baltimore: Paul H. Brookes Publishing Co.

Sainato, D.M., & Carta, J.J. (1992). Classroom influences on the development of social competence in young children with disabilities. In S.L. Odom, S.R. McConnell, & M.A. McEvoy (Eds.), *Social competence of young children with disabilities: Issues and strategies for intervention* (pp. 93–109). Baltimore: Paul H. Brookes Publishing Co.

Sainato, D.M., Goldstein, H., & Strain, P.S. (1992). Effects of self-evaluation on preschool children's use of social interactions strategies with their classmates with autism. *Journal of Applied Behavior Analysis, 25,* 127–141.

Schwartz, I.S., Carta, J.J., & Grant, S. (1996). Examining the use of recommended language intervention practices in early childhood special education classrooms. *Topics in Early Childhood Special Education, 16,* 251–272.

Shores, R.E. (1987). Overview of research on social interaction: A historical and personal perspective. *Behavior Disorders, 12,* 233–241.

Stokes, T.F., & Baer, D.M. (1977). An implicit technology of generalization. *Journal of Applied Behavior Analysis, 10,* 349–367.

Stokes, T.F., & Osnes, P.G. (1986). Programming the generalization of children's social behavior. In P.S. Strain, M.J. Guralnick, & H.M. Walker (Eds.), *Children's social behavior: Development, assessment, and modification* (pp. 407–443). San Diego: Academic Press.

Strain, P.S. (1983). Generalization of autistic children's social behavior change: Effects of developmentally integrated and segregated settings. *Analysis and Intervention in Developmental Disabilities, 3,* 23–34.

Strain, P.S., & Fox, J.J. (1981). Peers as behavior change agents for withdrawn classmates. In B.B. Lahey & A.E. Chasten (Eds.), *Advances in clinical child psychology* (Vol. 4, pp. 167–198). New York: Kluwer Academic/Plenum Publishers.

Strain, P.S., & Shores, R.E. (1977). Social reciprocity: Review of research and educational implications. *Exceptional Children, 43,* 526–531.

Strain, P.S., Shores, R.E., & Kerr, M.M. (1976). An experimental analysis of "spillover" effects on social interaction among behaviorally handicapped preschool children. *Journal of Applied Behavior Analysis, 9,* 31–40.

Strain, P.S., Shores, R.E., & Timm, M.A. (1977). Effects of peer social initiations on the behavior of withdrawn preschool children. *Journal of Applied Behavior Analysis, 10,* 289–298.

Timm, M.A., Strain, P.S., & Eller, P. (1979). Effects of systematic, response-dependent fading and thinning procedures on the maintenance of child–child interactions. *Journal of Applied Behavior Analysis, 12,* 308.

Tremblay, A., Strain, P.S., Hendrickson, J.M., & Shores, R.E. (1981). Social interactions of normally developing preschool children: Using normative data for subject selection and target behavior selection. *Behavior Modification, 5,* 237–253.

Twardosz, S., Nordquist, V.M., Simon, R., & Botkin, D. (1983). The effects of group affection activities on the interaction of socially isolated children. *Analysis and Intervention in Developmental Disabilities, 3,* 311–338.

Vincent, L.J., Salisbury, C.L., Strain, P., McCormick, C., & Tessier, A. (1990). A behavioral-ecological approach to early intervention: Focus on cultural diversity. In S.J. Meisels & J.P. Shonkoff (Eds.), *Handbook of early childhood intervention* (pp. 173–195). New York: Cambridge University Press.

Vygotsky, L.S. (1978). *Mind and society: The development of higher psychological processes.* Cambridge, MA: Harvard University Press.

Wahler, R.G. (1967). Child–child interactions in free field settings: Some experimental analyses. *Journal of Experimental Child Psychology, 5,* 278–293.

Wetherby, A.M., & Prizant, B.M. (1992). Profiling young children's communicative competence. In S.F. Warren & J. Reichle (Series & Vol. Eds.)

Communication and language intervention series: Vol. 1. Causes and effects in communication and language intervention (pp. 217–254). Baltimore: Paul H. Brookes Publishing Co.

Witt, J.C., & Elliott, S.N. (1985). Acceptability of classroom intervention strategies. In T.R. Kratochwill (Ed.), *Advances in school psychology* (pp. 251–288). Mahwah, NJ: Lawrence Erlbaum Associates.

Yan, X., Storey, K., Rhodes, L., Sandow, D., Petherbridge, R., & Lowewinger, H. (1990). Grouping patterns in a supported employment work setting: Clique analysis of interpersonal interaction. *Behavioral Assessment, 12,* 337–354.

7

Preschool Children
Putting Research into Practice

Maureen A. Conroy and William H. Brown

> Alexis, a 3-year-old child with spastic cerebral palsy, is enrolled in an inclusive early childhood program. Often during free play, Alexis sits with an adult and watches the other children play from a stationary place in the room. When her classmates approach her to play, she looks at them and wants to play but is unable to respond to their initiations. Alexis's peers want to play with her, but they don't know how. Alexis's significant communication, cognitive, and motor delays interfere with her ability to play with the other children in her class.
>
> Jacob, a 4-year-old with communication delays and behavior problems, is enrolled in a Head Start program. Jacob often fights with his peers during free play over play materials. When he wants to play with a toy, Jacob will grab the toy away from another child. If the child tries to regain possession of the toy, Jacob will hit him or her and scream. Because of his disabilities, Jacob cannot play well with his classmates.
>
> Both Alexis' and Jacob's teachers are concerned about the children's peer-related social-communicative competence. Alexis and Jacob need intervention to facilitate their peer-related social interactions, but their teachers are uncertain about how to encourage their social-communicative development.

The relationship between communication abilities and the development of social interactions among young children has been acknowledged by researchers (e.g., see Goldstein & Ferrell, 1987; Goldstein & Kaczmarek, 1992; Ostrosky, Kaiser, & Odom, 1993) as well as by practitioners. Chapter 6 provides a comprehensive review and analysis of the current research in this area as well as a discussion of an ecological framework for guiding future research efforts. This chapter presents 1) an overview of peer-related social-communicative competencies to target for intervention, 2) strategies for assessing peer-related social-communicative competencies, and 3) an intervention model for teaching peer-related social-communicative competencies to preschool-age children with developmental delays. The stories of Alexis and Jacob illustrate these strategies.

OVERVIEW OF PEER-RELATED SOCIAL-COMMUNICATIVE COMPETENCIES

An initial step in developing and implementing effective interventions in peer-related social-communicative competence is targeting critical and effective skills and competencies for intervention. Although researchers and practitioners agree that social and communicative competence are closely related, there is relatively little research that specifically identifies and examines effective peer-related social-communicative competencies. Therefore, we examined the skills and competencies identified in the areas of peer-related social interaction competence as well as social-communicative competence to provide an empirical basis for suggesting effective competencies to target for intervention in preschool-age children with developmental delays.

In general, many different skills and competencies that facilitate peer-related social interactions among children have been identified (e.g., Brown, Odom, & Holcombe, 1996; Strain, Shores, & Kerr, 1976; Tremblay, Strain, Hendrickson, & Shores, 1981). *Peer-related social interactions* are a "direct exchange of words, gestures, toys, or materials between two or more children" (Odom & Brown, 1993, p. 41). A critical component in peer-related social interactions is the *reciprocal exchange* between two or more children. The reciprocal nature of these behaviors has been globally categorized into several functional components including an initiation, a response to an initiation, or an ongoing social interaction (Fox, Shores, Lindeman, & Strain, 1986; Strain, Shores, & Timm, 1977).

In the 1980s and 1990s, specific types of initiation and responses were identified as being highly effective in facilitating and maintaining reciprocal social interactions in preschool-age children. Typically, these are verbal and/or gestural skills that suggest a specific action from the recipient. Examples of these skills include organizing play, showing affection, providing assistance, sharing play materials, engaging in rough-and-tumble play (Tremblay et al., 1981), engaging in conversations, dispensing information, responding to initiations (Odom & Ogawa, 1991), providing complimentary statements, requesting information or assistance (Odom, McEvoy, Ostrosky, & Bishop, 1987), commenting, and questioning (Guralnick & Paul-Brown, 1984).

Similar to the social interaction skills described, the use of specific social-communicative skills is likely to facilitate peer-related social-communicative competence in preschoolers with developmental delays. Therefore, practitioners need to consider targeting these competencies, as well. Social-communicative competencies effective in facilitating social interactions include establishing eye contact, establishing a joint focus of attention, using descriptive talk, responding appropriately to an initiation by repeating, expanding, or clarifying a peer's comments, suggesting joint play, prompting requests, redirecting play activities (Goldstein & Ferrell, 1987; Goldstein & Kaczmarek, 1992; Goldstein & Wickstrom, 1986; Goldstein, Wickstrom, Hoyson, Jamieson, & Odom, 1988), taking turns, and continuing topic maintenance (Ostrosky et al., 1993).

In summary, this literature provides an initial foundation for identifying social-communicative skills and competencies for preschool-age children that may be effective in facilitating peer-related interactions. Table 7.1 provides a list of peer-related social and social-communicative skills for practitioners to consider when identifying and targeting skills to teach preschoolers who demonstrate developmental delays in peer-related interactions. Practitioners should consider targeting particular skills for intervention depending on individual children's abilities and needs in the area of social-communicative competence as determined through assessment.

In addition to targeting effective peer-related social-communicative skills for intervention, practitioners should consider the following critical factors when targeting skills and designing interventions: 1) the forms or topographies of social-communicative skills and competencies, 2) the social-communicative functions and goals, 3) the contexts in which these abilities are demonstrated, 4) the appropriateness of the form of the skill in obtaining the goal (e.g., a gestural request versus aggressive behavior), 5) the reciprocal nature of the social-communicative exchange, and 6) the degree of success in attaining the goal of the social-communicative exchange.

Social-communicative abilities may represent different forms or topographies. These forms may range from simple (e.g., a smile to initiate social contact) to highly complex (e.g., a conversation), and different forms may occur simultaneously. For example, to request play materials from a peer, children may use a very simple form such as grabbing a toy from a peer or a more complex form such as asking the peer to share the toy. Both of these forms serve the same function—that is, obtaining a toy from a peer. Whether children use a simple, complex,

Table 7.1. Recommended peer-related social and communicative competencies

Organizing play with peers
Demonstrating affection toward peers
Providing assistance to peers
Sharing play materials with peers
Engaging in rough-and-tumble play with peers
Engaging in conversations with peers
Dispensing information to peers
Responding to peers' initiations
Providing complimentary statements to peers
Requesting information or assistance from peers
Commenting to peers
Asking peers questions
Establishing eye contact with peers
Establishing a joint focus of attention with peers
Verbally describing play to peers
Repeating, expanding, or clarifying a peer's comments
Suggesting joint play with a peer
Redirecting peer's play activities
Prompting responses from peers
Taking turns during play activities
Maintaining the topic of conversation with peers

or a combination of forms (which is often the case) is related to their cognitive, social, and communication abilities as well as the form that has been proven to be most effective in meeting the goal. A child may have the ability to request the toy verbally; however, grabbing the toy as opposed to asking for the toy may be more efficient and effective in meeting his or her goal.

Children's social-communicative interactions may serve a variety of functions or goals and are often appropriate or inappropriate depending on the specific context in which they occur. Some skills are more effective than others in accomplishing a particular goal. For example, suggesting joint play (e.g., a child says to a peer, "Let's play") may not be as effective for the child in obtaining a play partner as using a play organizer (e.g., a child says to a peer, "Let's play race cars. Here is your car"). In addition, the contexts of peer-related social-communicative interactions may have an impact on the form and function of the behaviors used by children. A variety of skills may be effective in facilitating peer-related interactions, but the appropriateness of demonstrating these skills may change depending on the context. Competencies demonstrated during free play may have many different forms and functions in comparison to competencies displayed during other activities in which children engage in peer-related interactions. For example, effective skills to facilitate sharing play materials during a free play environment may include directing or commanding a peer to share toys. At another time, such as during snack time, directing or commanding peers to share their food may be effective but would be less appropriate. In order to determine the effectiveness and appropriateness of the skill, an evaluation of the function according to the context in which the skill occurs needs to be examined. Practitioners need to be aware of the influence contexts may have on the effectiveness and appropriateness of the skill and determine the appropriateness of social-communicative forms, functions, and goals.

Another critical component of social-communicative interactions is to examine the effectiveness of the reciprocal nature of the exchange. Effective interactions tend to progress through a consistent sequence of four stages—initiations, responses, maintaining interactions, and terminating interactions (Strain et al., 1977). In addition, specific social-communicative skills are more likely to be differentially effective in initiating, maintaining, or terminating peer-related exchanges. For example, skills such as redirecting, prompting, and persisting may prove to be more effective for children to learn in order to facilitate maintenance of social-communicative exchanges; however, these skills may be less effective for children to use for terminating an exchange. Once again, the appropriateness of initiating, responding, maintaining, and terminating interactions in relation to the context in which they occur as well as the skills learned when using these strategies are important aspects for practitioners to consider.

A final factor to consider is the success of the social-communicative interactions. After establishing the function or goals, practitioners need to examine children's success in obtaining their goals. Consider the following example. A child uses a play organizer to initiate play and says to his peer, "Let's play house. You be the mommy; I'll be the daddy." The goal in this example is to initiate a play activity. To determine if the child's goal is successfully met, the practitioners need to observe whether the peer responds and if the two children begin playing house together.

In summary, when targeting social-communicative skills for intervention, practitioners need to consider the form as well as the function of the behavior based on the context in which the skill occurs. In addition, the goals outlined previously as well as the sequence of reciprocal exchanges and the effectiveness of these exchanges should be considered when targeting social-communicative competencies for intervention. Nevertheless, further research is needed to establish a more exhaustive and normative database of competencies that promote peer-related social-communicative competence in preschool-age children with developmental delays and their peers; however, this literature provides a logical foundation for practitioners to use when targeting skills to facilitate peer-related social-communicative competence in preschool-age children.

ASSESSMENT OF SOCIAL-COMMUNICATIVE COMPETENCIES

Identification of skills to target for instruction begins with an assessment of children's social-communicative competence (e.g., Bricker & Pretti-Frontczak, 1996). Researchers and practitioners have used a variety of techniques to assess both social (e.g., Odom & Munson, 1996) and communication skills (Wetherby & Prizant, 1992) that are also applicable to assessment of social-communicative skills. The most effective technique for conducting assessments is to observe children directly interacting in natural and familiar environments during typically occurring activities. Given the reciprocal nature of peer-related social-communicative interactions and the continuous and dynamic interactions among children and their social and physical environments (Peck, 1993), we suggest assessing these competencies from an ecological and interactive perspective.

Using an ecological approach, the assessment of social-communicative abilities may occur through a variety of techniques that evaluate children's interactions with both their physical and social environments. Critical to the assessment of these competencies is the evaluation of specific social-communicative skills as suggested in Table 7.1 as well as the contextual components that may influence children's demonstration of these abilities. Figure 7.1 represents a schematic view of the assessment and intervention process using an ecological perspective. As illustrated, after identifying familiar environments, activities, routines, and peers to target for observation, an assessment of the physical and social contexts is conducted. If factors that may facilitate children's use of social-communicative competencies (e.g., socially competent peers) are missing, the practitioner should make adaptations to rectify this problem before continuing the assessment process. The third step is conducting a direct assessment of the child's social-communicative skills and competencies. Finally, an evaluation of the effectiveness and appropriateness of these skills given specific contexts is examined. Each of these components is discussed further in the next section.

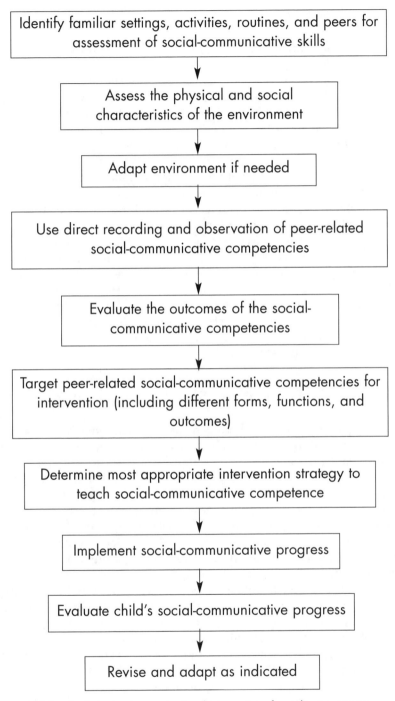

Figure 7.1. Ecobehavioral assessment and intervention of social-communicative competencies.

Targeting Familiar Activities, Peers, and Routines

Children engage in social-communicative interactions with their peers throughout the day during a variety of routines and activities (e.g., during snack time, free play, transitions). Therefore, the assessment of these skills should begin with the identification of several familiar activities and routines, as well as familiar peers to target for direct observation of social-communicative competencies. Direct observation should occur over several days and be scheduled at different times and locations during the day. In order to target these activities, routines, and peers, the practitioner may want to conduct an ecological analysis of the children's daily schedule and their friends by informally observing when these interactions are most likely to occur or asking the family of caregivers when they occur. Targeting several environments that require different types of social-communicative skills may provide the practitioner with a more representative sample of the children's social-communicative abilities. For example, the practitioner may want to target a structured activity such as morning circle to observe social greetings as well as free play or snack that has less structure and no specific social-communicative requirements.

Assessing the Physical and Social Characteristics

After targeting activities, routines, and peers, practitioners should assess the physical and social environments to determine the factors that may support and facilitate social-communicative skills. Researchers have suggested that specific contextual factors may set the stage for peer-related social interactions (Sainato & Carta, 1992). For example, the level of familiarity of the peers (Doyle, Connolly, & Rivest, 1980), the similarity in age and gender of the students (Hartup, 1983), and the size of the peer group (Asher & Erickson, 1979) are all likely to increase interactions among young children. In addition, pairing young children with mild disabilities with socially competent children may also increase interactions (Guralnick & Paul-Brown, 1984), but it may be necessary to train typical students how to interact with children with disabilities.

Similar to the identification of social factors, researchers have identified physical factors that facilitate social interactions among peers. Specific activities, such as free play, clean up (Odom, Peterson, McConnell, & Ostrosky, 1990) and snack (Kohl & Beckman, 1984) as well as the spatial density of the play space (Brown, Fox, & Brady, 1987) are more likely to encourage social interactions among preschoolers. Although the exact nature of the relationship still remains unclear, the structure (i.e., teacher versus child) of the activity is also likely to affect social interactions (DeKlyen & Odom, 1989; Shores, Hester, & Strain, 1976). Finally, it is critical to consider the types of toys and materials available and to examine the accessibility of social and familiar toys and play materials prior to assessing specific social-communicative abilities.

Assessment Using Naturalistic Procedures

Given the complex and reciprocal nature of these interactions, we suggest using direct observation procedures to assess social-communicative competence. Practitioners may want to consider using a snapshot assessment by directly observing specific social-communicative exchanges that occur naturally throughout various activities and recording the exact nature of those interactions. Figure 7.2 presents an observation form for practitioners to use to organize social-communicative observations into different components including 1) the type and form of the behavior, 2) the context surrounding the behavior and appropriateness of the behavior, 3) the goal of the behavior, 4) the reciprocal exchange of the behavior, and 5) the success of the exchange. Using a direct observation form that includes all these factors may assist the practitioner in identifying different components of social-communicative abilities to target for intervention.

In the case of Alexis, her teacher observed her interactions during free play and identified several social and social-communicative competencies to target for intervention (see the appendix at the end of this chapter). She determined through observation that Alexis demonstrated appropriate initiations and responses with a social goal; however, she was not able to attain her goals due to her limited social-communicative skills and her peers' inability to understand her cues. Therefore, the skills Alexis' teacher targeted for Alexis included sharing play materials, establishing eye contact, and responding to peers' initiations by smiling and reaching toward them. The teacher also targeted several competencies for Alexis' peers to learn that would facilitate Alexis' peer interactions including demonstrating affection to Alexis, providing assistance to her, sharing play materials with Alexis, and prompting responses from her.

After conducting an observational assessment, Jacob's teacher determined that although Jacob was highly successful in obtaining his goals, the forms of social-communicative behaviors he used were inappropriate. In addition, Jacob needed to learn more skills for playing

Child's name:		Date:		
Observer:		Activity:		
Time of observation:				

Type and form of behavior	Context and appropriate-ness of behavior	Goal of behavior	Reciprocity of exchange	Attainment of goal

Figure 7.2. Snapshot assessment of peer-related social-communicative skills.

with his peers. Therefore, his teacher targeted the following skills for intervention: organizing play, sharing play materials, responding appropriately to peer initiations, and asking peers questions about play.

In summary, there is no single or standardized technique or instrument available for assessing peer-related social-communicative competencies in preschool-age children. Rather, practitioners should approach assessment of these skills from an ecological perspective through direct observation of children's interactions with their peers within natural environments and routines. Direct observational assessment should include not only whether the children demonstrate the specific skills but also the qualitative aspects of these interactions—that is, the context and appropriateness of these interactions. After conducting a comprehensive assessment, the practitioner will need to target specific competencies for intervention and design intervention strategies to facilitate skill acquisition and maintenance.

INTERVENTIONS FOR PROMOTING PEER-RELATED SOCIAL-COMMUNICATIVE COMPETENCE

Given the critical nature of social-communicative competence in children's development, practitioners should facilitate these skills in all young children; however, it is particularly important for practitioners to target social-communicative skills and design intervention strategies to promote successful peer-related exchanges for children who may demonstrate developmental delays in this area. Often, young children demonstrate individual differences in acquiring skills. As with Alexis, children may demonstrate *competence* problems in acquiring skills (i.e., they do not know how or lack the ability to perform the skill) and/or they may demonstrate *performance* problems in demonstrating the skills (i.e., they know how to perform the skill, but they do not perform the skill) as with Jacob. As a result of individual differences, different children may benefit from different types and intensities of intervention and may acquire skills at different rates and in different sequences.

Several levels of intervention strategies have been developed to facilitate both social and communicative skills: 1) inclusion with socially responsive peers (Odom & Munson, 1996), 2) arrangement of developmentally appropriate and engaging environments (Bredekamp & Copple, 1997; Sainato & Carta, 1992), 3) use of incidental teaching strategies (McGee, Almeida, Sulzer-Azaroff, & Feldman, 1992), and 4) implementation of coaching interventions (English, Goldstein, Shafer, & Kaczmarek, 1997) (see Figure 7.3). Prior to implementing inter-

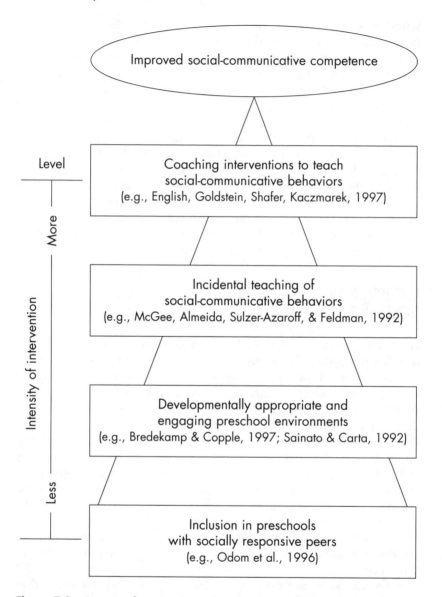

Figure 7.3.   Strategies for promoting and supporting preschool children's peer-related social-communicative competence. (From Brown, W.H., & Conroy, M.A. [1997]. *Inclusion of preschool children with developmental disabilities in early childhood education programs.* Little Rock, AR: Southern Early Childhood Association; adapted with permission from *Dimensions of Early Childhood,* Southern Early Childhood Association, 8500 W. Markham, Suite 105, Little Rock, AR 72205 1-800-305-7322.)

vention strategies, practitioners should be certain that the appropriate environmental context exists for facilitating social-communicative competencies. Therefore, when designing interventions it is critical to start from an ecological perspective.

Employing an Ecological Perspective for Planning Interventions

Designing interventions from an ecological perspective places children in an environment conducive to peer interaction. Practitioners should plan for and develop an appropriate social and physical context that facilitates social-communicative skills. The physical and social environment should be motivating in order to encourage exploration and peer-related interactions. It is important that the materials in the classroom are within an appropriate developmental range for the children and that peers are familiar and socially responsive. The physical and social environment should be responsive so that when children engage in social-communicative exchanges, these interactions are reciprocated and successful.

Because the ecological environment is critical, both Alexis' and Jacob's teachers have included toys and materials that are appropriate for their levels of development and abilities. Alexis' teacher has adapted materials (e.g., paint brushes, sponges, scoops) at the sand and art tables, two of Alexis' favorite areas, so that she can manipulate materials independently. Jacob's teacher has planned for there to be a sufficient number of toys for all children in the classroom to share. In addition, both teachers have made certain that peers in the classroom are socially responsive and model appropriate peer interaction skills.

Hierarchy of Intervention Techniques

As illustrated in Figure 7.3, several levels of interventions can be implemented to foster social-communicative competencies. These interventions vary according to intensity level and should be implemented based on the individual needs of the child as determined through observational assessment. Practitioners should begin intervention using the least intensive strategy and progress to more intense interventions if warranted. Typically, the more significant the needs of individual children, the more intensive intervention strategies are warranted (Odom, McConnell, & McEvoy, 1992). That is, if a child has significant delays in the areas of social and communicative skills, such as Alexis does, the practitioner will most likely need to employ more intensive intervention strategies.

Including children with developmental delays in preschool programs with socially responsive peers (Odom et al., 1996) and in environments that are developmentally appropriate and engaging (Bredekamp & Copple, 1997; Sainato & Carta, 1992) is the initial level of intervention that practitioners should use to facilitate social-communicative competencies. Practitioners should arrange the physical and social environments to facilitate social-communicative exchanges among children with disabilities and their peers. The activities and space should be arranged to encourage active engagement and exploration with peers. Peers should be socially responsive so that when children initiate social-communicative exchanges, their efforts are reciprocated. The materials should be developmentally appropriate for children in order to encourage active engagement. Developing an environment that is developmentally appropriate and fosters active exploration and engagement with socially responsive peers is the initial step for increasing children's social-communicative competencies. Although almost all children can benefit from this level of intervention, many children need a more intensive level of intervention, such as incidental teaching.

Incidental teaching is a naturalistic intervention strategy that practitioners can use to increase appropriate social-communicative competencies (McGee et al., 1992). There are typically four steps described in the literature for implementing incidental teaching strategies on social behaviors (Brown, McEvoy, & Bishop, 1991). The first step is to target unstructured activities that children with disabilities are showing interest in and are actively exploring. Once a practitioner observes a child with disabilities actively engaging, the next step is to prompt the child to engage in a social-communicative behavior. The third step is for the practitioner to elaborate on the child's response or to model an appropriate response (if needed). The final step is for the practitioner to provide positive feedback and praise to the child with disabilities. The following is an example of how Alexis' and Jacob's teachers use incidental teaching strategies to facilitate their peer-related interactions.

Rebecca and Tyrone are playing in the art area. Alexis' teacher, Ms. Jennifer, observes Alexis looking at Rebecca and Tyrone playing. Ms. Jennifer asks Alexis "Do you want to play at the art table?" Alexis looks at Ms. Jennifer and then at the art table. In response, Ms. Jennifer verbally prompts Alexis to point toward the art table and provides a gestural model to encourage her to smile indicating that she wants to play. Next, Ms. Jennifer physically guides Alexis to point toward the art table and moves Alexis over to the table. Ms. Jennifer asks Rebecca and Tyrone if they will share their art materials with Alexis. Rebecca says, "Alexis, you can have my sponge. We are making fall leaves." Alexis begins to make flowers with Rebecca and Tyrone. Ms. Jennifer says, "Alexis, it is nice to see you play with Rebecca and Tyrone."

Jacob's teacher, Mr. Timothy, observes Jacob approach his friend, Richard, who is riding a bike on the playground. Mr. Timothy says to Jacob, "Do you want to ride bikes with Richard?" Jacob says, "That is my bike!" Mr. Timothy prompts Jacob, "Ask Richard to share his bike." Jacob says, "Richard, can I ride the bike?" Richard gives Jacob the bike, and Mr. Timothy praises both Jacob and Richard for sharing their play materials.

Incidental teaching strategies have many advantages for use to facilitate social-communicative exchanges. They are relatively simple to use. The intervention strategies are primarily child directed and natural consequences reinforce and maintain appropriate behaviors. Table 7.2 provides practical suggestions for using incidental teaching strategies to facilitate social-communicative behaviors.

Some children who demonstrate significant developmental delays may need a more intensive intervention strategy than simply rearranging and enhancing the environment or implementing incidental teaching strategies. As illustrated in Figure 7.3, practitioners can also use adult and peer-mediated coaching strategies to teach social-communicative skills. Coaching strategies are intervention strategies that are highly planned, directed, and monitored by the practitioner. They include direct intervention between the practitioner and the children who are demonstrating social-communicative delays. In addition, the practitioner

Table 7.2. Incidental teaching suggestions for facilitating social-communicative skills

Identify children who will benefit from additional opportunities to interact with peers appropriately.

Identify common activities and circumstances that will allow the teacher to use incidental teaching strategies (e.g., free play, center time, snack time, arrival time).

Plan a variety of methods to encourage peer interactions through physical or verbal guidance. Provide encouragement and support when peer interactions occur.

Implement incidental teaching strategies when you have time to observe and intervene on children's behaviors. Often, less structured times are the best to target for incidental teaching.

Follow the child's lead when implementing incidental teaching. Children will usually indicate their interests and needs.

Provide teacher support by encouraging children to interact with their peers. Provide praise and support to the peers who are reciprocally interacting with the target children.

can teach coaching strategies to peers, and in return peers may play the role of an interventionist.

When implementing adult-mediated intervention techniques, the practitioner in the classroom may directly prompt children to use their social and communicative skills to interact with one another and provide positive feedback such as praise to children when they begin to interact. For example, when Alexis' teacher observes her and a peer playing at the water table side by side rather than cooperatively, her teacher suggests to the children to begin playing together. Once the children begin to share water toys and interact with one another, she praises them for sharing their toys and playing together.

A second adult-mediated strategy that practitioners may use is to conduct social-communicative peer-interaction training groups. The practitioner can lead role-playing groups or group games that facilitate social-communicative exchanges. For example, Jacob's teacher has chosen to conduct an affection activity to the song "The Farmer in the Dell" to facilitate positive peer-related social interactions among Jacob and his friends. In this activity, Mr. Timothy instructs all the children in the class to show affection toward each other (e.g., hug each other) as they sign the song. After conducting this activity, Mr. Timothy notices that Karin, a peer in Jacob's class, asks Jacob to share a book during free play, and Jacob responds in a positive manner.

Affection activities are another type of adult-mediated intervention strategy to facilitate social-communicative interactions. A thorough description of affection activities is beyond the scope of this chapter, but further description of affection activities can be found in Brown, Ragland, and Bishop (1989). In addition, the reader is referred to Odom and McConnell's (1993) *Play Time/Social Time* and Mize's (1995) *Cognitive-Social Learning Intervention Model* for further descriptions of adult- and peer-mediated intervention techniques.

Similar to adult-mediated interventions, peers can be used to teach social-communicative competencies to children with developmental delays. There are several steps practitioners need to consider in order to use peers as interventionists. First, targeting peers who are socially and communicatively sophisticated is important. Peers who have a high level of appropriate social interaction skills and are able to communicate successfully should be targeted as peer interventions. Not only should the practitioner target appropriate skills and strategies and plan the environment to support these skills, but the practitioner will also need to plan for and train peers to implement the interventions. That is, practitioners must train the peers to make social-communicative bids to children with disabilities and be responsive to the children's bids to social-communicative exchanges. In addition to being responsive, peers need to learn how to be persistent in their social bids. For example, if a peer suggests joint play to a child with disabilities and this child is unresponsive, it is important for the peer to persist with this child to further encourage a social-communicative exchange.

Providing positive feedback to the peers for making social bids to the children targeted for intervention is an important role of the practitioner when implementing this strategy. In addition to training the peers, the practitioner often will need to teach the children with disabilities specific appropriate social-communicative competencies to use when interacting with their peers. Role-playing sessions may be needed to practice and master these skills in a structured environment. After the environment is arranged and training is provided to both the peers and the target children, the practitioner will still need to use adult-mediated prompting and praising to facilitate social-communicative interactions. After structuring and adapting the environment and implementing incidental teaching strategies, Alexis' teacher observes that her social interactions still need improvement. She decides to implement a peer-directed coaching strategy.

Ms. Jennifer chooses several children in the class to become better friends with Alexis. Using role-playing, Ms. Jennifer teaches these children how to interact with Alexis by instructing them to "read" Alexis's communication skills such as looking and smiling. She also teaches the peers to encourage Alexis to respond to their initiations and persist at interacting with her. Following the role-play activity, Ms. Jennifer coaches the peers to ask Alexis to play house with them during free play. She prompts both the peers and Alexis to play together and provides feedback and praise as they begin to interact.

Coaching interventions have been demonstrated to successfully increase social and communicative behaviors in young children with developmental delays. There are a variety of techniques to use when implementing coaching interventions (e.g., English, Goldstein, Kaczmarek, & Shafer, 1996; English et al., 1997). Table 7.3 provides an overview of factors that the practitioner will want to consider when implementing peer-mediated interventions that facilitate social-communicative competencies.

CONCLUSION

Young children with developmental delays often have difficulties in the area of social-communicative competence that affect their ability to

Table 7.3.   Peer-mediated interventions to facilitate social-communicative competencies

Target competencies and goals to teach target children appropriate social-communicative behaviors.

Arrange the environment to facilitate peer interactions (e.g., toys, materials, space).

Teach the target child specific appropriate social-communicative competencies to use in the classroom with peers.

Teach the peers specific skills for initiating to, responding to, maintaining, or terminating interactions with the target child.

Use role-playing sessions to practice and master these skills in a structured setting.

Prompt the target child and peers to use social-communicative competencies that have been targeted and taught.

Provide praise when children demonstrate these skills.

Monitor progress and revise and adapt instructional strategies as needed.

interact successfully with their peers. The beginning of this chapter has reviewed the literature and outlines skills and competencies to target when working with young children who demonstrate social-communicative delays. When targeting skills, we have suggested that practitioners consider appropriateness, successfulness, and the context surrounding the skills. Next, we have provided strategies for practitioners to use when assessing social-communicative skills and competencies. Although practitioners can use a variety of techniques to assess these skills, we recommend the use of direct observational strategies to obtain information regarding the form and function, context, appropriateness, and successfulness of the social-communicative exchange. Finally, the chapter has outlined intervention techniques to use for ameliorating delays in this area. When designing an effective intervention program, the practitioner should choose from a menu of intervention techniques beginning with the least intrusive strategy to foster these skills. Practitioners need to approach the assessment and intervention of social-communicative competencies from an ecological perspective to provide children with the most appropriate environment for developing their social-communicative competence. With the implementation of effective intervention strategies, children such as Alexis and Jacob will improve their peer-related social-communicative abilities.

REFERENCES

Asher, K.N., & Erickson, M.R. (1979). Effects of varying child–teacher ratio and group size on day care children's and teacher's behavior. *American Journal of Orthopsychiatry, 49,* 518–521.

Bredekamp, S., & Copple, C. (Eds.). (1997). *Developmentally appropriate practice in early childhood programs* (Rev. ed.). Washington, DC: National Association for the Education of Young Children.

Bricker, D., & Pretti-Frontczak, K. (Eds.). (1996). *Assessment, evaluation, and programming system for infants and children: Vol. 3. AEPS measurement for three to six years*. Baltimore: Paul H. Brookes Publishing Co.

Brown, W.H., Fox, J.J., & Brady, M.P. (1987). Effects of spatial density on 3- and 4-year-old children's socially directed behavior during free play: An investigation of a setting factor. *Education and Treatment of Children, 10*, 247–258.

Brown, W.H., McEvoy, M.A., & Bishop, J.N. (1991). Incidental teaching of social behavior: A naturalistic approach to promoting young children's peer interactions. *Teaching Exceptional Children, 24*, 35–58.

Brown, W.H., Odom, S.L., & Holcombe, A. (1996). Observational assessment of young children's social behavior with peers. *Early Childhood Research Quarterly, 11*, 19–40.

Brown, W.H., Ragland, E.U., & Bishop, N. (1989). *A socialization curriculum for preschool programs that integrate children with handicaps*. Nashville: Vanderbilt University Press.

DeKlyen, M., & Odom, S.L. (1989). Activity structure and social interactions with peers in developmentally integrated play groups. *Journal of Early Intervention, 13*, 342–352.

Doyle, A.A., Connolly, J., & Rivest, L. (1980). The effects of playmate familiarity on the social interactions of young children. *Child Development, 51*, 217–223.

English, K., Goldstein, H., Kaczmarek, L., & Shafer, K (1996). "Buddy skills" for preschoolers. *Teaching Exceptional Children, 28*, 62–66.

English, K., Goldstein, H., Shafer, K., & Kaczmarek, L. (1997). Promoting interactions among preschoolers with and without disabilities: Effects of a buddy skills training program. *Exceptional Children, 63*, 229–243.

Fox, J.J., Shores, R., Lindeman, D., & Strain, P. (1986). Maintaining social initiations with withdrawn handicapped and nonhandicapped preschoolers through a response-dependent fading tactic. *Journal of Abnormal Child Psychology, 14*, 387–396.

Goldstein, H., & Ferrell, D. (1987). Augmenting communicative interaction between handicapped and nonhandicapped preschool children. *Journal of Speech and Hearing Disorders, 52*, 200–211.

Goldstein, H., & Kaczmarek, L. (1992). Promoting communicative interactions among children in integrated intervention settings. In S.F. Warren & J. Reichle (Series & Vol. Eds.), *Communication and language intervention series: Vol. 1. Causes and effects in communication and language intervention* (pp. 81–112). Baltimore: Paul H. Brookes Publishing Co.

Goldstein, H., & Wickstrom, S. (1986). Peer intervention effects on communicative interaction among handicapped and nonhandicapped preschoolers. *Journal of Applied Behavior Analysis, 19*, 209–214.

Goldstein, H., Wickstrom, S., Hoyson, M., Jamieson, B., & Odom, S.L. (1988). Effects of sociodramatic play training on social and communicative interactions. *Education and Treatment of Children, 11*, 97–117.

Guralnick, M.J., & Paul-Brown, D.P. (1984). Communicative adjustments during behavior request episodes among children at different developmental levels. *Child Development, 55*, 911–919.

Hartup. W.W. (1983). Peer relations. In P.H. Mussen & E.M. Hetherington (Eds.), *Carmichael's manual of child psychology* (Vol. 4, pp. 103–196). New York: John Wiley & Sons.

Kohl, F.L., & Beckman, P.J. (1984). A comparison of handicapped and nonhandicapped preschooler's interactions across classroom activities. *Journal of the Division of Early Childhood, 8*, 49–56.

McGee, G., Almeida, C., Sulzer-Azaroff, B., & Feldman, R.S. (1992). Promoting reciprocal interactions via peer incidental teaching. *Journal of Applied Behavior Analysis, 25,* 117–126.

Mize, J. (1995). Coaching preschool children in social skills: A cognitive-social learning curriculum. In G. Carledge & J.F. Milburn (Eds.), *Teaching social skills to children and youth: Innovative approaches* (3rd ed., pp. 237–261). Needham Heights, MA: Allyn & Bacon.

Odom, S.L., & Brown, W.H. (1993). Social interaction skills interventions for young children with disabilities in integrated settings. In C.A. Peck, S.L. Odom, & D.D. Bricker (Eds.), *Integrating young children with disabilities in community programs: Ecological perspectives on research and implementation* (pp. 39–64). Baltimore: Paul H. Brookes Publishing Co.

Odom, S.L., & McConnell, S.R. (1993). *Play time/social time: Organizing your classroom to build interaction skills.* San Antonio, TX: Communication Skill Builders.

Odom, S.L., McConnell, S.R., & McEvoy, M.A. (Eds.). (1992). *Social competence of young children with disabilities: Issues and strategies for intervention.* Baltimore: Paul H. Brookes Publishing Co.

Odom, S.L., McEvoy, M.A., Ostrosky, M., & Bishop, L. (1987, May). *Observing the functional classes of social interactions of preschool children.* Paper presented at the annual convention of the Association for Behavior Analysis, Nashville.

Odom, S.L., & Munson, L. (1996). Assessing social performance. In M. McLean, D.B. Bailey, & M. Wolery (Eds.), *Assessing infants and preschoolers with special needs* (pp. 398–434). Columbus, OH: Charles E. Merrill.

Odom, S.L., & Ogawa, I. (1991). Direct observation of young children's social interaction with peers: A review of methodology. *Behavioral Assessment, 14,* 407–441.

Odom, S.L., Peck, C.A., Hanson, M., Beckman, P.J., Kaiser, A.P., Lieber, J., Brown, W.H., Horn, E.M., & Schwartz, I.S. (1996). Inclusion of young children with disabilities: An ecological analysis. *Social Policy Report of the Society for Research in Child Development, 10,* 18–30.

Odom, S.L., Peterson, C., McConnell, S., & Ostrosky, M. (1990). Ecobehavioral analysis of early education/special classroom settings and peer social interaction. *Education and Treatment of Children, 13,* 316–330.

Ostrosky, M.M., Kaiser, A.P., & Odom, S.L. (1993). Facilitating children's social communicative interactions through the use of peer-mediated interventions. In S.F. Warren & J. Reichle (Series Eds.) & A.P. Kaiser & D.B. Gray (Vol. Eds.), *Communication and language intervention series: Vol. 2. Enhancing children's communication: Research foundations for intervention* (pp. 159–187). Baltimore: Paul H. Brookes Publishing Co.

Peck, C.A. (1993). Ecological perspectives on the implementation of integrated early childhood programs. In C.A. Peck, S.L., Odom, & D.D. Bricker (Eds.), *Integrating young children with disabilities into community programs: Ecological perspectives on research and implementation* (pp. 3–15). Baltimore: Paul H. Brookes Publishing Co.

Sainato, D.M., & Carta, J.J. (1992). Classroom influences on the development of social competence in young children with disabilities. In S.L. Odom, S.R. McConnell, & M.A. McEvoy (Eds.) *Social competence of young children with disabilities: Issues and strategies for intervention* (pp. 93–109). Baltimore: Paul H. Brookes Publishing Company.

Shores, R.E., Hester, P., & Strain, P.S. (1976). The effects of amount and type of teacher–child interaction on child–child interaction during free-play. *Psychology in the Schools, 13,* 171–175.

Strain, P.S., Shores, R.E., & Kerr, M.M. (1976). An experimental analysis of "spillover" effects on social interaction among behaviorally handicapped preschool children. *Journal of Applied Behavior Analysis, 9,* 31–40.

Strain, P.S., Shores, R.E., & Timm, M.A. (1977). Effects of peer social initiations on the behavior of withdrawn preschool children. *Journal of Applied Behavior Analysis, 10,* 289–298.

Tremblay, A., Strain, P.S., Hendrickson, J.M., & Shores, R.E. (1981). Social interactions of normally developing preschool children: Using normative data for subject selection and target behavior selection. *Behavior Modification, 5,* 237–253.

Wetherby, A.M., & Prizant, B.M. (1992). Profiling young children's communicative competence. In S.F. Warren & J. Reichle (Series & Vol. Eds.), *Communication and language intervention series: Vol. 1. Causes and effects in communication and language intervention* (pp. 217–254). Baltimore: Paul H. Brookes Publishing Co.

Appendix

Child's name:	*Alexis*
Age:	*3 years old*
Location:	*Inclusive early childhood program*

1. Snapshot assessment

Child's name: *Alexis*   Date: *September 7, 2000*
Observer: *Jennifer Logan*   Activity: *Free play*
Time of observation: *9:30 A.M. – 10:00 A.M.*

Type and form of behavior	Context and appropriateness of behavior	Goal of behavior	Reciprocity of exchange	Attainment of goal
After being asked to play "castle" by her friend Becky, Alexis *looks* at Becky *(makes eye contact)*	Block area Responsive peer Interesting play materials Appropriate response to an initiation	To play with a peer	Response to a peer initiation	Not successful; Alexis does not follow Becky as she moves across the block area
Alexis watches two of her friends play in the water table. She vocalizes, looks at the teacher, and reaches toward the table *(suggesting joint play with peers)*	Water table Interesting play materials Unresponsive peers Appropriate request for initiating play	To play with peers at the water table	Initiation	Successful; the teacher places Alexis in a prone stander at the water table

2. Social-communicative skills

Goals for Alexis:
Sharing play materials
Establishing eye contact
Responding to peers' initiations by smiling and reaching toward them

Goals for Alexis' peers:
Demonstrating affection toward Alexis
Providing assistance to Alexis
Sharing play materials with Alexis
Prompting Alexis to respond to initiations

3. Arrangement of the ecological environment to facilitate social-communicative interactions

Adapt art center with paintbrushes with Velcro that can be strapped to Alexis' hand
Adapt art center with rubber tablemat so paints will not move
Adapt art center with sponges so Alexis can use independently for painting
Place small scoops at the sand table so Alexis can manipulate them independently
Ensure socially responsive peers who can prompt social interactions with Alexis

4. Intervention Strategies

Implement incidental teaching strategies during free play activites indoor and outdoors
Implement coaching interventions including prompting and praise peers and teaching peers to be interventionists

Child's name:	Jacob
Age:	4 years old
Location:	Head Start classroom

1. Assessment of social-communicative skills

Child's name: _Jacob_____ Date: _September 10, 2000_____
Observer: _Timothy Richards_____ Activity: _Outdoor free play_____
Time of observation: _8:30 A.M.—9:00 A.M._____

Type and form of behavior	Context and appropriateness of behavior	Goal of behavior	Reciprocity of exchange	Attainment of goal
Jacob runs up to Manuel on the bike and says, "It's my turn," and Manuel gets off the bike (requesting play items)	Bikes on the playground Inappropriate behavior	Requesting play item	Initiation	Successful; Jacob obtained the bike and began to ride
Peer asks Jacob if she can play on the see-saw. Jacob says, "No, it is my turn" (response to a peer initiation)	Seesaw on the playground Responsive peer Inappropriate behavior	Obtaining play activity	Response	Successful; Jacob continued to play on the seesaw
Jacob approaches two peers playing balls and says, "I want to play ball" while grabbing the ball out of their hands. One boy grabs the ball back and says "No." Jacob pushes him down and grabs the ball (requesting play item)	Black top area of the playground with balls Inappropriate behavior	Obtaining play activity	Initiation	Unsuccessful; Jacob is told by the teacher to give the ball back and play elsewhere

2. Social-communicative competencies targeted for Jacob

Organizing play with his peers using verbal skills
Sharing play materials with his peers
Responding appropriately to peers' initiations
Asking peers questions during play

3. Arrangement of the ecological environment to facilitate social-communicative interactions

Ensure a sufficient number of blocks, trucks, balls, tricycles, and other materials
Ensure socially appropriate peers who are not aggressive
Train peers to be responsive to Jacob's attempts to share materials

4. Intervention strategies

Implement incidental teaching strategies during free play activites indoors and outdoors
Implement coaching interventions including affection activities

8

Social-Communicative
Strategies for School-Age Children

Debra M. Kamps, Tammy Kravits, and Michelle Ross

Educational environments provide a rich environment for students with developmental disabilities to learn social and communicative skills. Odom and McConnell in a special issue of the *Journal of Applied Behavior Analysis* devoted to social competence stated,

> Successful participation in social interaction is a hallmark skill of our species. Performing adequately in social situations defines our competence as individuals and establishes the necessary social history for future interactions. . . . Social competence is the effective and appropriate use of social behavior in interactions with an individual . . . a lack of social competence is marked by behavior that fails to produce, maintain, or enhance positive interactions with others or by a complete absence of behavior in contexts in which it is required. (1992, pp. 239–240)

A broader definition would propose that *social competence* is a general term to summarize children's quality of communication, interaction, and appropriate engagement, as observed by teachers, parents, peers, and others in real-life social environments. It evaluates the effectiveness (outcomes of the social task) and the appropriateness (amount, type, variety of behaviors) of the interactions in a particular environment. Thus, social competence and instruction include appropriate social, communicative, and behavior skills within the context of the environment, and assessment through direct observation of 1) reciprocity of interactions; 2) social status and networks; and 3) accomplishment of social tasks, that is, goals and actual performance of skills (Guralnick, 1990; Odom & McConnell, 1992; Odom, McConnell, & McEvoy, 1992; Walker, Hops, & Greenwood, 1988).

Clearly, a combined focus on social skills instruction and communication training, rather than sole reliance on separate programming, (e.g., therapy-based language intervention, after-school social events) is necessary to meet these outcomes. That is, communication training is irrelevant if it does not include a social or interactive component with generalization to naturalistic environments. Likewise, social skills training is irrelevant if it does not include an effective means of communication with teachers, parents, and peers. For some children with developmental disabilities, ongoing support, training, and structuring of the natural environment and inclusion with peers are critical to acquisition and maintenance of socially competent performance (Odom & McConnell, 1992). This chapter describes the literature supporting this multicomponent approach to social-communicative interventions, with a focus on elementary- and middle school–age children as participants in reported studies. We review the following intervention strategies for improving social competence via teaching of social and communicative skills for school-age children: 1) adult mediation using naturalistic strategies and direct instruction in social skills and play-group formats, 2) peer mediation in playgroup and social environments, 3) augmentative and alternative communication (AAC) systems within social structures, 4) self-management strategies for social behaviors, 5) peer mediation within tutoring and cooperative learning formats, and 6) peer networks systems for school environments.

ADULT-MEDIATED INSTRUCTION WITHIN INDIVIDUAL AND GROUP FORMATS

Adult mediation of social-communicative skills includes functional social-communicative training using naturalistic strategies and direct instruction within small-group environments with peers as models. Interventions have included both naturalistic teaching methods as well as direct instruction within clinical and school environments for school-age children with disabilities. Rowland and Schweigert (1993) described three major characteristics of functional communication: 1) occurs in everyday, natural environments, 2) results in real consequences whereby the communication affects the environment, and 3) includes spontaneous and directed language. Specific communicative functions that have a social component include greetings, requests for assistance, requests for objects, requests for information, protests, and commenting behaviors (Kaiser, Alpert, & Warren, 1987; Reichle, York, & Sigafoos, 1991).

Naturalistic Approaches to Teaching Social-Communicative Skills

Naturalistic instruction is largely child directed and builds on environmental arrangements designed to increase opportunities for children to use language (Koegel & Koegel, 1995; Koegel, O'Dell, & Koegel, 1987). Some of these teaching strategies include 1) following the child's lead (i.e., teaching occurs based on child preferences or interests), 2) providing multiple examples in the child's natural environment, 3) explicitly prompting language (i.e., delays are provided to allow children to use their language instead of having teachers ask direct questions), 4) using direct and natural consequences, 5) reinforcing communicative attempts, and 6) emulating natural interactions (e.g., turn taking). For example, milieu language teaching relies on a functional communication model and uses many of these teaching strategies when implementing child-directed modeling, mand-model, and time-delay procedures. Child-directed modeling entails waiting for the child to show interest in items before modeling an appropriate communicative act to request the item. In the mand-model procedure, the adult arranges a variety of interesting materials and cues to prompt the language. In the time delay procedure, the adult identifies occasions during which the child is likely to need assistance or want materials, establishes joint attention, waits for the child to initiate a request or models the request, and subsequently gives access for correct communication or for attempts (Hart & Risley, 1978; Kaiser et al., 1987).

In another example of naturalistic teaching, Dyer (1989) investigated the relationship between spontaneous language and child preferences of three children with autism ages 9–12 years. Spontaneous requesting was examined during two play conditions. In one condition, students were allowed access to preferred reinforcers (i.e., following the child's lead), and in the other condition, only nonpreferred items were available. Preferences were determined through an assessment of various edibles and toy items prior to each experimental session. During sessions, therapists sat and played with toy items or took bites of designated foods, and items were given to the student if a verbal request was made. Results indicated a higher frequency of spontaneous requesting for all students when preferred items or activities were available.

Charlop and colleagues also demonstrated the motivating power of child preferences (Charlop, Schreibman, & Thibodeau, 1985). These investigators used a time-delay procedure to teach 5- to 11-year-olds with autism to request desired items in the absence of verbal cues. Sessions were conducted in a therapy room with the preferred food and drinks available for snack time for the students. All seven children learned to make spontaneous requests and generalized across people, environments, and stimuli. Other researchers have used time-delay and child initiation procedures to teach 1) basic social language skills such as initiating greetings with parents and saying "thank you" and "please" with 4- to 9-year-olds with autism (Charlop & Trasowech, 1991; Matson, Sevin, Fridley, & Love, 1990), 2) information-seeking questions such as "What's that?" with 5- to 6-year-olds with autism (Taylor & Harris, 1995), and 3) more frequent social interaction and communication during ball playing with 5- to 6-year-olds with mental retardation (Coe, Matson, Fee, Manikam, & Linarello, 1990). Similarly, Camarata and Nelson (1992) found that targeted language structures were learned more rapidly when 4- to 5-year-olds with language impairments were allowed to select activities during speech-language therapy sessions.

Koegel, O'Dell, and Koegel (1987) developed another naturalistic procedure, the Natural Language Paradigm (NLP), to improve communication skills during play for children with developmental disabilities. The NLP combines traditional operant procedures and natural language procedures to increase motivation by incorporating child preferences into natural teaching situations (e.g., turn taking) and to reinforce all verbal utterances. In this study, the language learning of two children with autism, ages 4 and 5, was evaluated in a clinical environment using a more traditional teaching approach (i.e., similar to discrete trial format) followed by the NLP approach. In the NLP sessions, children selected items, adults modeled language and play with toys, and adults reinforced communicative attempts with access to toys. Both children demonstrated increases in immediate and deferred imitation, as well as spontaneous utterances when the NLP was implemented. These effects also generalized to probes taken outside of the clinic. In a second study (Koegel, O'Dell, & Koegel, 1987), the NLP was implemented with four children with autism ages 3–11. Reinforcement of all verbal attempts produced higher frequencies of correct verbal behavior as well as more positive affect.

"Structured joint action routines" is a similar strategy that has been used successfully with children with mental retardation to facilitate communication (Snyder-McLean, Solomonson, McLean, & Sack, 1984). Key components include a unifying theme or purpose (e.g., making a snack, fireman routine), interactive rather than parallel activities, specific roles for participants, structures for turn taking in a predictable sequence, and planned repetition with controlled variation to promote generalization. The authors stressed that the joint action routines must work as a vehicle for facilitating communication and must effectively engage the interest and participation of the student to maintain motivation. Increases in intentional communication and peer interaction (with other students with disabilities) for adolescents and preschoolers suggests that joint action routines are a promising approach for school-age students, as well (McLean, Snyder-McLean, Jacobs, & Rowland, 1981).

Adult-Mediated Instruction within Social Skills Groups and Peer-Inclusive Play

A growing literature indicates that adults can mediate the teaching of social interaction by using peers. Examples include the use of play-groups with peers for teaching social-communicative behaviors, direct instruction strategies including social skills lessons and scripts, and peer-administered reinforcement schedules to increase social interaction (Carr & Darcy, 1990; Gonzalez-Lopez & Kamps, 1997; Kamps et al., 1992).

Several investigators have used scripted lessons and direct instruction to improve social competence (Kamps et al., 1992; Odom, Chandler, et al., 1992; Pierce & Schreibman, 1997; Sasso, Melloy, & Kavale, 1990; Strain, Kerr, & Ragland, 1979). Scripted lessons have been used to teach key skills such as 1) greetings and social conventions (i.e., using names, saying hello, asking friends to play, asking questions, conversing, keeping it going), 2) imitation and following instructions, 3) sharing and taking turns, and 4) helping. More advanced skills have included complimenting and encouraging others, anger management, negotiating, and other problem-solving skills. Several published curricula (see Table 8.1) have helpful "scripted" lessons for teachers to follow. These curricula are particularly helpful for teaching initial play and social interaction skills (Odom & McConnell, 1997; Walker et al., 1988; Wilson, 1993). Some of these curricula provide lessons and role-plays for more advanced social interaction as well as problem-solving skills (Jackson, Jackson, & Monroe, 1983; Walker et al., 1988).

When using these lessons, it is critical that children with disabilities receive consistent, direct instruction of social skills with multiple opportunities to respond (i.e., repeated practice of specific skills) with siblings and peers (Kamps et al., 1992; Strain & Danko, 1995). Finally, other resources are listed for establishing communicative repertoires and expanding language—that is, skills that may enhance student performance within peer groups (Koegel et al., 1989; Quill, 1995). All materials are applicable to elementary-age students, and some relate to preschool ages as well.

Table 8.1. Sample curricula and programming guides

Carr, E.G., Levin, L., McConnachie, G., Carlson, J.I., Kemp, D.C., & Smith, C.E. (1994). *Communication-based intervention for problem behavior: A user's guide for producing positive change.* Baltimore: Paul H. Brookes Publishing Co.

Gray, C. (1993). *The social story book.* Jenison, MI: Jenison Public Schools.

Jackson, N., Jackson, D., & Monroe, C. (1983). *Getting along with others: Teaching social effectiveness to children.* Champaign, IL: Research Press.

Koegel, L.K., Koegel, R.L., & Dunlap, G. (1996). *Positive behavioral support: Including people with difficult behavior in the community.* Baltimore: Paul H. Brookes Publishing Co.

Koegel, L., Koegel, R., & Parks, D. (1992). *How to teach self-management to people with severe disabilities: A training manual.* Santa Barbara: University of California.

Koegel, R.L., & Koegel, L.K. (1995). *Teaching children with autism: Strategies for initiating positive interactions and improving learning opportunities.* Baltimore: Paul H. Brookes Publishing Co.

Koegel, R., Schreibman, L., Good, A., Cerniglia, L., Murphy, C., & Koegel, L. (1989). *How to teach pivotal behaviors to children with autism: A training manual.* Santa Barbara: University of California.

Lovaas, O. (1981). *Teaching developmentally disabled children: The me book.* Austin, TX: PRO-ED.

Maurice, C., Green, G., & Luce, S. (1996). *Behavioral intervention for young children with autism: A manual for parents and professionals.* Austin, TX: PRO-ED.

McClannahan, L., & Krantz, P. (1999). *Activity schedules for children with autism: Teaching independent behavior.* Bethesda, MD: Woodbine House.

Odom, S.L., & McConnell, S.R. (1997). *Play time/social time: Organizing your classroom to build interaction skills.* Minneapolis: University of Minnesota.

Pierce, K. (1997). *Teaching typical children to be social skills trainers for their schoolmates with autism.* San Diego: University of California.

Quill, K. (1995). *Teaching children with autism: Strategies to enhance communication and socialization.* New York: Delmar.

Quill, K. (2000). *DO-WATCH-LISTEN-SAY: Social and communication intervention for children with autism.* Baltimore: Paul H. Brookes Publishing Co.

Reichle, J., & Wacker, D.P. (1993). *Communicative alternatives to challenging behavior: Integrating functional assessment and intervention strategies.* Baltimore: Paul H. Brookes Publishing Co.

Walker, H., Hops, H., & Greenwood, C. (1988). *Social skills tutoring and games: A program to teach social skills to primary grade students.* Delray Beach, FL: Educational Achievement Systems.

Walker, H., McConnell, S., Holmes, D., Todis, B., Walker, J., & Golden, N. (1988). *The Walker social skills curriculum: The ACCEPTS program.* Austin, TX: PRO-ED.

Warren, S.F., & Reichle, J. (Series & Volume Eds.). (1992). *Communication and language intervention series: Vol. 1. Causes and effects in communication and language intervention.* Baltimore: Paul H. Brookes Publishing Co.

Warren, S., & Rogers-Warren, A. (Eds.). (1985). *Teaching functional language.* Austin, TX: PRO-ED.

Watson, L., Lord, C., Schaffer, B., & Schopler, E. (1989). *Teaching spontaneous communication to autistic and developmentally handicapped children.* Austin, TX: PRO-ED.

Wilson, C. (1993). *Room 14: A social language program.* East Moline, IL: LinguiSystems.

Several studies have demonstrated the effectiveness of direct instruction of social skills for students with disabilities. For example, Gonzalez-Lopez and Kamps (1997) taught social skills and toy play to kindergarten and first-grade students with developmental disabilities using reverse mainstreaming of same-age typical peers. Peers initially were taught to provide simple instructions, to imitate and model toy play, and to ignore and then redirect inappropriate behavior. Following isolated peer training, students participated in playgroups comprised of one student with autism and three typical peers. Ten minutes were devoted to direct skill teaching (toy play, sharing, helping), and ten minutes were devoted to free play with teacher prompting and reinforcement to promote social interaction. Students with disabilities demonstrated longer interactions and fewer disruptive behaviors during the social skills intervention conditions.

In another study, Kamps and colleagues (1992) examined the effects of a social skills intervention on the interactions of three students with autism in an inclusive first-grade classroom. In this study with higher functioning students, no isolated peer training was conducted. During the small groups, the students were instructed on specific social skills (e.g., greetings, taking turns, sharing) and the use of these skills was assessed in a 10-minute free play period that followed. More frequent and longer social interactions resulted for all students, and typical peers nominated students with disabilities as playmates more often. These studies extend the results of research reviewed by Brown and Conroy (Chapter 7) conducted with preschool to school-age children (e.g., English, Goldstein, Shafer, & Kaczmarek, 1997; Goldstein, Kaczmarek, Pennington, & Shafer, 1992; Goldstein & Wickstrom, 1986; Odom, Chandler, et al., 1992; Strain & Danko, 1995; Strain, Danko, & Kohler, 1995).

Only a few data-based studies in which parents taught social skills have been reported. Strain and Danko (1995) reported successful parent implementation of social skills training with three young children with autism. Parents conducted approximately 40 sessions over a 10-month period focusing on teaching their children to solicit attention of friends, share or ask for toys, give play ideas, help friends, and talk nicely. Parents' use of modeling and practice produced more frequent social interaction for children with autism with their peers.

In another study involving children with autism (Laski, Charlop, & Schreibman, 1988), parents used naturalistic teaching strategies to teach seven 5- to 9-year-old children to engage in symbolic play (see description of procedures in training manual, Koegel et al., 1989). The parent served as both trainer and playmate during hour-long treatment sessions conducted three times per week. Parents presented numerous preferred toys and modeled symbolic play actions. If the child did not respond, the parent repeated the model. The child was reinforced with the opportunity to play with the preferred toy contingent on a response or approximation. In addition, improving the amount and complexity of the symbolic play meant that the children engaged in more interactive play with their parents. The children did not improve their responding to peers, however, suggesting a need to include peers in the training. Nevertheless, the findings expand on communication training conducted in clinical environments (e.g., Koegel et al., 1987) by incorporating social-communicative teaching into children's home environments with parents as trainers.

Despite success with social skills groups, teacher intrusiveness may hamper peer interaction (Odom & McConnell, 1992). Meyer, Fox, Schermer, Ketersen, and Montan (1987) examined the effects of teacher intrusiveness on social interactions between children with autism and their typical peers. Eight 5- to 12-year-olds with autism were observed playing with a same-age peer. During the intrusive simulation, a teacher was seated at the table with the dyad and intruded once each minute (e.g., giving instructions, making corrections, modeling play activities, praising). During the nonintrusive simulation, the teacher was located at least 6 feet from the play area and was allowed to intrude no more than three times within the 15-minute play session and only if the children were not interacting. In the nonintrusive condition, the children with autism demonstrated significantly higher levels of toy contact, more reaching for toys, and more appropriate play. They also demonstrated small but significant increases in appropriate and inappropriate play and fewer spontaneous vocalizations. Odom and McConnell (1997) recommended that teachers wait for 30 seconds to lapse with the target student not engaged in a social interaction before prompting peers to initiate.

Summary

Similar to instruction in beginning language and other basic skills, these studies indicate that educators must directly teach social-communicative behaviors. Thus, social-communicative skills should be viewed as critical individualized education program (IEP) objectives if one wants to promote future independence and community participation for children with developmental disabilities. Direct instruction of social skills, in particular, is a powerful technique for improving students' interactions with their teachers and parents (Camarata & Nelson, 1992; Dyer, 1989; Laski et al., 1988; Matson et al., 1990). In addition, the inclusion and training of peers within social groups greatly enhances the ability of students to participate in peer interactions within structured playgroups and natural environments (Kamps et al., 1992; Odom, Chandler, et al., 1992; Pierce & Schreibman, 1997; Sasso et al., 1990). Table 8.2 provides a summary of steps for designing successful social skills and playgroups for children with developmental disabilities and their peers. As described previously, one must include critical elements such as direct skill instruction, repeated practice, reinforcement of skill usage, and generalization programming strategies.

PEER MEDIATION WITHIN SOCIAL AND PLAY ENVIRONMENTS

Peer mediation is similar to adult-mediated instruction in that communication partners serve as models and teachers of social-communicative skills. The intensity of intervention, however, varies widely ranging from peers placed in proximity in order for students to imitate appropriate behaviors to peers directly instructing skills in a tutorial format. The environments for peer mediation encompass playgroups as well as other social environments designated for a specific activity (i.e., recess, lunch). The following section discusses a range of peer-mediation strategies and environments.

Social Skills and Playgroup Formats with Peer Mediation

Roeyers (1995) implemented a peer-mediated proximity approach in which 5- to 13-year-olds with pervasive developmental disorders were paired with same-age typical peers during play. Peers were told about autism and what behaviors to expect, but they were not given any specific training to engage in interaction. Peers were simply instructed to stay "on the same level" with the child with disabilities (e.g., if the child was sitting, the peer should sit). The children with disabilities improved their rates of interaction. There were fewer negative interactions and inappropriate behaviors and more positive interactions and socially acceptable behaviors. The authors noted, however, that the children with autism still had difficulty managing social situations, indicating a need for specific skill training and more intensive peer training.

Other researchers have investigated the effects of peer modeling and activity engagement strategies. In an early study, Strain and colleagues (1979) taught an 11-year-old peer two techniques to engage 9- to 10-year-old children with autism in play. The first method, prompt

Table 8.2.   Steps in implementing social skills groups and playgroups

Step 1. Provide information regarding social development/competence of children including the involvement of teachers, parents, siblings, and peers as trainers, reinforcers, and monitors of social behaviors.

Step 2. Determine the physical setting and scheduling arrangements of social skills groups in natural settings; select materials that foster positive peer interaction and skill development complimentary to individual goals (e.g., preparing snacks, playing games, priming of school activities within social games).

Step 3. Select a social skills teaching curriculum as a guideline for teaching children specific skills (e.g., Odom & McConnell, 1997; Walker et al., 1988).

Step 4. Periodically review and add new materials and activities that are "interactive" in nature (e.g., dress up clothes for dramatic play for younger children, games and recreational activities that encourage sharing and turn taking for both younger and older children).

Step 5. Develop monitoring procedures for providing a rich schedule of reinforcement to children for using proactive skills. Use monitoring and reinforcement procedures in generalization settings (e.g., new leisure activities).

Step 6. Use feedback, correction, and incidental teaching procedures (skills charts, signals, peer prompting, common materials and other stimulus items, etc.) for redirecting inappropriate behaviors that occur within social skills groups and during other home and school activities.

Step 7. Use self-monitoring and self-instruction procedures to promote generalization of prosocial skills and student independence in managing behaviors in additional settings beyond activities mediated or supervised by the parents or teachers (as deemed appropriate based on functioning levels).

Step 8. Select and conduct assessments including a social validity measure; that is, provide teachers and parents with a "user friendly" and "efficient" way to evaluate improvements in the positive behaviors and peer interactions of their children.

and praise, involved the peer encouraging the children with autism to play with each other through prompt statements such as "Give the ball to _____" or "Say hello to _____," followed by verbal praise. The second method, social initiations, involved encouraging the children to play with the peer instructor (e.g., "Let's play blocks," "Come play"). Both interventions produced an immediate increase in the number of initiations by the peer and the number of social responses by the students with autism.

Carr and Darcy (1990) also taught peers to model play behaviors, to prompt responses, and to reinforce the imitation of play behaviors by 4- to 5-year-old students with autism. Their procedures consisted of a "follow the leader" format in which the student and a peer model rotated through a series of stations with set activities (e.g., stacking blocks, jumping, crawling through a barrel, rolling a car). Results indicated that children could imitate peer models with limited interference from adults. Imitation and play behaviors also generalized to new tasks. These findings support earlier work demonstrating that children with developmental disabilities will imitate peers modeling play behaviors during social activities and that peers are quite capable of prompting and praising their classmates with disabilities (Egel, Richman, & Koegel, 1981; Lord & Hopkins, 1986; Strain & Odom, 1986).

Others also have provided systematic peer training as a strategy for increasing social initiation and interaction skills for participants with disabilities within the context of playgroups. For example, Gunter, Fox, Brady, Shores, and Cavanaugh (1988) taught elementary-school peers to prompt and praise two students with autism while engaging in free-play dyads. Implementation of a multiple exemplar strategy in which several peers took turns intervening with each student was effective in increasing initiations (e.g., sharing, assisting, greetings, using names) by peers and students with disabilities during training sessions. In addition, one of the two students with autism generalized to untrained peers and across environments.

Oke and Schriebman (1990) presented another case study in which a high-functioning child with autism and two typical peers were taught to initiate play. At first, the peers were taught to initiate to the target child using sharing and play organizers and to "keep trying" if initial attempts were rejected. After several sessions, the peers also were taught to discriminate between parallel and interactive play in order to encourage interactions. In the final stage of intervention, the target child was taught via direct instruction and video feedback to initiate play using the same sharing and play organizing skills. These behaviors were reviewed prior to each play session. Each of these strategies resulted in increases in positive social interaction. The child's disruptive behavior decreased only after he was taught his initiation skills. This student also demonstrated generalization to an untrained peer.

Davis and Reichle (1996) used high-probability requests as an additional mediation strategy to increase play skills in kindergarten peer playgroups with students with developmental disabilities. In their study, the intent was to teach participants to respond to social bids that were typically low probability. Naturally, students did not want to share or engage cooperatively with peers (e.g., hand peer the soda, share pizza with peer, help build the city with peer, make peer a hamburger). The authors found that students were more likely to respond to the low-probability requests, if those requests were proceeded by high-probability sequences of requests, such as "Point to the soda fountain," "Get a chocolate doughnut," "Point to the cash register," or "Put some soda in the glass." High-probability requests were child specific and included engagement with preferred toys. Compliance was higher when requests were varied.

Some investigations of peer mediation have taught peers to model rather sophisticated language skills within social training contexts. For example, Ostrosky and Kaiser (1995) taught multiple elementary-school peers to use specific social-communicative behaviors (e.g., mirroring, offering assistance, choice making, play describing, redirecting) during playgroups to enhance the social skills and social interaction of classmates with disabilities. Pierce and Schreibman (1995, 1997) implemented an even more ambitious approach to peer training. They had peers implement pivotal-response training derived from earlier investigations of teacher and parent implementations of the NLP (Koegel et al., 1987; Laski et al., 1988). Four 10-year-old peer trainers were taught to use the pivotal strategies (i.e., paying attention, giving choices, modeling appropriate social behavior, reinforcing attempts, encouraging and extending conversation, taking turns, narrating play, and responding to child cues) using modeling and role play with the experimenter and other peers. Peers, who were then paired with students with autism, played for 10 minutes and later received feedback. Social interaction increased dramatically, but only one student demonstrated impressive generalization across environments, materials, and peers (Pierce & Schreibman, 1995). In a second study, effects were replicated when eight peers were taught pivotal-response strategies. Both participants demonstrated impressive generalization, maintaining their interactions and initiation rates with untrained peers. These findings suggest that multiple peer trainers may facilitate greater generalization of social-communicative skills (Pierce & Schreibman, 1997).

Peer Programs for Lunch, Recess, and Recreational Groups

Several investigations have successfully incorporated peer-mediation strategies into a greater variety of everyday activities. Sasso and his colleagues sought to include a 12-year-old student with severe disabilities in recess activities (Sasso, Hughes, Swanson, & Novak, 1987). Their novel approach entailed teaching typical peers to enlist the support of other peers. Initially, peers were paired with the student with disabilities and instructed to remain in contact. Second, peers were taught to praise other peers who interacted with the student. Finally, peers were taught to prompt other peers to interact with the student with disabilities in appropriate ways during recess. Thus, the role of the trained peers was to initiate to the student with disabilities and later to actively solicit additional play partners.

The highest percentage of positive interactions occurred during the final peer prompting condition. Additional research replicated the success of the peer initiation intervention during recess and showed that improved social interaction could be obtained and generalized to untrained peers regardless of the status or popularity of the peers (Sasso & Rude, 1987). Likewise, Knapczyk (1989) instituted peer mentoring for 9- to 10-year-old students with mental retardation to increase cooperative play at recess and in the classroom. Peers were asked to include the student with disabilities in their existing group, and peers were taught how to adapt play to the skills of the students with disabilities. Results showed substantial increases in cooperative play from low baseline levels.

Rynders, Schleien, and Mustonen (1990) implemented a peer-training program in an inclusive summer camp that included 9- to 11-year-olds with severe disabilities. Campers with severe disabilities were reinforced for displaying appropriate behavior and for interacting with peers. Typical peers were taught cooperative learning strategies using the Special Friends curriculum (Voeltz et al., 1983). Peers' roles as friends rather than as tutors were emphasized. Students worked in small, inclusive groups on camp activities, such as table setting, swimming, crafts, and outdoor play. The children with disabilities demonstrated improved skills in the activities, and peers increased their prosocial bids and friendship ratings. Staff members' perceptions of inclusive camp programs also improved. These authors have applied cooperatively structured activities to a variety of recreational programs (Rynders et al., 1993), including physical education classes for adolescents (Schleien, Heyne, & Berken, 1988) and leisure activities such as bowling and gallery trips (Rynders, Johnson, Johnson, & Schmidt, 1980; Schleien, Rynders, & Mustonen, 1988).

Peer-mediated programming also has focused on mealtimes in lunch, snack, and similar environments. Agran, Fodor-Davis, Moore, and Martella (1992), for example, investigated the effects of peer-delivered instruction on sack lunch preparation for three adolescents with developmental disabilities in a cafeteria. The peers taught the students how to follow their task analyses. Peer assistance was faded, and the students gradually became independent. Two of the adolescents learned to make the lunches and generalized skills to novel customers, whereas a third mastered the task with the addition of picture cues and adult instruction. In a similar study, peer tutors learned to apply incidental teaching procedures to social skills during lunch-making routines for young adults with developmental disabilities. Improved social skills were noted during training sessions at lunch and also during dinner (Farmer-Dougan, 1994).

In another study, Haring, Roger, Lee, Breen, & Gaylord-Ross (1986) taught communication skills immediately prior to lunch to three 10- to 13-year-old students with moderate mental retardation. The topics were derived from interviews with 80 typical peers. The students were taught how to initiate topics first and then how to continue conversations. Although adults did the training, generalization was programmed and measured using eight fifth graders who served as co-workers at lunchtime in a rotation every 3 weeks. All participants generalized both conversational skills to lunchtime with their peers (Haring et al., 1986).

Finally, Blew, Schwartz, and Luce (1985) had peers conduct training with students with autism (5 and 8 years old) in three environments: the library, a restaurant, and street intersections in the community. Peers first provided discrete trial teaching sessions on specific skills for their partners with autism, followed by participation in the actual environments. Peers provided prompts, models, and reinforcement for their partners. Improved social skills were noted in all environments.

Summary

These studies demonstrate distinct advantages to including peers as intervention agents over programs that teach play and communication skills within teacher–student or clinician–client dyads alone (e.g., Carr & Darcy, 1990; Pierce & Schreibman, 1997; Sasso et al., 1987). First, increased peer interaction is a natural outcome in peer-mediated interventions. Second, substantial generalization to natural environments and untrained peers is a common finding. Third, when measured, these interventions have produced greater acceptance and more positive attitudes toward students with disabilities among teachers and peers. Table 8.3 presents a summary of effective teaching procedures that have been found to be helpful for practitioners in implementing peer mediation to teach social-communicative strategies (e.g., Kamps, Potucek, Gonzalez-Lopez, Kravits, & Kemmerer, 1997).

SOCIAL PROGRAMS USING AUGMENTATIVE AND ALTERNATIVE COMMUNICATION SYSTEMS

Social and communicative interaction between children with disabilities and their teachers and peers has incorporated augmentative and visual aids such as signs, picture-pointing and AAC systems, scripts, communication books, photographs, picture schedules, and so forth (e.g., Krantz & McClannahan, 1993; Loveland & Tunali, 1991; Mirenda, 1985). These systems tend to enhance the ability of students to learn to communicate in social situations due to increased understanding of the content and the social intentions of students with and without disabilities (Mirenda, 1985). This section reviews studies that address the use

Table 8.3.   Guidelines for designing peer-mediated social interventions

Peer intervention sessions should occur regularly and often, with a minimum of 10 minutes per activity, scheduled three or four times per week.

At least one peer should be involved consistently, but two to five peers are preferred.

An adult must be available to train peers, supervise activities, reinforce participants, and provide feedback.

Activities should be social in nature, provide ample opportunities for peer interaction, be fun for peers, and involve preferred or motivating activities for children with disabilities.

Training of peers should be systematic (e.g., modeling, adult–student practice, peer–student practice) and should be multifaceted, addressing at least two social skills (see curricula).

Conspicuous reinforcement systems (e.g., tokens, star charts, etc.) should be instituted initially to establish high rates of peer interaction and social skill usage.

An adult should provide feedback to students at the end of sessions.

Generalization should be programmed and measured.

A number of components need to be considered in the planning process:
 Are peers available regularly?
 Are relevant materials present during additional times during the day?
 Are the selected skills pivotal or multipurpose in nature?
 Are the identified social activities naturally motivating for peers?
 Are target students likely to demonstrate necessary skills or can they be learned readily?
 Are they likely to encounter sufficient reinforcement to maintain appropriate social skills in the activities?

of AAC systems for teaching social-communicative skills to children with developmental disabilities.

Signing

Sign language has been documented as an effective alternative means of communication for many nonverbal individuals (e.g., Carr, 1979; Clark, Remington, & Light, 1988; Reichle, York, & Sigafoos, 1991). Simultaneous communication training (i.e., presenting a verbal identifier simultaneously with the manual sign) has been a technique that has been used most often when teaching sign language. As an exemplary study, Carr and Kologinsky (1983) conducted a study documenting the effectiveness of signing as an AAC system. Based on child preferences, 10 items and social activities (e.g., juice, balloons, tickles) were selected. Six children with autism (ages 9–14) were taught the signs for each item or activity. Following sign acquisition, the children were taught to use their sign repertoires to make spontaneous requests while in the presence of the preferred items and activities. This was accomplished using a variety of techniques including imitative prompting, fading, differential reinforcement, and some aspects of incidental teaching. Generalized sign requests were observed with different adults present in the training room and with the teacher in the classroom during other times of the day. In addition, reductions in stereotypic behavior accompanied increases in signing. Unfortunately, no measures of interaction with peers were reported.

Other studies have demonstrated the effectiveness of teaching signs to nonverbal children to initiate requests, to label items in their environment, and to communicate in natural environments (e.g., Partington, Sundberg, Newhouse, & Spengler, 1994; Remington & Clarke, 1983). Signing also has been used as a means of interacting in social play situations (ring toss, bean bag game) (Sommer, Whitman, & Keogh, 1988) and to communicate with classmates during peer network activities (Romer, White, & Haring, 1996).

Augmentative and Alternative Communication Systems

Communication systems using pictures and symbols are gaining popularity among language intervention specialists for teaching social-communicative skills to students with developmental disabilities (Shafer, 1993). AAC systems vary from picture or symbol boards and books to computer-operated devices that electronically produce voice output. Behavioral techniques such as shaping, prompting, and fading often have been utilized to teach picture communication systems. For example, in one study, an 8-year-old girl was taught to request via pictures using a shaping strategy in which physical guidance was faded until she was able to spontaneously request a variety of items (Mirenda & Santogrossi, 1985). Training was conducted in a clinical environment, and generalization was noted in both the student's home and school.

Bondy and Frost (1994) developed the Picture Exchange Communication System (PECS) to address the communicative and social impairments common to many children with developmental disabilities including autism. Children were taught to initiate to adults and peers using a picture from a communication board to request desired items (toys, food, school items). Thus, it was structured in a way that resembled a more naturalistic approach to teaching in that the adults received all of their cues from the children as opposed to providing the children with the cues (similar to following a child's lead in naturalistic teaching approaches). Thus, the PECS was developed to minimize the prompt dependency incurred using other AAC systems. The PECS was designed to teach children to initiate their wants and needs through an exchange of a picture for the corresponding item or activity. Bondy and Frost (1994) reported improved communication using the PECS as well as increases in spontaneous language and speech acquisition even though verbal language was not directly taught as part of the PECS training protocol. Bondy and Frost (1994) reported that reductions in maladaptive behaviors were associated with using PECS, possibly because the ability to communicate appropriately replaced the need to misbehave for attention, escape, and express wishes.

Kravits, Kamps, Kemmerer, and Potucek (1998) used the PECS system in combination with peer training to teach social-communicative skills to a 7-year-old girl with developmental disabilities. The communication system was effective for teaching spontaneous requesting, commenting, and expanding. The student learned to discriminate among icons and generalized her system use to other people and environments, including her kindergarten playgroup. Social interactions did not increase, however, until peer social skills training was implemented. Other researchers have extended the use of AAC systems to a variety of contexts, such as teaching reading and science content areas (e.g., Light & Binger, 1992; Light & Lindsay, 1991; Lindsay et al., 1992) and increasing communication in general education environments (Calculator & Jorgensen, 1991; Mirenda & Beukelman, 1990).

Additional studies have incorporated voice output systems into picture and symbol selection. Adamson and colleagues (1992), for example, taught 12 students with mental retardation to use computerized speech-output devices during mealtime and recreational activities. The students learned to select symbols representing nouns, such as BANANA, BREAD, and FRENCH FRIES, during mealtimes at home and school. Students were able to add social-regulative symbols to their AAC systems (e.g., NO, YES, HELP, STOP, I WANT, EXCUSE ME, THANK YOU), which enhanced their ability to converse with parents and teachers (Adamson et al., 1992; Romski, Sevcik, & Wilkinson, 1994). Others have noted that voice output communication aids are viable means for communication for young children with severe disabilities (Schepis, Reid, & Behrmann, 1996) and have suggested that voice output systems increase activity performance and interactions with peers (see Zangari, Lloyd, & Vicker, 1994).

Some researchers have compared various modes of communication. For example, Rotholz, Berkowitz, and Burberry (1989) found that two adolescents with autism were able to place orders in a fast-food restaurant using a communication book but not manual signing. Soto, Belfiore, Schlosser, and Haynes (1993) compared the use of a picture board and a voice output device. The participant, a young adult, was able to learn both systems but showed a preference for the voice output system. In addition, he was able to generalize his use of the system to different activities within the training environments and to additional environments and people.

Pictures, Photos, and Scripts to Teach Social-Communicative Skills

Picture prompts and scripts have been used repeatedly to teach social-communicative skills to students with developmental disabilities. Pierce and Schreibman (1994), for example, used photographs as prompts for selected steps in a task analysis of activities for three low-functioning students with autism. Children were taught to follow the six- or seven-picture sequence to complete daily living tasks selected by parents (i.e., setting the table, making the bed, doing laundry, getting dressed, making drinks, and fixing lunch). Children learned to complete the tasks successfully in the absence of the trainer and in new environments and learned to deliver their own reinforcers. Similar work taught children with developmental disabilities to follow sequences of photographs during after-school activities, such as eating snack, playing with toys, doing homework, playing games, doing puzzles, and watching TV (MacDuff, Krantz, & McClannahan, 1993). Students were able to engage independently in lengthy response chains and to change activities in the same and different environments without immediate supervision or prompts. Likewise, Kim and Lombardino (1991) used script-based routines to teach language skills while making popcorn, pudding, and milkshakes with 5- and 6-year-olds with mental retardation. These studies serve as examples of scripted activities to teach independence and self-management of behaviors during leisure time and daily activities, though without the benefit of peer participation.

To address social interaction specifically, Krantz and McClannahan (1993) used a script-fading procedure to teach four children with autism, ages 9–12 years, to initiate conversations with each other during art activities. Each child learned a script of 10 statements reflecting: 1) activities that they had recently completed, 2) activities that the children were planning, and 3) objects in the school environment (e.g., class materials, bowls of potato chips). The children were pretaught to identify all the words in the written script when necessary. Not only did each student maintain initiations as the script was faded, but also unscripted initiations increased and initiations generalized to new environments, times, and teachers.

Krantz and McClannahan (1998) extended the use of script-fading procedures to social interaction skills for 4- and 5-year-olds with autism. Textual cues, *Look* and *Watch me* were embedded in students' photographic activity schedules. Following script training, the children's verbal elaborations and unscripted interactions increased and generalized to unscripted topics. The authors noted that the procedures following script training were similar to incidental teaching in that teachers were instructed not to ask questions or give directions but to comment on children's activities and accomplishments and to model and expand utterances relevant to the interests of the children.

Rather than written scripts, Charlop and Milstein (1989) presented scripted conversations on videotape to teach conversation skills to three 6- to 7-year-old students with autism. Videotape modeling was effective in increasing conversational speech with the therapist and appropriate question asking. Spontaneous variations in responses were noted and the improved conversational skills generalized to unfamiliar people and to the siblings of the participants.

A limitation of many of the studies demonstrating success with scripts, picture schedules, communication books, and so forth has been the absence of peers without disabilities in the assessment and training of social-communicative skills. A few investigations have incorporated typical peers into script and picture interventions. Jolly, Test, and Spooner (1993) taught 10- and 11-year-old students with severe disabilities to initiate to peers during play by offering photographs of toys and games. The intervention produced more frequent play organizers, initiations, and sharing among students and their peers. Peers also have been incorporated into role-play situations using scripts for adolescents with mild mental retardation (O'Reilly & Glynn, 1995). The scripts taught social problem solving and decision-making skills for peer interaction. The steps included decoding (what's happening?), deciding (what should I do?), performing (initiate/respond), and evaluating (what happened and was it right?). The students with mild developmental disabilities were able to recognize the steps following practice with their peer tutors, to demonstrate the behaviors in training, and to transfer them to nontraining situations.

In a series of studies, Hunt and colleagues applied scripts and communication systems to students with developmental disabilities and typical peers. In one study, adolescents with developmental disabilities learned conversation skills by using topic menus, communication books, and initiation strategies within peer groups. Improvements in their conversation and turn-taking skills were accompanied by reductions in their inappropriate behaviors (Hunt, Alwell, & Goetz, 1988). In another study, communication books were used to facilitate conversation skills for adolescents; however, it was necessary to provide a minimal level of awareness training to novel peers for skills to generalize (Hunt, Alwell, & Goetz, 1991).

Although the data-based literature on augmentation (e.g., signs, picture-point systems, communication boards) within the context of social-communicative skills is in its infancy, its potential is apparent. AAC systems offer students with developmental disabilities an effective means of communicating with adults and peers. They have been used to improve learning opportunities for many individuals who are non-verbal or who have limited speech abilities (e.g., Bondy & Frost, 1994; Mirenda, 1985; Reichle, York, & Sigafoos, 1991; Shafer, 1993; Zangari et al., 1994).

SELF-MANAGEMENT OF SOCIAL-COMMUNICATIVE BEHAVIORS

Despite extensive research on the positive effects of self-management on enhancing on-task behavior and work production skills (Hughes & Boyle, 1991; Kapadia & Fantuzzo, 1988; McCarl, Svobodny, & Boare, 1991; Shapiro & Klein, 1980; Sugai & Rowe, 1984), only a few studies have used self-management to improve social and communicative be-haviors (Strain, Kohler, Storey, & Danko, 1994). In one example, Koegel and colleagues examined the effects of teaching four children with autism, ages 6–11 years, to self-monitor their rates of response to verbal initiations from others (Koegel, Koegel, Hurley, & Frea, 1992). All four children were taught to use wrist counters to record the num-ber of responses they made to others in 30-minute teaching sessions.

Prompting to record responses was completely faded for all chil-dren after approximately 3 hours of treatment. Then, reinforcement based on recorded responses was gradually thinned until 30–40 re-sponses were required to earn a reward. After use of the wrist counter was learned in training, its use was introduced into the community, home, and school environments. Findings demonstrated that the chil-dren increased their rate of responding with minimal adult presence. As the children's responsiveness improved, there was a decrease in their rate of disruptive behavior. The majority of interactions, however, took place with adults, parents, and teachers, and the participants were not taught to initiate interactions.

In a subsequent study, two adolescents were taught improved conversational skills in a community video arcade through a similar self-management procedure (Koegel & Frea, 1993). Another report demonstrated the success of self-management for increasing play be-haviors in students with autism, ages 7–13 years (Stahmer & Schreib-man, 1992). Social behaviors used when playing with dolls or toy rockets, games, and puzzles generalized to the home environment and also were associated with reductions in stereotypic behavior.

Newman, Buffington, and Hemmes (1996) used external reinforcement and self-reinforcement to increase the appropriate conversation of three older students with autism. Sessions began with the reading of a short story by a facilitator, followed by a request for any questions from the participants, as a prompt to begin conversations about the stories. The facilitator prompted the participants to respond if 3 seconds elapsed without any conversation. During baseline, tokens were delivered noncontingently at the end of the conversation period. During the external reinforcement phase, trainers provided one token for each appropriate response. During the self-reinforcement phase, the participants were responsible for taking a token after each appropriate response. Tokens could be exchanged for a variety of activities or edibles. Conversation skills improved for all participants across both types of contingent reinforcement. Notably, self-reinforcement was just as effective as external reinforcement.

The findings from these studies suggest that self-management is an effective strategy for improving social behavior in students with developmental disabilities (e.g., Koegel et al., 1992). Furthermore, self-management of appropriate social skills following appropriate modeling and teaching of interaction skills may greatly facilitate generalization and promote greater independence in participants.

PEER-MEDIATED ACADEMIC PROGRAMS FOR IMPROVING SOCIAL COMPETENCE

Peer tutoring programs have been shown to be an effective teaching strategy for improving academic and social skills for students in a variety of educational environments. There are three common tutoring arrangements:

1. Cross-age tutoring (e.g., Barbetta, Miller, Peters, Heron, & Cochran, 1991)
2. Classwide peer tutoring (Carlton, Litton, & Zinkgraf, 1985; Greenwood, 1991)
3. Typical peers as tutors for children with learning disabilities or behavioral disorders (e.g., Kamps, Locke, Delquadri, & Hall, 1989)

Peer tutoring and other student-to-student learning dyads have had positive effects on academic achievement for students with and without disabilities in general classroom environments (Barbetta et al., 1991;

Cooke, Heron, Heward, & Test, 1982; Fowler, 1988; Franca, Kerr, Reitz, & Lambert, 1990; Fuchs, Fuchs, Bentz, Phillips, & Hamlett, 1994; Greenwood, 1991; Maheady, Sacca, & Harper, 1988). Peer tutoring by its nature also is a peer interactive intervention with potential benefits for improving social performance. The peer tutoring studies reviewed in this chapter are examples that measured some aspect of social functioning, were designed as a tactic for successful inclusion with typical peers, or embedded social skills into the tutoring intervention.

Results of tutoring programs for children with developmental disabilities have been quite impressive. Peer tutoring has not only been effective in teaching basic skills to students with disabilities but also effective as a means for generalizing social responsiveness toward peers (Carr & Darcy, 1990). For example, Kamps, Barbetta, Leonard, and Delquadri (1994) noted both social and academic gains. They investigated classwide peer tutoring (CWPT) in three second- and third-grade classrooms that included students with autism. CWPT occurred three or four times per week and consisted of 30–35 minutes of structured peer tutoring in reading. Results showed higher reading comprehension scores for students with autism and their general education peers, with slight increases in oral-reading rates. CWPT also resulted in longer peer social interactions during subsequent free-time groups for students and for their peers. Others have reported reading gains as a result of tutoring programs (i.e., peers without disabilities tutoring students with mental retardation ages 8–18 years). Similar social benefits have been noted, including increased social interactions for students with and without disabilities in inclusive environments and appropriate interactions skills such as conversation skills and joking behaviors (Collins, Branson, & Hall, 1995; Wolery, Werts, Snyder, & Caldwell, 1994).

Adding a social component to the tutoring activity appears critical to promoting social as well as academic benefits. For example, in one study peers taught 7- and 8-year-olds with developmental disabilities to accurately perform response chains following peer modeling of the behaviors (i.e., adding with a calculator, spelling name with tiles, sharpening pencil, playing an audiotape) (Werts, Caldwell, & Wolery, 1996). No increases, however, were noted in social interaction time with peers following the intervention. In another study, changes in the quality of peer interactions were compared during game-playing activities with 8-year-old students with mental retardation (McMahon, Wacker, Sasso, Berg, & Newton, 1996). Initially peers taught students game skills by modeling, prompting, and reinforcing appropriate skills. For three of four participants, interactions that were both instructional and social in nature remained constant, interactions that were purely social increased, and interactions that were purely instructional decreased as students mastered the game. Positive social interactions also generalized to novel social situations for participants.

Other investigations have found cooperative learning groups effective. For example, in one study, cooperative activities promoted both friendship and caregiving roles on the part of the peers (Staub, Schwartz, Gallucci, & Peck, 1994). Peers' assistance was noted during nongroup activities as well as in transitions and recess. Peer tutoring within highly structured cooperative groups also seems to promote appropriate social interactions. Two studies used cooperative learning groups to include students with autism in a fourth-grade social studies program and third- and fifth-grade reading activities (Dugan, Kamps, & Leonard, 1995; Kamps, Leonard, Potucek, & Garrison-Harrell, 1995). Cooperative learning group procedures entailed peer tutoring in academic content as well as teacher monitoring and reinforcement for "social behaviors" (e.g., sharing ideas, offering praise, encouraging and helping others). Increases in positive peer interactions were demonstrated.

Hunt and colleagues (Hunt, Staub, Alwell, & Goetz, 1994) also showed that peers were effective tutors within cooperative learning groups for three students with severe disabilities. Students learned new communication skills (i.e., looking at peers when their names were called, responding to questions by activating switches or using communication symbols) and motor skills (i.e., receiving and passing items to peers). Furthermore, peers' math test performance was similar to that of peers who were not in cooperative learning groups with students with disabilities.

In summary, several researchers have shown that peer support through tutoring and other curricular adaptations provides both academic and social benefits for children in inclusive educational environments (Cushing & Kennedy, 1997; Kamps et al., 1995; Strayhorn, Strain, & Walker, 1993). Peer tutoring and cooperative peer learning are powerful strategies that should be integral to school environments that include children with developmental disabilities. Tutoring activities naturally increase interaction time with peers in activities typical of classroom environments. In addition, components of the structured peer and student training associated with tutoring programs address positive social interaction behaviors such as helping, responsiveness, and praising. Thus, they facilitate improved social competence in all participants. Other positive side effects may accrue, as well. For example, the process of peers observing high engagement and subsequent learning within tutoring arrangements for students with disabilities may have a secondary effect of improved status and acceptance for those students (Kamps et al., 1998).

PEER NETWORKS TO IMPROVE
SOCIAL-COMMUNICATIVE BEHAVIORS

Peer networks are an additional strategy for providing both social and academic support for students with disabilities in school environments (e.g., Garrison-Harrell, Kamps, & Kravits, 1997; Haring & Breen, 1992). Peer networks are based on several key principles. First, awareness training of disabilities for typical peers along with supervised joint activities enhances the acceptance of students with disabilities in school environments. Second, children with developmental disabilities can function and learn in group situations in school environments (e.g., Gast, Winterling, Wolery, & Farmer, 1992; Kamps, Dugan, Leonard, & Daoust, 1994; Kamps, Leonard, Dugan, Boland, & Greenwood, 1991). Third, children with disabilities also can learn from and participate with peer models (e.g., Carr & Darcy, 1990; Egel et al., 1981). Successful peer networks incorporate several peer-mediation strategies. For example, peers may be taught to be initiators of social interaction for the students with disabilities (e.g., Sasso & Rude, 1987; Strain & Odom, 1986), to be models of appropriate play and behavior (Carr & Darcy, 1990; Charlop, Schreibman, & Tryon, 1983; Knapczyk, 1989; McEvoy et al., 1988; Shafer, Egel, & Neef, 1984), and to be tutors or co-participants in social skills groups (Haring et al., 1987; Kamps et al., 1989; Kamps et al., 1992).

Awareness and Friendship
Training for Peer Support Networks

Providing information about disabilities through awareness activities has been promoted as an initial step in developing peer support networks (Sasso, Simpson, & Novak, 1985; Stainback & Stainback, 1989). Awareness activities have produced some positive effects, perhaps because typical peers are more likely to make themselves available, sit in closer proximity, and be more responsive to children with disabilities. Two models of peer training that foster acceptance and participation in inclusive environments have included the Special Friends programs (Sasso et al., 1985; Voeltz et al., 1983) and Circles of Friends groups (Forest, 1987). These programs provide awareness information regarding disabilities, specific information regarding individuals with disabilities in the identified school environment (communication strategies, personal likes and dislikes, preferred and competent activities), and ideas for social and environment-specific support from peers. In spite of reports of positive effects from these more naturalistic support programs, additional ongoing training for both peers and students with disabilities may be necessary to promote more active involvement. Indeed, some have noted that even with initial training and awareness activities such as those provided in inclusive environments, measurable changes in true participation or engagement in activities and acceptance by teachers and peers without disabilities may not result (e.g., Horner, Sprague, & Flannery, 1993; Sale & Carey, 1995).

Forest (1987) promoted Circles of Friends to build support systems of significant others at home and school. These friends attended regular meetings to discuss support needs and accomplishments. Her results have shown active participation in school activities and increases in friendship. Stainback and Stainback (1989) provided a parental perspective for "support networks" for children with severe disabilities and highlighted a number of operational considerations:

1. Supports should empower a person to assist him- or herself.
2. Support networking should be natural and ongoing, not episodic or reserved for use only in times of difficulty.
3. Support networking should be run by insiders (i.e., those individuals directly involved).
4. Support networking starts with an examination of the social interactions and supportive characteristics that naturally operate in classrooms and builds on these.

Haring and Breen offered some additional guidelines for establishing peer networks:

> (a) Existing social cliques incorporate the target child into their group; (b) the program provides a rationale for the peers as enabling improved quality of life and appropriate peer modeling for the new member; (c) members are selected based on common interests or from an expressed interest by the child with disabilities; (d) implementation of networks begins with mapping child and peer schedules and assigning interactive routines; and (e) specific commitments from peers and adults are required. (1992, p. 322)

Peer Networks Using Mediation for Social Support

Peer networks in school, home, and community environments have the potential to improve the social and behavioral performance of students as well as their ability to participate in lifelong neighborhood and community events. A few studies have documented the effects of peer networks. Haring and Breen (1992) recruited junior high peers to serve as a social support group for three students with moderate to severe disabilities. Students facilitated social interaction and activity participation during transition times in the hallways and during lunch. The intervention consisted of 1) having peers map their schedules to determine availability, 2) providing an interaction schedule for times to assist with one peer responsible for each transition, 3) introducing the student to his or her network, 4) teaching initiation and reinforcement strategies to peers to use to encourage interactions (i.e., establishing joint attention, showing persistence in obtaining a response, modeling appropriate responses, modifying the content, increasing motivation), and 5) weekly peer network meetings to provide feedback and reinforcement. Students increased their interactions and appropriate social responding within structured and unstructured contexts with the peer network.

Others have implemented peer interventions across multiple environments to increase social-communicative skills. Kamps and colleagues (1997) implemented peer networks across multiple school activities (e.g., reading, lunch, game time, work-time) for three students with autism. The peer network consisted of two to five peers per activity. Peers were taught to prompt and reinforce social skills as well as to tutor and help the students with autism. All students increased their interaction time with peers (Kamps, Potucek, Gonzalez-Lopez, Kravits, & Kemmerer, 1997). Garrison-Harrell and colleagues (1997) replicated these findings in a study in which the network of peers remained constant across three environments. More frequent and longer interactions among students, increased use of AAC systems, more expressive language production for two students, and an increased number of nominations of target students on a sociometric scale resulted (Garrison-Harrell et al., 1997).

To summarize, a primary goal of peer networks is to increase and enhance the social opportunities for children with developmental disabilities by making multiple peer activities available. When peers are added to networks of teachers and family members, they can provide effective training and potent reinforcement for improved social-communicative skills. Table 8.4 summarizes seven steps that should be considered when establishing peer networks. These suggested procedures are derived from a number of the studies that sought to facilitate social skill development and to improve social relationships for children with disabilities (e.g., Garrison-Harrell et al., 1997; Haring & Breen, 1992; Kamps et al., 1992; Pierce & Schreibman, 1995, 1997; Sasso et al., 1987; Strain et al., 1995). As depicted, implementation and monitoring of peer networks follow a similar process to implementation of social groups. Key elements include 1) setting aside time to plan with assistance from

Table 8.4. Steps in the implementation of peer networks

Step 1
Plan with teachers and parents regarding selection of specific activities for organizing a peer network or enhancing participation within existing school and community events. Steps should include
    selection of activities with many social opportunities (group activities, leisure, after school snacks, social clubs, music, cooking)
    selection based on age-appropriateness, peer interests, and target student preferences and choices
    organization and adaptations of materials, games, and so forth

Step 2
Select the type of role best suited to the child and activities including
    peers as monitors for behavior
    peers as prompters for social initiations and responses
    peers as role models and demonstrators for specific tasks and activities
    peers as reinforcement providers and feedback givers at regularly scheduled times

Step 3
Recruit and train peers for participation with children with disabilities in a variety of activities. Training for peers includes
    appropriate skills (e.g., modeling, giving directions, corrective feedback, prompting, praising)
    skills to assist target children in social and communicative functions (e.g., requesting, social amenities, attention seeking, protesting, commenting, encouraging, yes/no responding)

Step 4
Implement and monitor the peer network activities including
    schedule consistent social events with peer network members
    incorporate a reinforcement schedule for the target child and peers
    use peer monitoring (if determined as appropriate)

Step 5
Monitor the peer networks using several strategies including
    repeated measures of peer interaction during network activities
    reliability checks of peer monitoring systems
    feedback from peers regarding acceptability of activities with input for revisions as well as generating ideas regarding networks

Step 6
Include ongoing programming to incorporate new skills or improve social skills for the target children to maintain and increase their participation (e.g., systems to foster reciprocal interaction chains and social-communicative functions).

Step 7
As peer networks are functioning in a satisfactory manner with improvements noted in interaction skills, incorporate strategies to promote generalization such as
    rotate additional peers
    develop new networks for new settings
    increase the length of network time to include expanded activities (e.g., longer outings, overnights) or the location of network activities (e.g., homes of peers, relatives, other community persons)

multiple people (e.g., peers, school staff, parents, community participants), 2) supplying adult and peer modeling of successful interaction skills, 3) implementing functional reinforcement systems, and 4) providing feedback for the participating children.

CONCLUSION

Current research in teaching social-communicative skills has yielded promising results. There is general agreement that many children with developmental disabilities do not develop social competence through typical developmental experiences and ongoing encounters at home and in school. As with other basic skills, there is a need to provide systematic teaching and practice for children using a fairly well-established set of social and communicative skills as included in published programs (see Tables 8.1 and 8.2).

Several strategies are available to teach social-communicative skills to school-age children with developmental disabilities. First, adult-mediated direct instruction of social and communicative skills has been found to produce robust outcomes for students. For example, adult-mediated intervention has been used to teach greetings, social amenities, and information seeking in one-to-one clinical environments (e.g., Matson et al., 1990; Taylor & Harris, 1995); to enhance language and play skills (e.g., Camarata & Nelson, 1992; Dyer, 1989); and to promote communication during snack and leisure activities (e.g., Charlop et al., 1985). Likewise, much research has demonstrated the effectiveness of using naturalistic and milieu teaching techniques during social language training (Hart & Risley, 1978). Some important features of naturalistic teaching include incorporating child preferences into teaching sessions, reinforcing communicative attempts, using multiple exemplars and modeling of appropriate skills, varying tasks and including some known tasks or trials to ensure success, using time-delay prompts, and using direct and natural consequences (Kaiser et al., 1987; Koegel et al., 1987).

Second, teaching social and communicative skills within activity routines is a highly desirable approach, whether routines are naturally occurring or structured (Alwell, Hunt, Goetz, & Sailor, 1989; Snyder-McLean et al., 1984). School routines and social activities (e.g., imitation games, toy play, turn-taking games) are particularly effective at increasing social interaction when peers are included (Carr & Darcy, 1990; Kamps et al., 1992; Meyer et al., 1987; Sasso et al., 1990). Small peer groups (one student with a disability and 1–4 peers) and dyads (e.g., Gonzalez-Lopez & Kamps, 1997; Pierce & Schreibman, 1997) have been effective in promoting appropriate behaviors and interactions. Some of the skills taught have included initiating play, turn taking, sharing, conversing, and game playing (Oke & Schreibman, 1990; Strain et al., 1995).

A third finding is that peer mediation has been a highly effective approach for teaching social skills to students with disabilities. Examples have included peer teaching within play and social groups (e.g., Gunter et al., 1988; Ostrosky & Kaiser, 1995; Roeyers, 1995), as well as peer mediation to increase social interactions and engagement during specific school activities such as recess and lunch (Farmer-Dougan, 1994; Haring et al., 1986; Knapczyk, 1989; Sasso et al., 1987). Peer mediation has been shown to assist in the development of skill acquisition (e.g., sharing, turn taking, conversations). More importantly, it often appears to promote increased generalization to additional school environments and novel peers (e.g., Ostrosky & Kaiser, 1995; Pierce & Schreibman, 1997).

A fourth important conclusion is that peer tutoring (e.g., one-to-one teaching, cooperative learning groups), though primarily designed for practice in content areas such as reading and math, has also benefited social behavior. Investigators have found generalization of social interaction skills to free time following academic tutoring (Kamps, Barbetta, et al., 1994). Helping behaviors and social expansions generalized to transitions, recess, and other nontraining environments (Collins et al., 1995; Staub et al., 1994).

A variety of other supportive strategies may greatly facilitate the acquisition of social competence. Photos, communication books, and more sophisticated AAC systems have been shown to promote communication within social contexts (e.g., Bondy & Frost, 1994; Hunt et al., 1988; Johnson, Knowlton, Adams, & Swall, 1992; Mirenda & Santogrossi, 1985; Rotholz et al., 1989). Scripts and schedules can increase activity engagement as well as social interaction (Krantz & McClannahan, 1998). Social skills can be learned observationally from video modeling (Charlop & Milstein, 1989; Oke & Schreibman, 1990). Students with developmental disabilities have learned to self-manage their interaction skills in social contexts (e.g., Koegel & Frea, 1993). Self-assessment of social behaviors, self-recording of skill usage, and self-reinforcement or reporting of social interaction performance to others are all steps toward increasingly independent use of social skills in natural environments. In addition, positive behavioral support programs to treat disruptive and maladaptive behavior also facilitate the use of social interaction skills with peers (e.g., Oke & Schreibman, 1990).

The results from a multitude of data-based studies demonstrate the effectiveness of teaching social-communicative behaviors to school-age children with developmental disabilities. Positive outcomes are reflected in increased responsivity by students with disabilities, more social time with peers, enhanced communication skills, and often improved acceptance by peers (e.g., Goldstein & Cisar, 1992; Kamps et al., 1997; Odom, Chandler, et al., 1992). When intervention efforts combine multiple strategies with various environments and peer groups as in peer networks, student outcomes appear to be even greater (e.g., Garrison-Harrell et al., 1997; Haring & Breen, 1992; Kamps et al., 1997).

Despite these favorable outcomes, a need for additional research and more complete monitoring of effects attributable to social skills interventions remains. For example, skills do not generalize for all participants, suggesting a need for more intensive intervention, longer interventions, and better programming for generalization of prosocial skills to nontraining environments. In addition, longitudinal studies are needed to demonstrate the effects of continuous teaching of skills in multiple environments for longer time spans, as in the peer network programs (see Chandler, Fowler, & Lubeck, 1992; Sasso et al., 1990; Simpson, 1987; Walker, Schwartz, Nippold, Irvin, & Noell, 1994; Zaragoza, Vaughn, & McIntosh, 1991). As Strain, Danko, and Kohler (1995) argued, there is an immediate need for more intensive, longitudinal social skills interventions that are inclusive of home and community environments for children with developmental disabilities in order to prepare them for socially complex world demands.

Despite a rather vast compendium of effective strategies that could be devoted to this challenging endeavor, there is no guarantee that schools will view the development of social competence as a high priority. Although successful social skills interventions are quite rewarding for students with disabilities as well as their peers (Kamps et al., 1998), it is not uncommon for teachers to balk at requests to spend school time on social skills training, peer support networks, and the like. Therefore, recommendations include outreach training to adequately inform parents, teachers, and clinicians of the benefits of social competence training. In addition, the following steps may promote more widespread adoption: 1) determining social priorities for individual students, 2) inclusion of communication goals on IEPs to reflect social skills interventions, 3) careful analysis of the school environment and environments therein that may be conducive to peer programs, and 4) the use of multiple peer groups to support social-communicative programming and instruction across school, home, and community environments.

REFERENCES

Adamson, L.B., Romski, M.A., Deffebach, K., & Sevcik, R.A. (1992). Symbol vocabulary and the focus of conversations: Augmenting language development for youth with mental retardation. *Journal of Speech and Hearing Research, 35,* 1333–1343.

Agran, M., Fodor-Davis, J., Moore, S.C., & Martella, R.C. (1992, December). Effects of peer-delivered self-instructional training on a lunch-making work task for students with severe disabilities. *Education and Training in Mental Retardation and Developmental Disorders, 27,* 230–240.

Alwell, M., Hunt, P., Goetz, L., & Sailor, W. (1989). Teaching generalized communicative behaviors within interrupted behavior chain contexts. *Journal of The Association for Persons with Severe Handicaps, 14,* 91–100.

Barbetta, P.M., Miller, A.D., Peters, M.T., Heron, T.E., & Cochran, L.L. (1991). Tugmate: A cross-age tutoring program to teach sight vocabulary. *Education and Treatment of Children, 14,* 19–37.

Blew, P.A., Schwartz, I.S., & Luce, S.C. (1985). Teaching functional community skills to autistic children using nonhandicapped peer tutors. *Journal of Applied Behavior Analysis, 18,* 337–342.

Bondy, A., & Frost, L. (1994). The picture exchange communication system. *Focus on Autistic Behavior, 9,* 1–19.

Calculator, S., & Jorgensen, C. (1991). Integrating AAC instruction into regular education settings: Expounding on best practices. *Augmentative and Alternative Communication, 7,* 204–214.

Camarata, S., & Nelson, K. (1992). Treatment efficiency as a function of target selection in the remediation of child language disorders. *Clinical Linguistics and Phonetics, 6,* 167–178.

Carlton, M.B., Litton, F.W., & Zinkgraf, S.A. (1985). The effects of an intraclass peer tutoring program on the sight-word recognition ability of students who are mildly mentally retarded. *Mental Retardation, 23,* 74–78.

Carr, E.G. (1979). Teaching autistic children to use sign language: Some research issues. *Journal of Autism and Developmental Disorders, 9*(4), 345–359.

Carr, E.G., & Darcy, M. (1990). Setting generality of peer modeling in children with autism. *Journal of Autism and Developmental Disorders, 20,* 45–60.

Carr, E., & Kologinsky, E. (1983). Acquisition of sign language by autistic children: II. Spontaneity and generalization effects. *Journal of Applied Behavior Analysis, 16,* 297–314.

Chandler, L.K., Fowler, S.A., & Lubeck, R.C. (1992). An analysis of the effects of multiple setting events on the social behavior of preschool children with special needs. *Journal of Applied Behavior Analysis, 25,* 249–264.

Charlop, M.H., & Milstein, J.P. (1989). Teaching autistic children conversational speech using video modeling. *Journal of Applied Behavior Analysis, 22,* 275–285.

Charlop, M.H., Schreibman, L., & Thibodeau, M.G. (1985). Increasing spontaneous verbal responding in autistic children using a time delay procedure. *Journal of Applied Behavior Analysis, 18,* 155–166.

Charlop, M.H., Schreibman, L., & Tryon, A. (1983). Learning through observation: The effects of peer modeling on acquisition and generalization in autistic children. *Journal of Abnormal Child Psychology, 11,* 355–365.

Charlop, M.H., & Trasowech, J.E. (1991). Increasing autistic children's daily spontaneous speech. *Journal of Applied Behavior Analysis, 24,* 747–761.

Clark, S., Remington, B., & Light, P. (1988). The role of referential speech in sign language learning by mentally retarded children: A comparison of total communication and sign-alone training. *Journal of Applied Behavior Analysis, 21,* 419–426.

Coe, D., Matson, J., Fee, V., Manikam, R., & Linarello, C. (1990). Training nonverbal and verbal play skills to mentally retarded and autistic children. *Journal of Autism and Developmental Disabilities, 20,* 177–187.

Collins, B.C., Branson, T.A., & Hall, M. (1995). Teaching generalized reading of cooking product labels to adolescents with mental disabilities through the use of key words taught by peer tutors. *Education and Training in Mental Retardation and Developmental Disorders, 30,* 65–75.

Cooke, N.L., Heron, T.E., Heward, W.L., & Test, D.W. (1982). Integrating a Down's syndrome child in a classwide peer tutoring system: A case report. *Mental Retardation, 20,* 22–25.

Cushing, L.S., & Kennedy, C.H. (1997). Academic effects of providing peer support in general education classrooms on students without disabilities. *Journal of Applied Behavior Analysis, 30*(1), 139–151.

Davis, C.A., & Reichle, J. (1996). Variant and invariant high-probability requests: Increasing appropriate behaviors in children with emotional-behavioral disorders. *Journal of Applied Behavior Analysis, 29*(4), 471–482.

Dugan, E., Kamps, D., & Leonard, B. (1995). The effects of using cooperative learning groups to facilitate integration of students with autism into a fourth-grade social studies class, *Journal of Applied Behavior Analysis, 28,* 175–188.

Dyer, K. (1989). The effects of preference on spontaneous verbal requests in individuals with autism. *Journal of The Association for Persons with Severe Handicaps, 14*(3), 184–189.

Egel, A., Richman, G., & Koegel, R. (1981). Normal peer models and autistic children's learning. *Journal of Applied Behavior Analysis, 11,* 3–12.

English, C., Goldstein, H., Shafer, K., & Kaczmarek, L. (1997). Promoting interactions among preschoolers with and without disabilities: Effects of a buddy skills-training program. *Exceptional Children, 63*(2), 229–243.

Farmer-Dougan, V. (1994). Increasing requests by adults with developmental disabilities using incidental teaching by peers. *Journal of Applied Behavior Analysis, 27,* 533–544.

Forest, M. (Ed.). (1987). *More education/integration: A further collection of readings on the integration of children with mental handicaps into the regular school systems.* Downsview, Ontario, Canada: The G. Allan Roeher Institute.

Fowler, S.A. (1988). The effects of peer-mediated interventions on establishing, maintaining, and generalizing children's behavior changes. In R.H. Horner, G. Dunlap, & R.L. Koegel (Eds.), *Generalization and maintenance: Life-style changes in applied settings* (pp. 143–171). Baltimore: Paul H. Brookes Publishing Co.

Franca, V.M., Kerr, M.M., Reitz, A.L., & Lambert, D. (1990). Peer tutoring among behaviorally disordered students: Academic and social benefits to tutor and tutee. *Education and Treatment of Children, 13,* 109–128.

Fuchs, L., Fuchs, D., Bentz, J., Phillips, N., & Hamlett, C. (1994). The nature of student interactions during peer tutoring with and without training and experience. *American Educational Research Journal, 31,* 75–103.

Garrison-Harrell, L., Kamps, D., & Kravits, T. (1997). The effects of peer networks on social-communicative behaviors for students with autism. *Focus on Autism and Other Developmental Disabilities, 12,* 241–257.

Gast, D.L., Winterling, V., Wolery, M., & Farmer, J.A. (1992). Teaching first aid skills to students with moderate handicaps in small group instruction. *Education and Treatment of Children, 15,* 101–124.

Goldstein, H., & Cisar, C.I. (1992). Promoting interaction during sociodramatic play: Teaching scripts to typical preschoolers and classmates with disabilities. *Journal of Applied Behavior Analysis, 25,* 265–280.

Goldstein, H., Kaczmarek, L., Pennington, R., & Shafer, K. (1992). Peer-mediated intervention: Attending to, commenting on, acknowledging the behavior of preschoolers with autism. *Journal of Applied Behavior Analysis, 25,* 289–305.

Goldstein, H., & Wickstrom, S. (1986). Peer intervention effects on communicative interaction among handicapped and nonhandicapped preschoolers. *Journal of Applied Behavior Analysis, 19,* 209–214.

Gonzalez-Lopez, A., & Kamps, D. (1997). Social skills training to increase social interactions between children with autism and their typical peers. *Focus on Autism and Other Developmental Disabilities, 12,* 2–14.

Greenwood, C.R. (1991). Longitudinal analysis of time, engagement, and achievement in at-risk versus non-risk students. *Exceptional Children, 57,* 521–535.

Gunter, P., Fox, J.J., Brady, M.P., Shores, R.E., & Cavanaugh, K. (1988). Non-handicapped peers as multiple exemplars: A generalization tactic for promoting autistic students' social skills. *Behavioral Disorders, 13,* 116–126.

Guralnick, M. (1990). Social competence and early intervention. *Journal of Early Intervention, 14,* 3–14.

Haring, T.G., & Breen, C. (1992). A peer-mediated social network intervention to enhance the social integration of persons with moderate and severe disabilities. *Journal of Applied Behavior Analysis, 25,* 319–334.

Haring, T.G., Breen, C., Pitts-Conway, V., Lee, M., & Gaylord, R. (1987). Adolescent peer tutoring and special friend experiences. *Journal of The Association for Persons with Severe Handicaps, 12,* 280–286.

Haring, T.G., Roger, B., Lee, M., Breen, C., & Gaylord-Ross, R. (1986). Teaching social language to moderately handicapped students. *Journal of Applied Behavior Analysis, 19,* 159–172.

Hart, B., & Risley, T. (1978). Promoting productive language through incidental teaching. *Education in Urban Society, 10,* 407–429.

Horner, R., Sprague, J., & Flannery, K. (1993). Building functional curricula for students with severe intellectual and severe problem behaviors. In R. Van Houten & S. Axelrod (Eds.), *Behavior Analysis and Treatment* (pp. 47–58). New York: Kluwer Academic/Plenum Publishers.

Hughes, C.A., & Boyle, J.R. (1991). Effects of self-monitoring for on-task behavior and task productivity on elementary students with moderate mental retardation. *Education and Treatment of Children, 14,* 96–111.

Hunt, P., Alwell, M., & Goetz, L. (1988). Acquisition of conversation skills and the reduction of inappropriate social interaction behaviors. *Journal of The Association for Persons with Severe Handicaps, 13,* 20–27.

Hunt, P., Alwell, M., & Goetz, L. (1991). Establishing conversational exchanges with family and friends: Moving from training to meaningful communication. *The Journal of Special Education, 25*(3), 305–319.

Hunt, P., Staub, D., Alwell, M., & Goetz, L. (1994). Achievement by all students within the context of cooperative learning groups. *Journal of The Association for Persons with Severe Handicaps, 19,* 290–301.

Jackson, N., Jackson, D., & Monroe, C. (1983). *Getting along with others: Teaching social effectiveness to children.* Champaign, IL: Research Press.

Johnson, T.E.B., Knowlton, H.E., Adams, S.E., & Swall, R. (1992). The effects of personal photographs on verbal responses to figural stimuli by students with moderate mental retardation: A Brunerian approach. *Education and Training in Mental Retardation and Developmental Disabilities, 27,* 367–378.

Jolly, A.C., Test, D.W., & Spooner, F. (1993). Using badges to increase initiations of children with severe disabilities in a play setting. *Journal of The Association for Persons with Severe Handicaps, 18,* 46–51.

Kaiser, A.P., Alpert, C.L., & Warren, S.F. (1987). Teaching functional language: Strategies for language intervention (pp. 247–272). In M.E. Snell (Ed.), *Systematic instruction of persons with severe handicaps.* Columbus, OH: Charles E. Merrill.

Kamps, D., Barbetta, P.M., Leonard, B.R., & Delquadri, J. (1994). Classwide peer tutoring: An integration strategy to improve reading skills and promote peer interactions among students with autism and regular education peers. *Journal of Applied Behavior Analysis, 27,* 49–61.

Kamps, D., Dugan, E.P., Leonard, B.R., & Daoust, P.M. (1994). Enhanced small group instruction using choral responding and student interaction for children with autism and developmental disabilities. *American Journal on Mental Retardation, 99,* 60–73.

Kamps, D., Gonzalez-Lopez, A., Potucek, J., Kravits, T., Kemmerer, K., & Garrison-Harrell, L. (1998). What do the peers think? Social validity of integrated programs. *Education and Treatment of Children, 21,* 107–134.

Kamps, D., Leonard, B.R., Dugan, E.P., Boland, B., & Greenwood, C.R. (1991). The use of ecobehavioral assessment to identify naturally occurring effective procedures in classrooms serving students with autism and other developmental disabilities. *Journal of Behavioral Education, 1,* 367–397.

Kamps, D., Leonard, B., Potucek, J., & Garrison-Harrell, L. (1995). Cooperative learning groups: An integration strategy to improve academic and social performance for students with autism and regular education peers. *Behavioral Disorders, 21,* 88–108.

Kamps, D., Leonard, B., Vernon, S., Dugan, E., Delquadri, J., Gershon, B., Wade, L., & Folk, L. (1992). Teaching social skills to students with autism to increase peer interactions in an integrated first grade classroom. *Journal of Applied Behavior Analysis, 25,* 281–288.

Kamps, D., Locke, P., Delquadri, J., & Hall, R.V. (1989). Increasing academic skills of students with autism using fifth grade peers as tutors. *Education and Treatment of Children, 12,* 38–51.

Kamps, D.M., Potucek, J., Gonzalez-Lopez, A.G., Kravits, T., & Kemmerer, K. (1997). The use of peer networks across multiple settings to improve social interaction for students with autism. *The Journal of Behavioral Education, 7,* 335–357.

Kapadia, S., & Fantuzzo, J.W. (1988). Training children with developmental disabilities and severe behavior problems to use self-management procedures to sustain attention to preacademic/academic tasks. *Education and Training in Mental Retardation and Developmental Disabilities, 23,* 59–69.

Kim, Y.T., & Lombardino, L.J. (1991). The efficacy of script contexts in language comprehension intervention with children who have mental retardation. *Journal of Speech and Hearing Research, 34,* 845–857.

Knapczyk, D.R. (1989). Peer-mediated training of cooperative play between special and regular class students in integrated play settings. *Education and Training in Mental Retardation and Developmental Disabilities, 24,* 255–264.

Koegel, L., Koegel, R., Hurley, C., & Frea, W. (1992). Improving social skills and disruptive behavior in children with autism through self-management. *Journal of Applied Behavior Analysis, 25,* 341–353.

Koegel, R.L., & Frea, W.D. (1993). Treatment of social behavior in autism through the modification of pivotal skills. *Journal of Applied Behavior Analysis, 26,* 369–377.

Koegel, R.L., & Koegel, L.K. (Eds.). (1995). *Teaching children with autism: Strategies for initiating positive interactions and improving learning opportunities.* Baltimore: Paul H. Brookes Publishing Co.

Koegel, R., O'Dell, M., & Koegel, L. (1987). A natural language teaching paradigm for nonverbal autistic children. *Journal of Autism and Developmental Disorders, 17,* 187–200.

Koegel, R.L., Schreibman, L., Good, A., Cerniglia, L., Murphy, C., & Koegel, L.K. (1989). *How to teach pivotal behaviors to children with autism: A training manual.* Berkeley: University of California Press.

Krantz, P., & McClannahan, L. (1993). Teaching children with autism to initiate to peers: Effects of a script-fading procedure. *Journal of Applied Behavior Analysis, 26,* 121–132.

Krantz, P., & McClannahan, L. (1998). Social interaction skills for children with autism: A script-fading procedure for beginning readers. *Journal of Applied Behavior Analysis, 31,* 191–202.

Kravits, T., Kamps, D., Kemmerer, K., & Potucek, J. (1998). Increasing communication skills for an elementary-aged student with autism using the picture exchange communication system. Manuscript submitted for publication.

Laski, K.E., Charlop, M.H., & Schreibman, L. (1988). Training parents to use the natural language paradigm to increase their autistic children's speech. *Journal of Applied Behavior Analysis, 21,* 391–400.

Light, J., & Binger, C. (1992). Story reading experiences of preschoolers using AAC systems [Abstract]. *Augmentative and Alternative Communication, 8,* 148.

Light, J., & Lindsay, P. (1991). Cognitive science and augmentative and alternative communication. *Augmentative and Alternative Communication, 7,* 186–203.

Lindsay, P., McNaughton, S., Vanderheiden, M., Ellis, V., Krogh, K., & McNamara, A. (1992). A model of literacy acquisition in the AAC user [Abstract]. *Augmentative and Alternative Communication, 8,* 148–149.

Lord, C., & Hopkins, J.M. (1986). The social behavior of autistic children with younger and same-aged nonhandicapped peers. *Journal of Autism and Developmental Disorders, 16*(3), 249–263.

Loveland, K.A., & Tunali, B. (1991). Social scripts for conversational interactions in autism and Down syndrome. *Journal of Autism and Developmental Disorders, 21,* 177–186.

MacDuff, G.S., Krantz, P.J., & McClannahan, L.E. (1993). Teaching children with autism to use photographic activity schedules: Maintenance and generalization of complex response chains. *Journal of Applied Behavior Analysis, 26,* 89–97.

Maheady, L., Sacca, M.K., & Harper, G.F. (1988). Classwide peer tutoring with mildly handicapped high school students. *The Council for Exceptional Children, 55,* 52–59.

Matson, J., Sevin, J., Fridley, D., & Love, S. (1990). Increasing spontaneous language in three autistic children. *Journal of Applied Behavior Analysis, 23,* 227–233.

McCarl, J., Svobodny, L., & Boare, P. (1991). Self-recording in a classroom for students with mild to moderate mental handicaps: Effects on productivity and on-task behavior. *Education and Training in Mental Retardation and Developmental Disabilities, 26,* 79–88.

McEvoy, M.A., Nordquist, V.M., Twardosz, S., Heckaman, K.A., Wehby, J.H., & Denny, R.K. (1988). Promoting autistic children's peer interaction in an integrated early childhood setting using affection activities. *Journal of Applied Behavior Analysis, 21,* 193–200.

McLean, J.E., Snyder-McLean, L.K., Jacobs, P., & Rowland, C.M. (1981). *Process-oriented educational programming for the severely-profoundly handicapped adolescent.* Lawrence: University Press of Kansas.

McMahon, C., Wacker, D., Sasso, G., Berg, W., & Newton, S. (1996). Analysis of frequency and type of interactions in a peer-mediated social skills intervention: Instructional vs. social interactions. *Education and Training in Mental Retardation and Developmental Disabilities, 31,* 339–352.

Meyer, L.H., Fox, A., Schermer, A., Ketersen, D., & Montan, N. (1987). The effects of teacher intrusion on social play interactions between children with autism and their nonhandicapped peers. *Journal of Autism and Developmental Disorders, 17,* 315–322.

Mirenda, P. (1985). Designing pictorial communication systems for physically able-bodied students with severe handicaps. *Augmentative and Alternative Communication, 1,* 143–150.

Mirenda, P., & Beukelman, D.R. (1990). A comparison of intelligibility among natural speech and seven speech synthesizers with listeners from three age groups. *Augmentative and Alternative Communication, 6,* 61–68.

Mirenda, P., & Santogrossi, J. (1985). A prompt-free strategy to teach pictorial communication system use. *Augmentative and Alternative Communication, 1,* 143–150.

Newman, B., Buffington, D.M., & Hemmes, N.S. (1996, December). Self-reinforcement used to increase the appropriate conversation of autistic teenagers. *Education and Training in Mental Retardation and Developmental Disabilities, 31,* 304–309.

Odom, S.L., Chandler, L.K., Ostrosky, M., McConnell, S.R., & Reaney, S. (1992). Fading teacher prompts from peer-initiation interventions for young children with disabilities. *Journal of Applied Behavior Analysis, 25,* 307–318.

Odom, S.L., & McConnell, S.R. (Eds.). (1992). Improving social competence: An applied behavior analysis perspective. *Journal of Applied Behavior Analysis, 25,* 239–243.

Odom, S.L., & McConnell, S.R. (1997). *Play time/social time: Organizing your classroom to build interaction skills.* Minneapolis: University of Minnesota.

Odom, S.L., McConnell, S.R., & McEvoy, M.A. (1992). Peer-related social competence and its significance for young children with disabilities. In S.L. Odom, S.R. McConnell, & M.A. McEvoy (Eds.), *Social competence of young children with disabilities* (pp. 3–35). Baltimore: Paul H. Brookes Publishing Co.

Oke, N., & Schreibman, L. (1990). Training social initiations to a high functioning autistic child: Assessment of collateral behavior change and generalization in a case study. *Journal of Autism and Developmental Disabilities, 20,* 479–497.

O'Reilly, M.F., & Glynn, D. (1995). Using a process social skills training approach with adolescents with mild intellectual disabilities in a high school setting. *Education and Training in Mental Retardation and Developmental Disabilities, 30,* 187–198.

Ostrosky, M.M., & Kaiser, A.P. (1995). The effects of a peer-mediated intervention on the social communicative interactions between children with and without special needs. *Journal of Behavioral Education, 5,* 151–171.

Partington, J.W., Sundberg, M.L., Newhouse, L., & Spengler, S.M. (1994). Overcoming an autistic child's failure to acquire a tact repertoire. *Journal of Applied Behavior Analysis, 27,* 733–734.

Pierce, K.L., & Schreibman, L. (1994). Teaching daily living skills to children with autism in unsupervised settings through pictorial self-management. *Journal of Applied Behavior Analysis, 27,* 471–481.

Pierce, K., & Schreibman, L. (1995). Increasing complex social behaviors in children with autism: Effects of peer-implemented pivotal response training. *Journal of Applied Behavior Analysis, 28,* 285–295.

Pierce, K., & Schreibman, L. (1997). Multiple peer use of pivotal response training to increase social behaviors of classmates with autism: Results from trained and untrained peers. *Journal of Applied Behavior Analysis, 30,* 157–160.

Quill, K. (1995). *Teaching children with autism: Strategies to enhance communication and socialization.* New York: Delmar.

Reichle, J., York, J., & Sigafoos, J. (1991). *Implementing augmentative and alternative communication: Strategies for learners with severe disabilities.* Baltimore: Paul H. Brookes Publishing Co.

Remington, B., & Clarke, S. (1983). Acquisition of expressive signing by autistic children: An evaluation of the relative effects of simultaneous communication and sign-alone training. *Journal of Applied Behavior Analysis, 16,* 315–328.

Roeyers, H. (1995). A peer-mediated proximity intervention to facilitate the social interactions of children with a pervasive developmental disorder. *British Journal of Special Education, 22,* 161–164.

Romer, L., White, J., & Haring, N. (1996). The effect of peer mediated social competency training on the type and frequency of social contacts with students with deaf-blindness. *Education and Training in Mental Retardation and Developmental Disabilities, 31,* 324–338.

Romski, M.A., Sevcik, R.A., & Wilkinson, K.M. (1994). Peer-directed communicative interactions of augmented language learners with mental retardation. *American Journal on Mental Retardation, 98,* 527–538.

Rotholz, D.A., Berkowitz, S.F., & Burberry, J. (1989). Functionality of two modes of communication in the community by students with developmental disabilities: A comparison of signing and communication books. *Journal of The Association for Persons with Severe Handicaps, 14*(3), 227–233.

Rowland, C., & Schweigert, P. (1993). Analyzing the communication environment to increase functional communication. *Journal of The Association for Persons with Severe Handicaps, 18,* 161–176.

Rynders, J., Johnson, R., Johnson, D., & Schmidt, B. (1980). Effects of cooperative goal structuring in producing positive interaction between Down syndrome and nonhandicapped teenagers: Implications for mainstreaming. *American Journal of Mental Deficiency, 85,* 268–273.

Rynders, J., Schleien, S., Meyer, L., Vandercook, T., Mustonen, T., Colond, J., & Olson, K. (1993). Improving integration outcomes for children with and without severe disabilities through cooperatively structured recreation activities: A synthesis of research. *The Journal of Special Education, 26,* 386–407.

Rynders, J.E., Schleien, S.J., & Mustonen, T. (1990). Integrating children with severe disabilities for intensified outdoor education: Focus on feasibility. *Mental Retardation, 28*(1), 7–14.

Sale, P., & Carey, D.M. (1995). The sociometric status of students with disabilities in a full-inclusion school. *Exceptional Children, 62,* 6–19.

Sasso, G., Hughes, G., Swanson, H., & Novak, C. (1987). A comparison of peer initiation interventions in promoting multiple peer initiators. *Education and Training in Mental Retardation and Developmental Disabilities, 22,* 150–155.

Sasso, G.M., Melloy, K.J., & Kavale, K. (1990). Generalization, maintenance, and behavioral covariation associated with social skills training through structured learning. *Behavioral Disorders, 16,* 9–22.

Sasso, G., & Rude, H. (1987). The effects of social status on interactions with severely handicapped children: Generalization of nontreated peers. *Journal of Applied Behavior Analysis, 20,* 35–44.

Sasso, G.M., Simpson, R.L., & Novak, C.G. (1985). Procedures for facilitating integration of autistic children in public school settings. *Analysis and Intervention in Developmental Disabilities, 5,* 233–246.

Schepis, M., Reid, D., & Behrmann, M. (1996). Effects of acquisition and use of voice output communication by individuals with profound multiple disabilities. In M. Behrmann (Chair), *Alternative means of enhancing communication for persons with severe disabilities.* Symposium conducted at the 22nd Annual Convention for Behavior Analysis, San Francisco.

Schleien, S., Heyne, L., & Berken, S. (1988). Integrating physical education to teach appropriate play skills to learners with autism: A pilot study. *Adapted Physical Activity Quarterly, 5,* 182–192.

Schleien, S., Rynders, J., & Mustonen, T. (1988). Art and integration: What can we create? *Therapeutic Recreation Journal, 22,* 18–29.

Shafer, E. (1993). Teaching topography-based and stimulus selection-based verbal behavior to developmentally disabled individuals: Some considerations. *The Analysis of Verbal Behavior, 11,* 117–134.

Shafer, M., Egel, A., & Neef, N. (1984). Training mildly handicapped peers to facilitate changes in the social interaction skills of autistic children. *Journal of Applied Behavior Analysis, 17,* 461–476.

Shapiro, E.S., & Klein, R.D. (1980). Self-management of classroom behavior with retarded/disturbed children. *Behavior Modification, 4,* 83–97.

Simpson, R.L. (1987). Public school integration of autistic pupils. *Focus on Autistic Behavior, 1,* 1–12.

Snyder-McLean, L.K., Solomonson, B., McLean, J.E., & Sack S. (1984). Structuring joint action routines: A strategy for facilitating communication and language development in the classroom. *Seminars in Speech and Language, 5,* 213–228.

Sommer, K.S., Whitman, T.L., & Keogh, D.A. (1988). Teaching severely retarded persons to sign interactively through the use of a behavioral script. *Research in Developmental Disabilities, 9,* 291–304.

Soto, G., Belfiore, P., Schlosser, R., & Haynes, C. (1993). Teaching specific requests: A comparative analysis on skill acquisition and preference using two augmentative and alternative communication aids. *Education and Training in Mental Retardation and Developmental Disabilities, 28,* 169–178.

Stahmer, A.C., & Schreibman, L. (1992). Teaching children with autism appropriate play in unsupervised environments using a self-management treatment package. *Journal of Applied Behavior Analysis, 25,* 447–459.

Stainback, S., & Stainback, W. (1989). Facilitating merger through personnel preparation. In S. Stainback, W. Stainback, & M. Forest (Eds.), *Educating all students in the mainstream of regular education* (pp. 121–128). Baltimore: Paul H. Brookes Publishing Co.

Staub, D., Schwartz, I.S., Gallucci, C., & Peck, C.A. (1994). Four portraits of friendship at an inclusive school. *Journal of The Association for Persons with Severe Handicaps, 19,* 314–325.

Strain, P., & Danko, C. (1995). Caregivers' encouragement of positive interaction between preschoolers with autism and their siblings. *Journal of Emotional and Behavioral Disorders, 3,* 2–12.

Strain, P., Danko, C., & Kohler, F. (1995). Activity engagement and social interaction development in young children with autism: An examination of free effects. *Journal of Emotional and Behavioral Disorders, 3,* 108–123.

Strain, P., Kerr, M., & Ragland, E. (1979). Effects of peer-mediated social initiations and prompting/reinforcement procedures on the social behavior of autistic children. *Journal of Autism and Developmental Disorders, 9,* 41–53.

Strain, P.S., Kohler, F.W., Storey, K., & Danko, C.D. (1994). Teaching preschoolers with autism to self-monitor their social interactions: An analysis of results in home and school settings. *Journal of Emotional and Behavioral Disorders, 2,* 78–88.

Strain, P.S., & Odom, S. (1986). Peer social initiations: Effective intervention for social skills development of exceptional children. *Exceptional Children, 52,* 543–552.

Strayhorn, J.M., Strain, P.S., & Walker, H.M. (1993). The case of interaction skills training in the context of tutoring as a preventive mental health intervention in schools. *Behavioral Disorders, 19,* 11–26.

Sugai, G., & Rowe, P. (1984). The effect of self-recording on out-of-seat behavior of an EMR student. *Education and Training of the Mentally Retarded, 19,* 23–28.

Taylor, B.A., & Harris, S.L. (1995). Teaching children with autism to seek information: Acquisition of novel information and generalization of responding. *Journal of Applied Behavior Analysis, 28,* 3–14.

Voeltz, L., Hemphill, N., Brown, S., Kishi, G., Klein, R., Furehling, R., Collie, J., Levy, G., & Kube, C. (1983). *The special friends program: A trainer's manual for integrated school settings* (Rev. ed.). Honolulu: University of Hawaii Press.

Walker, H., Hops, H., & Greenwood, C. (1988). *Social skills tutoring and games: A program to teach social skills to primary grade students.* Delray Beach, FL: Educational Achievement Systems.

Walker, H.M., Schwartz, I.E., Nippold, M.A., Irvin, L.K., & Noell, J.W. (1994). Social skills in school-age children and youth: Issues and best practices in assessment and intervention. *Topics in Language Disorders, 14,* 70–82.

Werts, M., Caldwell, N., & Wolery, M. (1996). Peer modeling of response chains: Observational learning by students with disabilities. *Journal of Applied Behavior Analysis, 29,* 53–66.

Wilson, C. (1993). *Room 14: A social language program.* East Moline, IL: LinguiSystems.

Wolery, M., Werts, M.G., Snyder, E.D., & Caldwell, N.K. (1994). Efficacy of constant time delay implemented by peer tutors in general education classrooms. *Journal of Behavioral Education, 4,* 415–436.

Zangari, C., Lloyd, L.L., & Vicker, B. (1994). Augmentative and alternative communication: An historic perspective. *Augmentative and Alternative Communication, 10,* 27–59.

Zaragoza, N., Vaughn, S., & McIntosh, R. (1991). Social skills interventions and children with behavior problems. *Behavioral Disorders, 16,* 260–275.

9

School-Age Children
Putting Research into Practice

Debra M. Kamps,
Adriana Gonzalez Lopez, and Christine Golden

As evidenced in the literature, there are a multitude of strategies to enhance the social and communicative skills of students with disabilities (e.g., Kamps et al., 1992; Ostrosky & Kaiser, 1995; Pierce & Schreibman, 1997). The following case studies illustrate peer mediation and direct instruction programs for two elementary-age students with developmental disabilities. The cases were selected to provide 1) intervention descriptions that are appropriate for verbal students with moderate cognitive delays (Jimmy), 2) social-communicative interventions as well as peer inclusive instruction for nonverbal or limited-language students with more severe cognitive delays (Billy), and 3) program descriptions that highlight interventions across multiple school environments including classrooms, playgrounds, play areas, and cafeterias (both cases).

JIMMY

Jimmy was a fourth-grade student with autism who was included in the general education classroom. He was able to read at the second-grade level but needed assistance for comprehension; he could recall basic factual information but was not able to draw inferences from

Procedures described in this chapter were developed through support by a grant from the Office of Special Education and Rehabilitation Services, U.S. Department of Education, #H023C30055 to the University of Kansas. The opinions expressed herein do not necessarily reflect the position of that agency, and no official endorsement should be inferred. For their assistance in procedural development and teacher training activities, the authors thank Jessica Potucek, Tammy Kravits, Linda Garrison-Harrell, Jorge Garcia, Betsy Leonard, Patricia Barbetta, Leslie Morrison, Daniel Parker, Kristi Ortiz, and Kristi Frissen.

readings. He also grasped basic math facts and number concepts with the assistance of manipulatives and produced three- to four-word sentences but not always with appropriate syntax. Jimmy requested needs and choices spontaneously but rarely initiated conversations with peers or adults. He typically understood language receptively and was able to request additional information when needed to complete tasks. Jimmy exhibited stereotypic gestures (finger waving) when overstimulated or when there were changes in his routine. He perseverated on particular topics (e.g., cartoon characters, time for activities in the classroom schedule). Nevertheless, Jimmy was generally compliant unless he was upset, and he liked to complete assignments.

A network of peers was established to help Jimmy maintain and improve his social competence. Although all the typical peers in Jimmy's class were involved, two to five peers at a time typically participated in activities with Jimmy (Garrison-Harrell, Kamps, & Kravits, 1997; Kamps, Potucek, Gonzalez-Lopez, Kravits, & Kemmerer, 1997). The peers were selected based on 1) age-appropriate play skills, 2) socially active roles as play partners (e.g., talkers, players), 3) good receptive/expressive communication, 4) reliability in following instructions, 5) ability to pay attention for 15 minutes, and 6) willingness to participate within or join an existing clique of peers (Haring & Breen, 1992; Odom & McConnell, 1997). In addition, parents were informed about the rotation of peers and classwide participation. They were asked to give permission for their children to be taken out of class to participate in social groups. Other helpful criteria for peers included good attendance, good academic records, and popularity, which all enhanced the probability of the acceptance of students with disabilities into peer groups.

Jimmy's skill level allowed for inclusion in a variety of general education classroom activities. Thus, social programs were designed to encompass both instructional (reading and math activities, independent work-time), and social environments (recess, lunch, free time). A primary goal was to increase opportunities to engage in interactions with peers and interventions that promoted appropriate verbalizations. Educators sought to improve Jimmy's social competence in the following contexts:

1. Games group (free time) during which students in the group practiced leisure and social skills as well as social interaction skills
2. Peer tutoring in which all students in the class engaged in reading practice, each assigned to rotating partners
3. Small-group math peer tutoring, again with rotating dyads
4. Lunch bunch in which four to five peers participated in conversation practice
5. Recess buddies in which students practiced specific outdoor games

6. Work groups of four students in which students assisted with independent work assignments
7. Monthly community-based field trips with Jimmy and two to six peers participating in age-appropriate leisure activities

Table 9.1 presents a summary of the peer programs designed to facilitate acquisition and maintenance of social competence for Jimmy, as well as information about the schedule, adults responsible for implementation, and the social goals addressed. Descriptions of the activities, the training process, and tips for implementation are provided in the sections that follow.

Games Group

Jimmy's games group occurred three times per week for 30 minutes with four peers typically participating. The teacher selected these students because they modeled appropriate social skills. The peers remained the same for the first 3 months of the school year and then rotated on a monthly basis so that all students could participate. Games included those appropriate for upper elementary-age students and those that appeared motivating for all participants. Examples included memory games, puzzles, Topple, Uno, Kerplunk, and Trouble.

Peer and Target Student Training

The skills selected for initial training for Jimmy and his peers were selected from two published curricula: *Social Skills Tutoring and Games: A Program to Teach Social Skills to Primary Grade Students* (Walker, Hops, & Greenwood, 1988), and *Play Time/Social Time: Organizing Your Classroom to Build Interaction Skills* (Odom & McConnell, 1997). Specific social skills taught were 1) playing and sharing (using names, asking and agreeing to play, sharing materials, taking turns), 2) giving help (offering help, asking for help, giving simple instructions, modeling, demonstrating), 3) keeping it going (extending play, routines), 4) conversations (talking about toys and games, asking and answering questions), 5) compliments (saying nice things about playing together, praising participation), and 6) problem solving (negotiating play activities and turns, dealing with problem behaviors).

The training format involved four steps. First, the adult presented the skill, defined it, and provided examples. One skill was presented per session, with frequent review of prior skills. Second, the adults and students practiced the skill in role plays. Third, the students practiced the role plays (five to six per session) with adult feedback. Fourth, the stu-

Table 9.1. Jimmy's peer programs for improving social competence

Peer program	Description	Social goals	Supervision
Games group	Three to five peers (rotate) play games (cards, memory, Kerplunk) for 20–30 minutes, three times weekly	Leisure skills, conversations, sharing, helping, keeping it going, compliments	Paraprofessional and speech-language therapist monitor
Peer tutoring: reading	Classwide reading in dyads from readers with point sheets for 30 minutes, three to four times weekly	Oral reading, awarding points, complimenting, helping, asking and answering questions	Teacher and paraprofessional supervise
Peer tutoring: math	Three peers and Jimmy are tutored by sixth graders on math facts for 10 minutes, three to four times weekly	Math facts, answering questions, following directions from peers	Paraprofessional monitors; teacher selects materials
Lunch bunch	Four to six peers and Jimmy describe pictures and use conversation topics for 15 minutes, three times weekly	Conversations, initiating, asking and answering questions, commenting	Paraprofessional monitors; speech-language therapist selects materials
Recess buddies	Multiple peers and Jimmy play kickball and practice functional language for 15 minutes at noon recess daily	Functional language, kicking/ running to bases, following directions from peers	Paraprofessional monitors
Peer helpers in work group	Three peers (rotate) in Jimmy's quad assist with work using script cards (help me/I need ____) daily during seatwork	Academic skills, requesting help, following directions, initiations to peers	Teacher and paraprofessional monitor assignment completion
Community field trips	Two to four peers (rotate) go on outings in community (fast food, bowling, miniature golf, shopping mall) once a month	Leisure skills, conversations, initiations to peers and community adults	Mother/paraprofessional monitor; teacher assists with skills

dents participated in the games group using different games and toys, with the adult providing prompting and feedback for an additional 10–15 minutes. The initial training lasted approximately 2 weeks. Thereafter, social skills were reviewed briefly at the beginning of games groups. This process is a typical training format for students with mild disabilities and those with higher-functioning autism (Kamps et al., 1992; Odom, Chandler, Ostrosky, McConnell, & Reaney, 1992; Pierce & Schreibman, 1997); however, this training format differed from many programs in which interaction skills focus on training peers independently of the student with disabilities (e.g., Ostrosky & Kaiser, 1995; Pierce & Schreibman, 1995, 1997). Similar outcomes for target students have been reported. For example, Pierce and Schreibman (1995) taught students with autism complex play actions (e.g., acting out a script with dolls), conversation skills (e.g., asking for toys from peers and narrating play, "I'm cooking the hamburger"), conversation expansions (e.g., "I like pizza; do you like pizza or ice cream?"), and turn taking. These researchers have developed a social skills training manual with scripts for peer training procedures (Pierce, 1997).

In addition to social skills training within the games group, additional training was necessary on an intermittent basis to help Jimmy learn how to play some of the games. This training used "social stories" (Gray, 1991), which were descriptive narratives of factual information about the games and expected student behaviors. Table 9.2 presents a social story for memory games. Initially, the teacher read the social story, and later peers reread the story. This strategy was quite useful because the student was primed for the activity and prompts were readily available, so the peers could reread the story or parts of the story as well as model the desired behaviors. Two procedures were especially helpful for teaching turn-taking skills within the games group. The first procedure was a written prompt for turn taking, a 3-inch by 5-inch card that said, "My turn." Students passed the card to the next person in the turn-taking sequence as a prompt to either wait (when another peer has the card) or to take a turn. A second procedure was a verbal prompt in which each student said the name of the next peer to take a turn "Jimmy's turn," "LaToya's turn," and so forth. This practice not only facilitated appropriate turn taking but also the use of peers' names.

Reinforcement for the games group consisted of stars on a chart for the use of skills that promoted interaction during the games. The adult initially provided reinforcement, but later the students practiced self-monitoring and peer-monitoring by awarding stars to each other on the chart for interactions (see Koegel, Koegel, Hurley, & Frea, 1992, and Koegel, Koegel, & Parks, 1989, for details on self-monitoring procedures). This procedure was coached by the adult and incorporated to

Table 9.2.   Social story for teaching and reviewing memory games

The Memory Game
I can play memory games with my friends.
I can play games during indoor recess or during game time at 3:30
  on Monday, Wednesday, Friday.
To play memory we take turns.
To take turns one person plays at a time:
  Turn over 2 cards.
  If a match (same), go again.
  If not a match (different), the next person takes a turn.
I only turn over the cards when it is my turn.
When it is not my turn, I watch my friends play.
I talk to my friends during the memory games.
I can talk about the game and say,
  Ty, it's your turn *or* Melissa, it's your turn.
  That's a match. Two birthday cakes!
  That's a match. Two pizzas!
  That's not a match. They are different.
  Too bad. Not a match.
I like to play memory with my friends.

To Play the Memory Game:
1. Put all the cards on the table:
_ _ _ _*   All students help place cards on table, pictures down.

2. Take turns:
_ _ _ _   One person at a time takes a turn.
_ _ _ _   Watch each person take a turn.

3. For your turn:
_ _ _ _   Turn over 2 cards
_ _ _ _   If a match (same), take another turn.
_ _ _ _   If not a match (different), the next person takes a turn.

4. At the end of the game:
_ _ _ _   All the cards are turned over. Count the number of matches.
The player with the most matches wins the game.

5. When finished:
_ _ _ _   All players help put the pictures back in the box.

---

*The teacher records as the target student completes/helps with each component of the game. The teacher places one mark in each blank as the student performs the skill.

promote independence by the students. Students also received stickers for participation in the games group each session. Figure 9.1 presents a model for the star chart used during games. This same monitoring chart can be used with students to promote generalization and reinforcement of conversation skills during additional social activities. Generalization was also promoted by providing games group practice for other games available during free time and indoor recess.

Peer Tutoring for Reading

The reading peer tutoring program was implemented on a classwide basis in Jimmy's fourth-grade class three times per week. The tutoring program provided practice in an important skill area (reading aloud to a peer) and was a mechanism for promoting appropriate social interaction.

The training procedures followed the Juniper Gardens Children's Project classwide peer tutoring format (CWPT) as published in the teacher manual (Greenwood, Delquadri, & Carta, 1997). These procedures have been implemented effectively in a study with three high-functioning students with autism (Kamps, Barbetta, Leonard, &

MONITORING CHART		
DID WE . . .	YES	NO
USE OUR FRIENDS' NAMES		
TALK NICELY TO OUR FRIENDS		
ASK OUR FRIENDS QUESTIONS		
ANSWER OUR FRIENDS		
HAVE CONVERSATIONS		
TALK TO EVERYBODY		
TAKE TURNS		
LET EVERYONE PLAY		

Figure 9.1. Sample monitoring chart for use in social skills group.

Delquadri, 1994). Students were assigned a partner who changed every week or two. These partners read to each other orally, provided points for reading, helped with unknown words, and asked comprehension questions. Students also reversed roles so that each student in the class served as both a tutor and a tutee within each 30-minute session. Points could be totaled for class teams; however, the teacher in Jimmy's class preferred to add all points as a "class total" to beat each consecutive tutoring session for the week.

Jimmy was able to read aloud to his partner and answer some comprehension questions that were factual. He also was able to provide points while his partner read but was not able to correct his partner's errors consistently. When his partner asked, "What is this word?" he was sometimes able to assist. Often, the peer prompted Jimmy to be sure he or she received points for each sentence read, and the paraprofessional also spent more time monitoring Jimmy and his partner than other pairs.

The teacher's role during tutoring was to rotate among students awarding bonus points for correct tutoring. The reading peer-tutoring program was initially trained in two class sessions (approximately 40 minutes in length), with individual retraining for students as necessary. An advantage to the CWPT program (Greenwood et al., 1997) was that the structured program included components identified as necessary for a successful social peer program (i.e., training, structured procedures, consistent opportunities for peer interaction, reinforcement). Consistent with many data-based studies documenting academic benefits for participants (see Greenwood, 1991), Jimmy's teacher applauded the benefits of the tutoring program for all students in the class.

Peer Tutoring for Math

The math peer tutoring was implemented as an individual program for Jimmy and three other students who had not mastered their math facts. Selected peers provided one-to-one tutoring in addition and subtraction facts for the students. Procedures followed the routine outlined by Greenwood and colleagues (1997), except they were implemented for the small group only, rather than classwide. The teacher assigned partners for the week and scheduled 10-minute tutoring sessions three times per week. When it was time for tutoring, the tutors retrieved the folders containing math facts preselected by the teacher. Students gathered in an alcove in the room for tutoring, each one sitting on carpet squares. Then, tutors presented the fact card to the student, provided praise, put two points on the tutoring score card for correct answers, and repeated the set until the timer sounded (7–8 minutes). When the student made an error, the tutor stated the fact (e.g., "3 times 5 equals 15"). The tutee then repeated the equation two times, and the tutor awarded one point. Points were graphed on a bar chart that was kept in the folder. Stickers were placed in a sticker book for the students for completing tutoring sessions. During math tutoring, a paraprofessional supervised students and gave prompts and reinforcement to all participants.

Lunch Bunch

Lunchtime is one of the more social times during students' school days. For students with autism or developmental disabilities, however, conversation skills may be limited and thus their social participation may be diminished or inappropriate. For Jimmy, peers used a *lunch bunch* routine to provide practice in conversation skills with lunch serving as a time for prompting and reinforcing language skills. The lunch bunch program used 1) picture or picture-word cues, 2) modeling and practice of question-and-answer routines and question-answer-comment routines, 3) advanced scripts (list of comments, questions followed by the target student to guide peer interaction), and 4) topic cards and reinforcement charts.

Peer and target student training consisted of modeling and practice of conversation skills. The skills included identifying appropriate conversation topics, making comments, asking and answering questions, and taking turns. An early procedure for Jimmy consisted of having a stack of note cards (3-inch by 5-inch index cards) with pictures from magazines and line drawings of items for making comments and asking questions. Fellow students were taught to select a note card from the pile, show it to a friend, and make a comment or ask a question. Examples of comments and questions were printed on the back of the cards. During training, using cards and taking turns were practiced in 10-minute sessions immediately prior to lunch.

As Jimmy and peers progressed with the note cards during lunch bunch, the students then advanced to using student-generated topics for conversations. The training procedure then consisted of students naming topics (e.g., field trips, pets, community activities, school projects, favorite activities during recess). The teacher or students wrote a list of three or four topics on a laminated 8½-inch by 11-inch sheet (topic card), and peers took turns making comments and asking questions. The teacher and students modeled examples.

A simple reinforcement procedure was used during the lunch bunch. Small stickers were placed on a reinforcement chart for each student's turn (e.g., each comment, each question-answer sequence). These stickers were tallied at the end of the lunch bunch time. Initially, the teacher placed stickers on the chart, but as students progressed with the game, peers took over the role of being the "sticker person" during each session (rotated among peers). All participants also received a piece of candy at the end of the lunch period. When students advanced to using the topic card, checks were placed on a monitoring sheet that listed each language skill on a separate row (comments, questions, answers). As each student took a turn, a check was placed in the appropriate row. Checks were tallied at the end of the session, with increasing checks as a goal for the activity. In some lunch bunch or conversation groups, students earn rewards for meeting the designated criterion. Rewards included 10 minutes of computer time, use of special toys at recess, and listening to music.

Recess Peer Programs

Recess is another socially active period for elementary school students. For students with autism who do not have a structured peer program, however, typical recess behaviors may include walking the perimeter of the playground repetitively, swinging on the same swing at every recess, engaging in stereotypic behavior using sticks or sand, and generally not participating in typical games and activities with peers. Peer network programming during recess involves 1) modeling and teaching simple games (e.g., kickball, tag), 2) teaching more advanced games (e.g., soccer, basketball), and 3) using scripts to teach age-appropriate participation.

Two procedures were used to increase Jimmy's peer interactions during recess. First, peer prompting and reinforcement were implemented. Kickball was a preferred game for Jimmy's classmates and thus selected for his participation. The targeted skills included waiting in line, kicking the ball when it was his turn, running to a base, following the peer coach's prompt at each base (run to next base, stop), repeating the sequence, and catching the ball in the outfield and throwing it to a peer. Student training occurred during the kickball game. Peers were prompted by the adult to prompt Jimmy to engage in each skill and to praise his participation (e.g., "Jimmy, you're waiting in line; good teamwork!" "Jimmy, your turn; get ready to kick," "Good kick; run to first base fast!"). Initially, two peers were designated as helpers, but as Jimmy learned the routine, all his classmates participated as "coaches" when next to him in line. An arrangement that facilitated success was placing a peer coach at each base including home base. Thus, a peer was readily available to direct the next action (e.g., going to the next base when a new person kicked the ball). Peer coaches were volunteers and were first kickers when their team was at home plate.

Second, script cards were used during the second half of the school year to encourage Jimmy's language expression during the games. The paraprofessional spent several sessions transcribing peers' comments during the kickball game and then wrote script cards to prompt Jimmy to use similar phrases. Examples of comments for kickball included "Kick the ball," "Run fast," "Great kick!" "Home run!" and "Go team!" The paraprofessional would wait for an opportunity to use a scripted line, then show the script to Jimmy, have him read it aloud, and say it to a peer. All scripted interactions were praised, and spontaneous language was noted on a reinforcement chart.

Peer Helpers During Work Groups

A final classroom procedure was designed to help Jimmy request assistance from peers when necessary during independent work time. Script cards were placed on Jimmy's desk as a visual cue to request help appropriately. Two cards were used, "Help me, please" and "I need _____" (e.g., pencil, paper, glue, book). Peers were taught to respond to Jimmy's initiations by asking him to show them what he needed help with (e.g., by pointing to directions or a word and then reading it to him) or by supplying the requested item or directing him to the location of the item (e.g., "Look in your pencil box"). Peers also were taught to ask the paraprofessional what they should do to provide assistance, if they were unsure. Generally, the paraprofessional would model two or three examples of ways to help Jimmy in his work group at the beginning of the activity. The teacher also changed the class groupings periodically so that students learned to work cooperatively with all class members. No formal training or reinforcement was provided for this program. Only a few examples were needed at the onset of independent tasks.

Community Field Trips

Jimmy had no formal home socialization programs; however, monthly field trips were scheduled after school to provide both reinforcement to peers and additional social skills practice in novel environments.

Jimmy's mother coordinated the activities with a paraprofessional who participated in the outings. The planning and implementation of outings included 1) generating a list of possible activities with peers at school, 2) scheduling the events for the next month, 3) drawing names for two to four peers to accompany Jimmy on each trip, 4) calling parents to coordinate dates and times (done by Jimmy's mother), 5) picking up the designated peers at the end of the school day when the field trip was planned, 6) going on the field trip, and 7) dropping students off after the trip.

Initially, parent information and permission letters were sent home to all peers in Jimmy's class. Twelve students' parents signed permission forms that they were agreeable to the field trips, and additional peers joined as the year progressed. From this pool of students, names were randomly drawn so that all students would have multiple opportunities to participate. Jimmy's mother and the paraprofessional decided in advance how many peers would participate depending on the requirements of the activity and their ability to supervise. With the number of peer programs in place at school, minimal training was necessary to promote successful field trips.

Two strategies were helpful, however, in facilitating interaction during the activities. First, Jimmy and his mother and siblings participated in the activity prior to including the peers at school, if it was a novel activity. This test run served to prime Jimmy for the activity, ensured that he was comfortable with the setting and requirements, and allowed his mother to determine appropriate accommodations in advance. Second, during the weeks of the field trips, the paraprofessional practiced role plays related to the activity during the social skills group at school. Thus, Jimmy and his peers practiced some of the required behaviors (ordering from the menu) and generated some conversational topics about the activity. These two procedures facilitated social interaction and successful participation during the field trips and provided additional social experiences for Jimmy with peers from school in new environments.

BILLY

Billy was a second-grade student with moderate mental retardation and some autistic-like behaviors. He participated in activities with second- and third-grade peers for approximately a third of his school day. He participated in intensive one-to-one and small-group instruction in a special education classroom for the remainder of the time. Billy used single word or simple phrases to communicate but generally did so only to request preferred items (i.e., ball, music, juice). He was able to play with several toys appropriately (balls, cars, tape player), could label several foods appropriately, and addressed many self-care needs (eating, washing hands, dressing with pull-over/pull-up clothes). He learned to match pictures, to sort by size and color, and to follow simple picture schedules. His instructional program targeted expressive communication training (sound production for common objects, requesting items using a communication board), functional item use (toys, mealtime items, classroom materials), following one- and two-part commands, self-care skills, and preacademic skills (e.g., sorting, matching, one-to-one correspondence). Behavior problems included occasional tantrums and crying, typically when Billy was tired, sick, or frustrated; stereotypic behaviors, such as rocking and jumping repetitively; and task avoidance in new situations (running, falling out of his chair). Billy was generally happy and responsive to positive reinforcement including a token system (chips on a token board exchanged for preferred activities and edibles) and hugs and smiles from adults.

Similar to Jimmy, social programs for Billy occurred throughout the school day and included multiple peers from his school (see Table 9.3). Because Billy spent approximately two thirds of his day receiving one-to-one and small-group instruction, peers were recruited from two classrooms for social programs, and some peer activities were conducted in a reverse mainstreaming format (peers went to the special education classroom). Programs were designed, similar to Jimmy's, to include both instructional activities (e.g., following directions, language training) as well as social times (e.g., free time, lunch, recess). Billy's programs focused on peer interactions that best fit his ability level and thus included peers as helpers, as well as playmates with social activities including the use of imitation, picture schedules, communication board icons, and simple gross motor activities. Educators sought to improve Billy's social competence in the following contexts:

• Playgroup with one to three peers practicing appropriate use of toys and social interaction skills
• Games in play stations (free time) during which peers engaged Billy in imitating actions and functional object use
• Lunch helpers with rotating peers who monitored his use of a picture activity schedule, encouraged his use of words, and practiced simple matching activities

Table 9.3. Billy's peer programs for improving social competence

Peer program	Description	Social goals	Supervision
Playgroup	Three to five peers (rotate) play with toys (cars, animals, blocks) for 20–30 minutes, three times weekly	Playing with toys, sharing, help-ing, initiating and responding to peers, making one- to two-word requests	Paraprofessional, speech-language therapist monitor
Play stations	Two or three third-grade peers rotate among six to eight tables in the gym, modeling play and use of picture schedule for 20 minutes, two or three times weekly	Playing with toys, imitation and incidental learning, responding to peers	Paraprofessional assists
Lunch helpers	Two peers (rotate) monitor Billy's use of picture schedule, prompt words, and do match/sort games three times weekly during lunch	Using a picture schedule, practic-ing language skills, matching and sorting, independence	Paraprofessional monitors
Recess buddies	Two to four peers (rotate) complete obsta-cle course, assist with kickball, or play affection activities (indoor recess) for 15 minutes daily during recess	Using leisure skills, following visual prompts and peer direc-tions, playing imitation games, singing, showing affection	Paraprofessional, occupational therapist monitor
Picture Exchange Communication System (PECS)	Two to four peers (rotate) in free time model use of communication board and toys with Billy for 10–15 minutes daily	Initiating to peers, using PECS, sharing, requesting, utilizing play skills	Training by speech-language therapist; special education teacher, paraprofessional monitor
Snack group	Two peers (rotate) help Billy practice greetings and asking for snack using PECS for 10 minutes daily	Initiating to peers, requesting, say-ing hi, using PECS	Speech therapist monitors
Sibling activity	One or two siblings use PECS to have snack and to play with toys with Billy during snack for 15 minutes daily and during playgroup for 30 minutes, two or three times per week	Initiating to siblings, requesting, using PECS, playing	Mother monitors

- Recess buddies who engaged in an obstacle course routine, affection activities, and playing ball
- Picture Exchange Communication System (PECS; Bondy & Frost, 1994) training with both the teacher and peers as language partners to promote initiation skills
- Snack group to promote peer initiation
- Home socialization activities with siblings

Playgroup

Playgroup activities were drawn from the Play Time/Social Time curriculum (Odom & McConnell, 1997), which consists of five key social skill areas: sharing, requesting to share, play organizing, agreeing, and assisting. Embedded within the skill areas were instrumental behaviors for learning initial social interaction (i.e., looking at peers, using names, playing with toys, giving and accepting toys by placing items in a peer's hand, and taking turns). The skills were designed for ages 4–8 years and had been validated with preschoolers, kindergartners, and first-grade children with autism and their typically developing peers.

The training program utilizes script training with specific and general prompts, modeling and partner practice during training, play after training with happy face charts for token reinforcement, play routines with examples of social skills and interactions, and a fading plan to reduce prompt levels and reinforcement (generalization phase). The 25 basic scripts and materials focus on age-appropriate activities and toys. Examples include a birthday party, cooking and eating, a car garage, fishing, a puppet show, zoo animals, and building a road for car and truck play. Table 9.4 illustrates a lesson for farm animals and blocks. Table 9.5 provides examples of prompting strategies from the curriculum.

Billy's social skills group was composed of one to three peers and occurred three times per week, lasting approximately 20 minutes. The speech-language therapist alternated leading the group with the paraprofessional. Scripts were sometimes simplified to match Billy's receptive language level. In addition, the speech-language therapist provided one-to-one instruction using the same materials as used in the playgroup. This language instruction covered object identification, functional use of items (e.g., driving toy car into garage), or the teaching of single words and requests. These direct instruction sessions served to develop expressive and receptive language skills and to prepare Billy for communication with his peers (see Wilde, Koegel, & Koegel, 1992).

Token reinforcement was delivered to the playgroup contingent on a predetermined number of correct responses and initiations (or

Table 9.4.   Sample social skills lesson: Farm animals and blocks

Materials: blocks, food bowls, blue paper for ponds, 6–8 farm animals

Children's Play: Children build a barn and use the animals in sociodramatic play in the barn.

Teacher's Role:

1. Arrangement: Place the blocks between the two children in each dyad and give each dyad some farm animals and one food bowl. Blue paper is used for ponds.

2. Introduction: Greetings (children say hi, using names). Introduce play—tell the children to build a big barn for the animals. Show them how to stack the blocks. Explain that the animals can live in the barn, drink from the pond, and eat from the bowls. Show them how the animals eat, talk to the other animals, and so forth.

3. Set timer: Remind children to play until timer rings (10 minutes).

4. Conduct the activity: Remember to prompt toy play and peer social interaction as necessary.

Prompts for Social Interaction:

1. Sharing
   "____, give ____ a block to put on the barn."
   "____, ask ____ if she wants the cow."

2. Requesting to Share
   "____, ask ____ to give you a block. Point to the one you want."
   "____, ask ____ if your cow can share the food bowl."

3. Play Organizing
   "____, tell ____ to put his horse in the barn."
   "____, tell ____ to take her pig swimming with your pig."

4. Agreeing
   "____, say 'yes, my dog is thirsty.'"
   "____, make your cow follow ____'s cow."

5. Assisting and Requesting Assistance
   "____, help ____ build a barn."
   "____, ask ____ to help you put some hay in the bowls for the cows."

Alternative play ideas: the animals get sick and go to the vet; animal parade

From Odom, S., & McConnell, S. (1997). *Play time/social time: Organizing your classroom to build interaction skills.* Minneapolis: University of Minnesota Press; adapted by permission.

approximations to correct responses). The reinforcement system varied in the number of responses required to earn each token and the number of tokens required for the reinforcer based on difficulty of the tasks. For example, initiating to a peer by saying his or her name or by tapping a shoulder was more difficult than imitating an action with a toy. All initiations to peers were reinforced with a token, whereas two or three play actions were required for a token.

Play Stations

Play stations served as a second type of playgroup for Billy during which he practiced imitation and following directions with two to three older peers, rather than dramatic play routines as in the social skills groups. This activity was based on an intervention evaluated by Carr and Darcy (1990) in which peers modeled gross motor skills and simple actions to children with autism to teach them to imitate a series of actions and to promote spontaneous imitation or observational learning in novel situations. Students were paired with a peer at different locations. The peer directed students to "watch me," and then demonstrated an action. Target students were prompted to imitate, if needed, with an adult providing occasional assistance and modeling. Carr and Darcy's (1990) results revealed high levels of generalized imitation in novel environ-

---

Table 9.5. Specific prompting strategies from the Play Time/ Social Time curriculum

---

Asking to play and giving toys:
    Look at your friend. Say, "Mike, let's play."
    Look. Tell your friend what to do: "Get the green fish."
    Look at your friend. Say, "Here, Julie." and put the toy in her hand.
Asking to share:
    Look at your friend. Hold out your hand. Say, "Give me __."
    Say, "Look, hand please." (hold out hand)
    Ask for a different toy.
    Use a picture of the toy to ask.
Persistence:
    Keep on trying if your friend doesn't play at first.
    Share a different toy.
    Touch your friend on the shoulder. Look at your friend.
    Talk a little louder.
    Try to share again.
    Try a new way. ("Play like this"; model.)
Prompting rules:
1. Prompt if the target student is not engaged in peer interaction for 30 seconds.
2. Prompt either the initiation or the response, not both.
3. After three prompts fail, wait, try another way/action/toy.
Play Time/Social Time is available from
Dr. Scott McConnell/University of Minnesota
Early Childhood Research Institute
215 Patee Hall
150 Pillsbury Drive SE
Minneapolis, MN 55455

From Odom, S., & McConnell, S. (1997). *Play time/social time: Organizing your classroom to build interaction skills.* Minneapolis: University of Minnesota Press; adapted by permission.

Table 9.6. Sample imitation activities for use with play stations

Item	Activity modeled by peer
Cup, can	Place cup in can Place cup on top of can
Hat, cone	Place hat on plastic cone Place hat on head
Ball	Kick ball or bounce ball
Tunnel	Crawl through tunnel Walk beside tunnel
Hurdle	Jump over hurdle Crawl under hurdle
Desk, mug	Put mug in desk Put mug on desk

From Carr, E., & Darcy, M. (1990). Setting generality of peer modeling in children with autism. *Journal of Autism and Developmental Disorders, 20,* 45–60; adapted by permission.

Additional items for Billy include more toys (e.g., basketball hoop, Toss Across, hammer and pegboard, whiteboard and dry erase marker).

ments following 8–25 training sessions. Table 9.6 provides examples of activities to teach imitation of peer models and activities probed for generalization.

Billy's play stations activities initially were similar to the activities in the Carr and Darcy study. Later, new activities were added to maintain interest in the activities. During the activities (20 minutes, three times per week), Billy accompanied the peers to the gym area. The peers placed items on several tables in the lunchroom to correspond to a small photo album with a picture schedule depicted with the play materials or the student using the materials. The paraprofessional prepared the photo album and picture schedule in advance. When it was time to begin, a peer gave the photo album to Billy, who then moved from station to station and engaged in the actions modeled by peers in earlier sessions. When new items were added, the peers demonstrated the action for Billy. If Billy did not complete the action at each station, a peer said, "Watch me," and modeled the play behavior. During the play stations activities, the adult observed and supervised but generally allowed the peers to lead the activity. Peers organized the stations, provided directions when necessary, offered praise and tokens at each station as Billy completed the actions, and prompted completion if needed. Thus, the activity was designed to work on several skills for Billy: using a picture schedule to complete a sequence and imitating models and following directions from peers. The training sequence was initially taught to peers without Billy present, with the adult providing additional guidance during play stations sessions as necessary.

Lunch Helpers

Because lunchtime was short, peers were asked to help Billy 1) follow a picture schedule for obtaining his lunch and utensils and cleaning up afterward, 2) name items to eat or drink, and 3) play simple matching games during the last 5 minutes when students were generally finished eating but waiting for the lunch period to end.

Two picture schedules were used for the lunch routine. These followed routines used to teach picture schedules developed by MacDuff and colleagues (e.g., MacDuff, Krantz, & McClannahan, 1993). To start lunch, the sequenced picture steps were children waiting in line, placing the ticket in the holder, collecting silverware from a bin, collecting milk from a bin, accepting the lunch tray from the cafeteria worker, and sitting at the table. The teacher worked with Billy using a simulated lunch routine to teach the steps of the activity and initially prompted him during lunch to follow the schedule. As Billy became independent with most steps in the sequence, peers were asked to monitor his completion of the schedule. They observed his completion of each step, checked off the step on the schedule, and praised Billy after every step or two.

During lunch, peers were taught to make five communication initiations to Billy and monitor his performance by making a check on a data sheet in the center of the table. The paraprofessional modeled examples of initiations during the first few minutes of lunch (e.g., "I like juice" before a drink, "good cake" after taking a bite, "pickles and ketchup" while looking at a hamburger). Peers prompted Billy by saying, "Look, Billy," prior to their initiations, gently touching his wrist as a delay tactic to prompt his imitation prior to a bite or a drink, pointing to the juice box, and so forth as gestural prompts, or providing a verbal prompt (e.g., "Say 'good juice'").

Simple matching games were played only when Billy completed lunch before the end of the period (one to two times per week for about 5 minutes). Billy was asked to match photos of toys used in the playgroups (both exact matches and similar matches such as different types of cars) and action pictures (e.g., jumping, climbing, playing ball). This matching activity was designed as a maintenance task to stimulate interaction (peers gave the photos to Billy and took turns) and as a deterrent to inappropriate behavior that occurred when Billy was bored.

A second picture schedule was used at the end of lunch and included the following steps: place items on tray, walk to trash bin in line with peers from table, throw away trash, place tray on cart, and follow peers in line to doorway.

Eating was an enjoyable activity for Billy. Thus, completing the picture schedule to obtain lunch was highly motivating. Initially, Billy received tokens on his reinforcement chart for learning the picture sequence. He eventually progressed to one token after the sequence was completed. Also, spontaneous verbal imitations were reinforced with tokens (prompted imitations were praised but not reinforced with a token). All spontaneous communication (labels, requests) was acknowledged and praised by peers and the paraprofessional placed a token on his reinforcement chart.

Recess Buddies

Peer intervention was conducted during three recess activities: an obstacle course with three to four peers, kickball, and affection activities (small group of peers singing songs and playing movement games) during indoor recess. During the morning recess, Billy could choose to join an activity in progress or practice gross motor skills in a parallel play fashion with the paraprofessional prompting skills (kicking the ball, climbing). The occupational therapist assisted one day per week, modeling skills for Billy and the paraprofessional. The recess buddies program was initiated daily during the afternoon recess.

All peers in Billy's homeroom class participated in the recess buddies program with rotations of three to four peers each week. The obstacle course consisted of a sequence of gross motor activities in a designated area of the playground. This activity was similar to the play stations in the cafeteria, except that outdoor equipment was used and Billy followed the lead of peers rather than a picture schedule. Peers took the materials to the playground, set up the obstacle course, chose a partner for the activity (one peer was with Billy), and took turns running the course. Obstacle course activities included relay races (teams), scooter board races (teams), split races (half running/half scooter boards), use of the playground equipment as part of the course, and incorporation of items into routines such as balls, jump ropes, balloons, or tunnels. As with the play stations, the adult initially taught the class the "system" and recruited ideas from peers for obstacle course activities. The adult also demonstrated ways to model and prompt Billy's participation, with assistance, directions, and feedback faded over time.

Billy was just beginning to learn kickball skills. Therefore, during some recesses when he was not running the obstacle course, Billy practiced kicking the ball (peers volunteered to roll him the ball) and running to bases. He engaged in approximately eight trials of kicking and running with the adaptive physical education coach supervising one recess per week with Billy and several classmates. The goal was to have Billy join in real kickball games with peers similar to Jimmy's case study.

Billy and his peers also engaged in affection activities (e.g., McEvoy et al., 1988). The affection activities were group songs and games that included an affection behavior as part of the routine (e.g., "If you're happy and you know it, hug a friend," "Simon says, give a high five.") Additional affection behaviors included patting someone on the back, shaking hands, winking at a friend, and clapping games. These activities were used with Billy during indoor recess and occasionally as part of morning routines.

The paraprofessional who supervised the obstacle course game initially used Billy's token system to reinforce completion of each part of the course, with a candy jar at the end of the course (each student took a piece of candy as they finished). As Billy learned the routines, he was motivated to engage in the obstacle course with peers without the token system; however, the candy jar was maintained. In addition, the recess buddies for the week went for a soda with the paraprofessional after the Friday recess. Intermittent token reinforcement was provided during the kickball practice and affection activities.

Picture Exchange Communication System

PECS (Bondy & Frost, 1994) was one of the primary language-training programs in Billy's daily instructional program. The program is designed to teach an alternative, nonverbal means for students to communicate using picture symbols on a communication board. PECS also promotes verbal skills for many of the students who receive training, as verbal models are provided as part of the program (Bondy & Frost, 1993). Other investigators have incorporated incidental teaching and initiation strategies into the teaching of augmentative and alternative communication systems (e.g., Mirenda & Iacono, 1988).

The training protocol has a number of phases: 1) physically assisted exchange (teaching students to initiate by giving a picture to an adult in exchange for an item), 2) expanding spontaneity (creating opportunities to initiate with the pictures to obtain desired items using an incidental teaching procedure), 3) discrimination of pictures (making choices among the pictures), 4) sentence structure (creating a series of pictures to make more complex requests), 5) responding to "What do you want?", and 6) commenting in response to a question. Billy advanced to Phase 3 of the program and thus was able to discriminate desirable items, choose the matching picture from the communication board, present the picture to his teachers and speech-language therapist, and receive the item. During free time activities, peers were taught to accept pictures from Billy, make the appropriate verbal response ("You want the bubbles!"), and give him the item. Thus, with minimal training, peers served as natural agents to reinforce communication initiations and engage in preferred play with Billy.

The PECS system has a built-in component for reinforcer assessment (conducted at the beginning of PECS training and intermittently when the system was in use). Thus, preferred items (highly motivating choices) constituted the majority of pictures on the communication board. Free time items that were depicted in Billy's system included toys providing sensory feedback as Billy preferred these (e.g., rubber balls, kaleidoscope viewers, musical toys, bubbles, and a small water tub with floating toys). No additional reinforcers (tokens, stickers) were necessary during the PECS training with peers.

Snack Group

Billy's snack group also used the PECS system. Snack group occurred for approximately 10 minutes every afternoon, and two to three peers participated. During this time Billy practiced two skills, saying "hi" to peers and requesting snack items using the PECS.

The procedure consisted of the paraprofessional and Billy approaching the snack table with the peers already seated, Billy waving and saying "hi," and Billy sitting at the table. The PECS communication board was on the table, and Billy took a snack item picture (potato chips, popcorn, raisins, and juice) and handed it to a peer, to which the peer replied, "You want the popcorn," and gave him a small bite. When Billy did not initiate with a picture, the peer prompted by holding out his or her hand. If this failed, the paraprofessional seated behind Billy gently pushed his arm toward the communication board to prompt Billy to pick up a picture and prompted handing the picture to the peer if necessary. Physical assistance was used to promote spontaneous initiations from the student rather than dependence on verbal requests by others (e.g., "What do you want to eat?"). The routine of saying "hi" and requesting snacks with the PECS was repeated for the four to six trials. Billy and peers then stayed at the table for a few extra minutes to allow Billy time to make multiple requests using the communication board. As during other PECS training times, the items received served as the reinforcer.

Home Socialization Procedures with Siblings

Corresponding home activities for Billy consisted of use of the PECS system during two scheduled times, snack and play. Billy's siblings participated in a snack routine similar to the school activity during which snack items were visible and shared with Billy upon initiation with the picture. This activity included at least one sibling when Billy first arrived home from school. In addition, a 30-minute play period was conducted two or three times per week during which the PECS system was used with toys available in their playroom (cars, musical toys, blocks) or outside (balls, sand toys, small trampoline). Phases in the PECS training and generalization programming were coordinated at monthly team meetings. This ensured that all people involved were requiring the same level of performance.

CONCLUSION

These case studies illustrate structured social programs for two students. Many of the programs have been experimentally validated in research studies with student-outcome data documenting benefits for students with mild to severe disabilities (e.g., Carr & Darcy, 1990; Garrison-Harrell et al., 1997; Gonzalez-Lopez & Kamps, 1997; Haring & Breen, 1992; Kamps et al., 1997; Krantz & McClannahan, 1993; Ostrosky & Kaiser, 1995; Pierce & Schreibman, 1995, 1997; Sasso, Hughes, Swanson, & Novak, 1987). The variety of programs incorporated into students' daily schedules attests to the viability of implementing multiple programs to maximize outcomes and ensure acquisition of behaviors. Much planning is needed to address social skills within students' instructional programs; however, relying on naturally occurring opportunities to teach social interaction skills is unlikely to be sufficient to promote successful relationships with school peers. These case studies are intended to demonstrate the degree of structure necessary initially to teach social skills to students with severe communicative and social impairments, including students with autism. Keep in mind that strict adherence to scripts, prompting procedures, and reinforcement schedules is faded as social competence is acquired. Learning social-communicative skills is an ongoing process similar to sequential curriculum programming in other developmental domains, such as language, reading, math, and self-care.

Data collection is necessary to monitor advancement in skills and social programs for students. Data collection may take several forms. One can use social skills checklists that are included in some curricula or other standardized social-behavior checklists (e.g., Gresham & Elliott,

SOCIAL INTERACTION DATA SHEET

Child's name:_____   Date:_____
Number of peers:_____   Observer:_____
Location:_____   Reliability:_____
Activity:_____
Condition (circle one):   Baseline   Training   Posttraining   Generalization

1	2	3	4	5	6
VERB ACT	VERB ACT	VERB ACT	VERB ACT	VERB ACT	VERB ACT
PI TI B	PI TI B	PI TI B	PI TI B	PI TI B	PI TI B
+ −	+ −	+ −	+ −	+ −	+ −
7	**8**	**9**	**10**	**11**	**12**
VERB ACT	VERB ACT	VERB ACT	VERB ACT	VERB ACT	VERB ACT
PI TI B	PI TI B	PI TI B	PI TI B	PI TI B	PI TI B
+ −	+ −	+ −	+ −	+ −	+ −
13	**14**	**15**	**16**	**17**	**18**
VERB ACT	VERB ACT	VERB ACT	VERB ACT	VERB ACT	VERB ACT
PI TI B	PI TI B	PI TI B	PI TI B	PI TI B	PI TI B
+ −	+ −	+ −	+ −	+ −	+ −
19	**20**	**21**	**22**	**23**	**24**
VERB ACT	VERB ACT	VERB ACT	VERB ACT	VERB ACT	VERB ACT
PI TI B	PI TI B	PI TI B	PI TI B	PI TI B	PI TI B
+ −	+ −	+ −	+ −	+ −	+ −
25	**26**	**27**	**28**	**29**	**30**
VERB ACT	VERB ACT	VERB ACT	VERB ACT	VERB ACT	VERB ACT
PI TI B	PI TI B	PI TI B	PI TI B	PI TI B	PI TI B
+ −	+ −	+ −	+ −	+ −	+ −

VERB = Verbal Behavior____%   PI = Peer Initiation____%
ACT = Activity Engagement____%   TI = Target Initiation____%
                                     B = Inappropriate Behavior____%
+ = Engaged in Social Interaction____%   − = Not Engaged in Social Interaction____%

Figure 9.2.   Sample interval data sheet for assessing peer interactions.

1990; Walker & McConnell, 1988). Data could be derived from ongoing monitoring of achievement of individualized education program (IEP) objectives. Language samples could be collected and analyzed to assess changes in the quantity and quality of social communication during peer programs. Figure 9.2 shows an interval recording system used to provide a global measure of social interaction for students. It is used to assess the percentage of intervals in which students engage in interaction (scored as + or −), as well as other related behaviors (e.g., activity engagement, appropriate verbalizations, target or peer initiations, inappropriate behaviors).

Problems and Solutions

Although the peer programs described previously have been used successfully with many students with disabilities, social skills are sometimes difficult to teach, and one is likely to encounter roadblocks when designing or implementing these programs. Examples of common issues and potential solutions follow.

Peer Avoidance

If peers are reticent initially, start with one or two peers and keep social skills sessions brief. Try to use preferred items and materials and use powerful reinforcers.

Lack of Play Skills

If the target student has limited play skills, start by using small segments of games. You may need to teach toy play in individual sessions and ask parents to teach play using the same toys.

Low Interactions

If interaction rates are too low, you may need to arrange the situations to increase interactions (e.g., asking for each piece needed for an activity). You may need to teach turn taking directly. Try to avoid overuse of instructions to the target student by emphasizing the use of comments about ongoing activities. As soon as possible, try to promote independence by using peer and student self-monitoring procedures.

Scheduling Problems

Teachers, parents, and administrators understandably are quite protective of intensive instruction time. To maximize times for social skill training, you may be able to use strategies that are appropriate for instruction time, such as classwide peer tutoring. You may need to recruit peers from multiple classrooms and look for other available blocks of time, such as before school routines, lunch and recess blocks, and special classes, such as physical education, library, music, and art times.

Personnel Assignments

Social skills teaching duties can be shared among many individuals, for example, paraprofessionals, speech and occupational therapists, and volunteers, as well as teachers. Some flexibility may be required to schedule activities and breaks. It may be possible to include older peers as well as same-age classmates.

Troubleshooting

It is important to include social skills objectives on the IEP. This will help ensure that time is devoted to planning, implementing, monitoring progress, and reporting results to the IEP team. One also may be able to request assistance from inclusion facilitators.

Generalization of Social Competence

Teaching social skills is unlikely to yield widespread maintenance, independence, and generalization unless teaching programs are systematic and comprehensive. The following strategies are likely to promote generalized and elaborated social skill usage (Kamps et al., 1997):

- Training mimics natural social situations.
- Similar situations are used across peer programs.
- Structured training occurs in close time proximity to natural environments or at the beginning of a social period (e.g., first 10 minutes of recess).
- Similar materials are incorporated in training and natural contexts
- Multiple peers and adults are trained and available during non-training times (environments).
- Multiple social interventions are scheduled across the day.

In summary, teaching social skills across multiple environments at school, at home, and in the community, with the inclusion of peers and siblings, will increase generalized skill use for students with disabilities (Strain, Kohler, Storey, & Danko, 1994). To accomplish this, parents, teachers, and peers alike must be committed to the value of social-communicative skills because active programming is needed to promote participation and to maximize benefits for all.

REFERENCES

Bondy, A., & Frost, L. (1993). Mands across the water: A report on the application of the picture-exchange communication system in Peru. *The Behavior Analyst, 16,* 123–128.

Bondy, A., & Frost, L. (1994). *The picture exchange communication system (PECS): Application with young children with autism.* Cherry Hill, NJ: Pyramid Educational Consultants.

Carr, E., & Darcy, M. (1990). Setting generality of peer modeling in children with autism. *Journal of Autism and Developmental Disorders, 20,* 45–60.

Garrison-Harrell, L., Kamps, D., & Kravits, T. (1997). The effects of peer networks on social-communicative behaviors for students with autism. *Focus on Autism and Other Developmental Disabilities, 12,* 241–254.

Gonzalez-Lopez, A., & Kamps, D. (1997). Social skills training to increase social interaction between children with autism and their peers. *Focus on Autism and Other Developmental Disabilities, 12,* 2–14.

Gray, C. (1991). *The social story book.* Jenison, MI: Jenison Public Schools.

Greenwood, C. (1991). Classwide peer tutoring: Longitudinal effects on the reading, language, and mathematics achievement of at-risk students. *Reading, Writing, and Learning Disabilities, 7,* 10–123.

Greenwood, C., Delquadri, J., & Carta, J. (1997). *Together we can! Classwide peer tutoring to improve basic academic skills.* Longmont, CO: Sopris West.

Gresham, F., & Elliott, S. (1990). *Social Skills Rating System (SSRS).* Circle Pines, MN: American Guidance Service.

Haring, T., & Breen, C. (1992). A peer-mediated social network intervention to enhance the social integration of persons with moderate and severe disabilities. *Journal of Applied Behavior Analysis, 19,* 319–333.

Kamps, D., Barbetta, P., Leonard, B., & Delquadri, J. (1994). Classwide peer tutoring: An integration strategy to improve reading skills and promote peer interactions among students with autism and general education peers. *Journal of Applied Behavior Analysis, 27,* 49–61.

Kamps, D., Leonard, B., Vernon, S., Dugan, E., Delquadri, J., Gershon, B., Wade, L., & Folk, L. (1992). Teaching social skills to students with autism to increase peer interaction in an integrated first-grade classroom. *Journal of Applied Behavior Analysis, 25,* 281–288.

Kamps, D., Potucek, J., Gonzalez-Lopez, A., Kravits, T., & Kemmerer, K. (1997). The use of peer networks across multiple settings to improve social interaction for students with autism. *Journal of Behavioral Education, 7,* 335–357.

Koegel, L., Koegel, R., Hurley, C., & Frea, W. (1992). Improving social skills and disruptive behavior in children with autism through self-management. *Journal of Applied Behavior Analysis, 25,* 341–353.

Koegel, L., Koegel, R., & Parks, D. (1989). *How to teach self-management to people with severe disabilities.* Berkeley: University of California Press.

Krantz, P., & McClannahan, L. (1993). Teaching children with autism to initiate to peers: Effects of a script fading procedure. *Journal of Applied Behavior Analysis, 26,* 121–132.

MacDuff, G., Krantz, P., & McClannahan, L. (1993). Teaching children with autism to use photographic activity schedules: Maintenance and generalization of complex response chains. *Journal of Applied Behavior Analysis, 26,* 89–97.

McEvoy, M., Nordquist, V., Twardosz, S., Heckaman, K., Wehby, J., & Denny, R. (1988). Promoting autistic children's peer interaction in an integrated early childhood setting using affection activities. *Journal of Applied Behavior Analysis, 21,* 193–200.

Mirenda, P., & Iacono, T. (1988). Strategies for promoting augmentative and alternative communication in natural contexts with students with autism. *Focus on Autistic Behavior, 3,* 1–15.

Odom, S., Chandler, L., Ostrosky, M., McConnell, S., & Reaney, S. (1992). Fading teacher prompts from peer-initiation interventions for young children with disabilities. *Journal of Applied Behavior Analysis, 25,* 307–317.

Odom, S., & McConnell, S. (1997). *Play time/social time: Organizing your classroom to build interaction skills.* Minneapolis: University of Minnesota Press.

Ostrosky, M., & Kaiser, A. (1995). The effects of a peer-mediated intervention on the social communicative interactions between children with and without special needs. *Journal of Behavioral Education, 5,* 151–171.

Pierce, K. (1997). *Teaching typical children to be social skills trainers for their schoolmates with autism: A training manual.* Berkeley: University of California Press.

Pierce, K., & Schreibman, L. (1995). Increasing complex social behaviors in children with autism: Effects of peer implemented pivotal response training. *Journal of Applied Behavior Analysis, 28,* 285–295.

Pierce, K., & Schreibman, L. (1997). Multiple peer use of pivotal response training to increase social behaviors of classmates with autism: Results from trained and untrained peers. *Journal of Applied Behavior Analysis, 30,* 157–160.

Sasso, G., Hughes, G., Swanson, H., & Novak, C. (1987). A comparison of peer initiation interventions in promoting multiple peer initiators. *Education and Training in Mental Retardation and Developmental Disabilities, 22,* 150–155.

Strain, P., Kohler, F., Storey, K., & Danko, C. (1994). Teaching preschoolers with autism to self-monitor their social interactions: An analysis of results in home and school settings. *Journal of Emotional and Behavioral Disorders, 2,* 78–88.

Walker, H., Hops, H., & Greenwood, C. (1988). *Social skills tutoring and games: A program to teach social skills to primary grade students.* Delray Beach, FL: Educational Achievement Systems.

Walker, H.M., & McConnell, S.R. (1988). *Walker-McConnell Scale of Social Competence and School Adjustment.* Austin, TX: PRO-ED.

Wilde, L., Koegel, L., & Koegel, R. (1992). *Increasing success in school through priming: A training manual.* Berkeley: University of California Press.

10

Promoting Social-Communicative Interactions in Adolescents

Craig H. Kennedy

Social interaction has emerged as a defining aspect of human experience. From both phylogenetic and ontological perspectives, there is evidence for the central role of social affiliation in psychological development (Darwin 1871/1989; Gewirtz & Petrovich, 1983; Hoffman, 1997; Piaget, 1971). Early aspects of development, such as a preference for orienting toward human faces, provide insight into the infants' predisposition to social stimuli (Cohen, DeLoache, & Strauss, 1979; Kagan, 1970). These social influences continue as children are taught a language and are enculturated into specific societal practices (Guerin, 1994; Moerk, 1992). As children mature, the influence of social interactions becomes increasingly pervasive. Until late childhood, those influences are largely derived from family members; however, by early adolescence a transfer of social influence occurs that increasingly involves peer group members (Buhrmester, 1990; Patterson, Reid, & Dishion, 1992).

Although the interaction partners may change, the influence of others' reinforcing social behavior remains central in determining a person's pattern of behavior, sometimes referred to as *personality* (Meehl, 1986; Thompson & Lubinski, 1986). This critical role for social interaction, with its biological and cultural bases, also is important for the social support it provides (Kennedy, Horner, & Newton, 1989; Pierce, Sarason, & Sarason, 1996). The behaviors that are exchanged between two or more individuals not only shape future responding but also provide meaningful assistance in a person's daily life. Social interactions serve a utilitarian purpose (Cook, 1987; Hamblin & Kunkel, 1977; Homans, 1974). For example, providing a pencil to a person who has requested it not only reinforces his or her request (Skinner, 1957) but also enables the speaker to act on his or her environment with enhanced competence. This social support component of social interaction began to interest researchers studying the social development of people with severe disabilities in the 1990s (Haring, 1991; Kennedy & Shukla, 1995; Storey, 1993).

Interest in social support behavior comes from the promise it holds for improving a person's quality of life and, conversely, from concerns regarding the bleak outcomes documented for individuals who lack social supports. From the 1970s to the year 2000, researchers documented the positive health and psychological effects of social supports and the negative impact resulting from the absence of social supports (Gottlieb, 1997). Because social support is derived through social interaction, understanding what occurs during social interactions as well as extended patterns of affiliation may provide important insights into enhancing the lives of people with severe disabilities.

This chapter focuses on adolescents with severe disabilities and the strong and evolving research literature documenting various aspects of their social development. We begin by asking what the smallest unit of measure should be for social interaction research. A review of research literature suggests that social development should be analyzed using a triadic perspective involving students with disabilities, their peers, and their teachers. Given such a conceptualization, multiple methods for assessing the participation of adolescents with severe disabilities are necessary, and a discussion of the field's current status is provided. Finally, strategies that have been developed to increase the frequency and quality of adolescent social interactions are presented, along with data illustrating their effects for students with severe disabilities.

THE NATURE OF SOCIAL INTERACTIONS

A common conceptualization is that social interactions are based on dyads of individuals. Perhaps this perspective derives from our many observations of long-term interactions occurring in pairs (e.g., dating, marriage). Indeed, most studies on social development have focused on dyads. Along with an intuitive appeal, such pairings also reveal our goal of facilitating friendships between students with disabilities and their peers. Friendships are, after all, between two individuals.

With adolescents, however, the focus of social interaction expands from an emphasis on the specific activity being engaged in with some other person, a pattern indicative of younger children's interactions (Selman, 1980), into a larger social context. This raises an interesting question: When analyzing social interactions and the social relationships that emerge from those interactions, should the focus be on just two people? The answer proposed in this chapter is no; dyads are not enough.

The field of *network analysis* suggests a quantitatively derived answer to studying social structure that is based on triads (Cartwright & Harary, 1956; Holland & Leinhardt, 1971; Johnson, 1985). The left panel of Figure 10.1 illustrates a set of dyads composed of a student with disabilities, the two peers she interacts with, and a teacher. Such an analytic tactic allows for the study of interaction between the student and Peer 1, the student and Peer 2, and the student and teacher but only as discrete pairings. Although each dyad can be studied separately, dyadic analyses do not permit the larger network of relationships to be revealed. The right panel of Figure 10.1, however, shows the integrative effect of using a triadic analysis. With triads, relationships among each of the individuals can be revealed without the need for larger analyti-

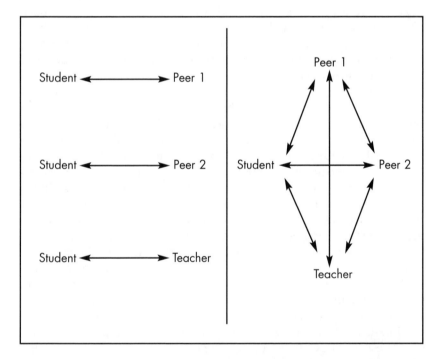

Figure 10.1. Two perspectives on analyzing social interaction. The left-hand panel shows a pattern of analysis that emphasizes dyadic interactions between a student with severe disabilities and her peers and teacher. The right-hand panel shows a pattern of analysis that focuses on triadic interactions among the student, peers, and teacher. The triadic approach allows for the analysis of social connections among the entire constellation of individuals, rather than only pairs of individuals.

cal structures (e.g., quadratic). Such a change in focus allows for an analysis of relationships among each of the individuals in relation to the other three participants.

Along with providing a mathematical vehicle for quantitative analysis (Hallinan, 1978/1979), examining social interactions as triads permits the study of additional social relationships that might bear on the development and maintenance of student–peer relationships (Moreno, 1953). Such analyses are particularly desirable for adolescents who, as noted previously, are coming under the influence of increasingly complex sets of social variables. Since the early 1980s, researchers have studied adolescent social interactions between students with severe disabilities and peers without disabilities. These studies have revealed important facets of dyadic social interactions, such as the importance of reciprocal sharing and age-appropriate activities (e.g., Gaylord-Ross, Haring, Breen, & Pitts-Conway, 1984). Because of the dyadic structure of the analyses, however, such studies have not been able to reveal the expanded social context of additional peers and adults.

A 1997 study by Cushing and Kennedy illustrated the importance of an expanded analytical scope. These authors studied the influence of teachers on peer support groups comprised of a student with severe disabilities and a peer without disabilities. The authors' findings demonstrated the important influence that adults can have on the classroom behavior of peers without disabilities, suggesting that adults also need to be included in social interaction research (a suggestion requiring triadic social structures). Similarly, Shukla, Kennedy, and Cushing (1998) found that peer-to-peer relationships could affect social interactions between a peer without disabilities and student with disabilities. Shukla and colleagues studied peer support groups comprised of two peers without disabilities and one student with severe disabilities. Social interactions among the three adolescents were frequent and of high quality; however, when one peer terminated his participation in the peer support group, substantial reductions occurred in the frequency and quality of social interactions between the remaining peer without disabilities and the student with disabilities. These results suggest the importance of studying peer-to-peer relationships as part of a larger network of social interactions involving students with severe disabilities.

These findings lend empirical support to the theoretical suggestion of expanding social interaction analysis to triadic structures. By expanding the scope of social interaction analyses, new dynamics of social participation may be revealed for study. Such an expanded conceptualization of social interactions may be necessary when dealing with the increased array of social influences that emerge in the social life of adolescents. An expansion also may reveal new functional influences on individual social relationships that previously have gone undetected. This suggestion has important consequences not only for how researchers conceptualize adolescent social interactions but also for how those interactions are measured.

MEASURING ADOLESCENT SOCIAL INTERACTIONS

Without adequate and dependent measures, no phenomenon can be understood, regardless of whether the method of study is quantitative or qualitative. To begin with, measures need to be reliable. Most important, that means that under constant conditions, repeated measures will yield similar results. If measures are not reliable, then unwanted variability is introduced (Sidman, 1960). If a measure is reliable, then the complex issue of validity, in this case defining *social interaction*, is encountered. The problems encountered when defining social interaction can be illustrated by asking a room full of adults to each write down his or her definition of *friendship*. The typical outcome of such an exercise is to encounter as many definitions as there are definers.

Despite the observation just made, some consensus has emerged across researchers about differing levels of social interaction. Not all researchers will agree with any conceptualization of social interaction, but the following conceptualization draws from many different literatures and sources to offer a reasonably integrative picture of a student's social life. Such a conceptual unit can be a useful heuristic because it suggests differing levels of social interaction that can be defined and studied in their own right, or the levels defined as distinct can be studied to see how they are integrated within particular contexts.

Figure 10.2 presents one possible conceptual model that is used by a variety of academic disciplines, including psychology, education, sociology, anthropology, health science, and mathematics. The figure illustrates three levels of social interaction within the context of various environments. At the macro-level, *social networks* organize social interactions along large spatio-temporal dimensions. The concept of a social network is an abstraction attempting to summarize the connections a group of people have with each other (Cartwright & Harary, 1956). The particular connections depend on the question being asked by researchers. In previous studies, for example, connections have been defined as friendships (e.g., Suitor & Keeton, 1997), classroom interactions (e.g., Jansson, 1997), peer cliques (e.g., Kirke, 1996), and family influences on problem behavior (e.g., Samualson, 1997). The social net-

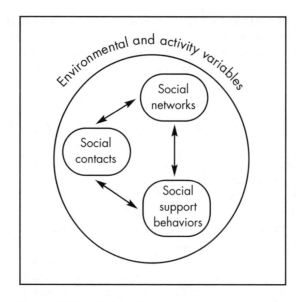

Figure 10.2. A conceptual approach to assessing adolescent social interactions.

work concept is useful as it can describe a pattern of interrelationships among a group of people that is not directly observable from one moment to the next because of the scope of the activities.

The next level shows an intermediate degree of analysis. *Social contacts* are interactions among individuals or groups of individuals. This construct encompasses interactions of 1 second or greater in length. Documenting social contacts describes who interacts with a student with disabilities, as well as the frequency and duration of those interactions (Bijou, Peterson, & Ault, 1968; Odom, McConnell, & McEvoy, 1992; Strain, 1990). Such data can identify students' social affiliation patterns at the level of discrete interactions. Argyle (1969, 1993) and Barker (1978), for example, made extensive use of social contacts as a descriptive means of documenting people's interactions. Such patterns can document how frequently particular individuals interact, whether that pattern is affected by the time of the day, the extent to which the interaction is mediated by other individuals, and whether the communication is embedded within a particular activity or environment.

The third level in Figure 10.2 is referred to as *social support behaviors*. This level of analysis focuses on the actions of participants. Put another way, social support behaviors occur during social interactions. These behaviors often have been combined into broad reciprocal classes (e.g., initiations or expansions) of social interaction (e.g., Goldstein,

Kaczmarek, Pennington, & Shafer, 1992; Haring, Roger, Lee, Breen, & Gaylord-Ross, 1986; Kamps et al., 1992). The concept of reciprocity (Strain, Odom, & McConnell, 1984) and the reinforcement entrapment that the process entails (McConnell, 1987) has proven an important vehicle for understanding social interaction processes. Because of the fruitfulness of reciprocal-interaction classes, researchers have attempted to decompose these broad classes into fine-grained classes based on the consequences of behavior and the topography of responding involved (e.g., Fryxell & Kennedy, 1995; Hughes, Lorden, & Scott, 1997; Hunt, Staub, Alwell, & Goetz, 1994). Behavioral groupings emerging from such analyses include giving physical assistance, hanging out together, providing companionship, and sharing information about current events.

Finally, *environments* are important, if for nothing else, as stimulus controls for various repertoires (Bronfenbrenner, 1979; Keller & Schoenfeld, 1950; Skinner, 1953). A person interacts differently with others in a synagogue than in a Thai restaurant or on the dance floor at a county fair. Environments also are important because they allow access to specific activities that often are dependent on the situation. People ride roller coasters, eat fast food, watch various performances, and play video games at amusement parks; they engage in very different activities in an algebra class. These contextual variables are of interest because they allow individuals to interact based on commonly preferred activities within mutually accessible environments (Newton & Horner, 1993).

This conceptual model of social interaction allows for multiple, integrated levels of analysis and encompasses a great deal of what interests researchers, practitioners, and families about an adolescent's social life. Multilevel systems require multiple measures and approaches to information collection (Bijou et al., 1968). The value of a diverse approach to data collection is the possibility of discovering phenomena or interrelations among events that were previously undocumented. Following this perspective for conceptualizing and measuring social interactions, the next section discusses differing approaches to improving interactions and the results that have been encountered by researchers.

VARIABLES INFLUENCING THE QUALITY OF ADOLESCENT SOCIAL INTERACTIONS

The remainder of this chapter focuses on various approaches to facilitating quality social interactions for adolescents with severe disabilities. Unlike younger children with severe disabilities, there does not appear to be a correlation between the severity of an adolescent's disabilities and his or her social participation and relationship development (Fryxell & Kennedy, 1995; Kennedy, Shukla, & Fryxell, 1997; Newton & Horner, 1993). Research findings for this group of students seem to support this nonexclusionary perspective. Because of this, this section focuses on strategies that work for a variety of learners with severe disabilities and does not presume any prerequisites for social interactions and relationship development. This literature review follows the time span of social-relationship development. The emphasis is on teacher- and peer-oriented strategies for producing meaningful outcomes. Given the various strategies that are emerging for documenting social interactions, a variety of effects can be documented that are associated with specific support strategies. The current literature can, by no means, tell a practitioner or family member how to *produce* friendships between adolescents with and without severe disabilities; however, the current literature offers some specific techniques that, when used at specific times, have been demonstrated to facilitate the development of social interactions.

An inductively derived sequence of "critical" phases based on a series of analyses of relationship development (e.g., Jackson & Rodriguez-Tomé, 1993; Kennedy, Cushing, & Itkonen, 1997) is proposed. Figure 10.3 presents an example of three such phases for Dan, a high school student with severe and multiple disabilities: 1) initial encounters, 2) additional interactions, and 3) sustained interactions. The numbers in the figure represent the number of individuals without disabilities who Dan interacted with at least once for an extended period of time (i.e., 15 minutes or greater) during the first 3 months of the school year. Along the *x*-axis is the number of school weeks that elapsed from their first interaction to the last interaction for that particular school year. The *y*-axis shows the number of different activities that Dan and each peer engaged in during the school year.

A set of social interaction patterns typically emerges across the course of a school year that are reflected in Dan's data. Pattern 1 represents a group of peers who interacted with Dan only once (lower left-hand corner). These peers were introduced to Dan, their interactions were supported by adults, and no further interactions occurred (30% of the total number of peers). Pattern 2 is exemplified by peers who continued to interact with Dan for a few weeks, engaged in several different activities, and then stopped interacting (59% of the total). Pattern 3 includes a final group of peers (11% of the total) who continued their social interactions with Dan throughout the school year and engaged in a large variety of activities with him (upper right-hand corner).

These patterns of social interaction suggest differing phases along which social contacts develop. The first phase is the initiation of interactions: who interacts with whom, where they interact, and what activ-

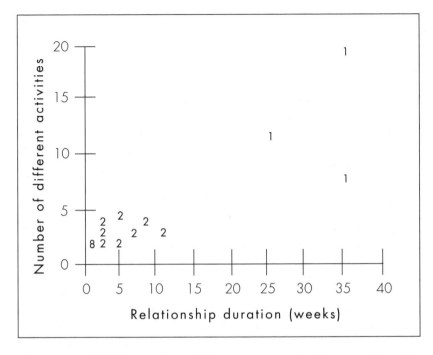

Figure 10.3. Social contact patterns for Dan across one school year. The data points are the numbers that correspond to how many individual peers without disabilities Dan interacted with for at least 15 minutes. The vertical axis represents the number of different activities Dan and a peer engaged in during the year. The duration of each social relationship is arrayed along the horizontal axis.

ities they do. If the initial interaction is not properly supported, then further opportunities for interaction may be avoided by one or more of the individuals involved. For social contacts that continue beyond the first or second interaction, however, a second pattern emerges in which a variety of activities are typically engaged in (moderated by environmental variables, of course). At this point, a bifurcation emerges within 5–10 weeks of repeated interactions. Most peers terminate their interactions, while a smaller subgroup moves on to sustained interactions with the student with severe disabilities (the third pattern). Each phase is discussed next, along with the research literature that suggests particular approaches for facilitating social interactions at each point in time.

Initial Social Encounters

One fundamental finding keeps being replicated in the research on initiating social interactions—the more typical the environment and activities engaged in, the more peers without disabilities and adolescents with severe disabilities are likely to meet (Fryxell & Kennedy, 1995; Kennedy, Shukla, & Fryxell, 1997; Logan & Keefe, 1997; Schnorr, 1997). There are two broad approaches to initiating social interactions for adolescents with severe disabilities. First, peers without disabilities can be brought into environments in which adolescents with severe disabilities have been traditionally supported (i.e., special education classrooms). This typically entails providing incentives for peers to participate in environments that they would not otherwise encounter. A second general approach is to have students with severe disabilities participate in environments in which adolescents without disabilities are typically educated (i.e., general education classrooms).

Very different levels of social contact will occur as a result of these approaches. For example, middle school students with severe disabilities will meet an average of one new peer without disabilities every 3 weeks using special education–based approaches; however, middle school students with severe disabilities will meet an average of two new peers without disabilities each week using general education–based approaches (Kennedy, Cushing, et al., 1997; Kennedy, Shukla, et al., 1997). This statistic means a difference of 12 versus 70 new peers interacted with each year for the special and general education–based approaches, respectively.

Students can be introduced into general education environments in a number of ways (Downing, 1996; Falvey, 1995; Gaylord-Ross & Pitts-Conway, 1984). Ecological inventories offer an effective entry into general education environments (e.g., Rainforth & York-Barr, 1997). Ecological inventories allow practitioners to assess what activities occur within a general education environment (e.g., chemistry, art) and identify potential matches with a student's individualized educational program. This approach can facilitate participation of the student with severe disabilities in typical routines and activities of the general education classroom and thereby increase opportunities for initial social interaction (Hunt, Farron-Davis, Beckstead, Curtis, & Goetz, 1994; Kennedy & Itkonen, 1994).

The network of individuals involved in the initial contact a student has with peers without disabilities needs to be considered. Previously in the chapter, a case was made understanding how multiple individuals interact with the student with disabilities and others involved in those interactions. Although this fact is not well documented in the research literature, there is an implicit suggestion that multiple individuals are involved in the initiation of social interactions. Typically those initial interactions involve an adult (e.g., general education teacher, special education instructional assistant), the student with severe disabilities, and one or more peers without disabilities. If peers and students are not familiar with each other, then the role of an adult as facilitator may be important in structuring interactions (Gaylord-Ross & Pitts-Conway, 1984; Hunt, Staub, et al., 1994); however, if students and peers have a history of interacting, then the role of adults may be more peripheral.

Finally, social support behaviors appear to be higher when participation in general education is the strategy used to initiate social interactions. For example, Fryxell and Kennedy (1995) observed that students with severe disabilities were more likely to engage in social support behaviors toward their peers within the context of general education classrooms, relative to special education–based environments. Although the occurrence of social support behaviors overall tends to be higher within general education environments, whether those levels result from simply being introduced into those environments or from a gradual shaping process that may occur over time is unclear (see Guralnick, Connor, Hammond, Gottman, & Kinnish, 1995). Further research is necessary to understand the initial impact of general education participation on students' social support behaviors and the social support behaviors they receive from their peers without disabilities.

There is growing evidence that a normative, or general education, focused approach to initiating social interactions is preferable to previous alternatives. Clearly, there are benefits to general education participation at the levels of social networks, social contacts, and social support behaviors. Because these are only introductory encounters, it appears that an ecological perspective focusing on participation in typical activities leads to more interactions. Although these initial contacts are important, as was exemplified in Dan's case, what occurs after may be far more influential in improving the prospects of durable social interaction patterns.

Facilitating Additional Social Interactions

Several issues emerge when an adolescent with severe disabilities initiates social interactions with his or her peers. Assessment of the roles and activities the student with disabilities will engage in within the general education environment is necessary. In addition, the interests and needs of peers without disabilities need to be estimated and integrated into an ongoing support plan. Finally, teachers and instructional assistants need to assess their roles in supporting students with disabilities and peers without disabilities. Each of these issues appears influential in the establishment of quality social interactions.

The context for facilitating social interactions in general education environments—whether it be art, calculus, physical education, vocational training, or English classes—is the establishment of a *support system*. A support system is typically composed of 1) the activities a student with disabilities will engage in, 2) people who will interact with the student while he or she engages in the activities, 3) the curricular adaptations that will occur, 4) information on how the support system is structured, and 5) the person who is responsible for monitoring the system's integrity. Each of the three constituencies mentioned previously—teachers, students, and peers—typically contribute to the establishment of a support system. Such peer-mediated strategies (Odom et al., 1992) at the middle and high school level are often referred to as *peer support programs* (Haring & Breen, 1992; Hughes et al., 1997; Hunt, Staub, et al., 1994; Kennedy & Fisher, 2001). A framework for establishing peer support programs is presented next.

Research on peer support programs has revealed that a student with severe disabilities might expect to have approximately 23 interactions with six different typical peers across four different environments and six activities per school day (Fryxell & Kennedy, 1995; Kennedy, Shukla, & Fryxell, 1997). In other words, peer support programs can be an effective means of facilitating social interactions within general education contexts. Peer support programs also appear to facilitate friendship development. Fryxell and Kennedy (1995) and Kennedy, Shukla, and Fryxell (1997) have found that students participating in general education classrooms via peer support programs have between 7 and 12 friends (versus 1 or 2 in more traditional arrangements). In addition, Shukla and colleagues (1998) have demonstrated that students with disabilities engage in more frequent and diverse social support behaviors within the context of peer support programs. The remainder of this section focuses on a detailed discussion of the various parameters of peer support programs.

Selecting Activities

The first element of establishing a peer support program is to specify the activities that the student with disabilities will engage in. Although this component has been an integral part of previous analyses of peer supports, no study has directly compared differing approaches to activity identification and selection. Indeed, as noted in the previous section on initiating social interactions, the use of ecological inventories has become ubiquitous for this purpose. Whether this aspect of developing peer supports influences subsequent social interactions remains an unanswered question.

Recruiting Peer Supports

The second component of peer support programs is the identification and use of peers without disabilities to participate in the groups. Some of the strategies proposed have included 1) circles of friends, 2) peer buddy systems, 3) lotteries or random selection, and 4) peer volunteers. Circles of friends introductions present the student with disabilities to the class and illustrate the impoverished nature of his or her social network when compared with peers in the classroom. Typically, after this introduction, a peer or peers are asked to help the student with disabilities participate in class activities. Perhaps because the student with disabilities is placed within the context of an outsider to the general education classroom, rather than an integral component, circles of friends introductions have largely been supplanted by other approaches.

Peer buddy systems focus on recruiting peers within the larger school context (Gaylord-Ross & Pitts-Conway, 1984; Haring & Breen, 1992; Hughes, Harmer, Killian, & Niarhos, 1995). Often announcements or presentations are made recruiting peers without disabilities to be "buddies" for students with disabilities. The focus is then on matching a peer or peers with a student to engage in interactions within particular school environments. Sometimes those environments include general education classes in which the peers can serve as peer supports. To date, these approaches have been demonstrated to be an effective means of recruiting peers and retaining them as peer supports for more than one school semester (Gaylord-Ross et al., 1984; Haring & Breen, 1992; Hughes et al., 1995).

Another approach that is proving viable is to use a probabilistic system of peer selection. Referred to as lotteries or random selection, these approaches allow each peer in a class to serve, at least temporarily, as a peer support (e.g., Gaylord-Ross et al., 1984). Peers without disabilities are selected on a daily or weekly rotation to provide support to a student with disabilities. Advantages of this system include the opportunity for each peer in the class to interact with the student with disabilities. Its primary disadvantages are that some peers may not want to interact with the student with disabilities and the strategy precludes long-term support by a particular peer. Overall, however, this approach has been demonstrated to be effective for adolescents (Kennedy & Fisher, 2001).

The final approach to recruiting peer supports is based on volunteerism. Generally, a special or general education teacher makes an announcement at the start of the semester that peers without disabilities are needed to assist a student with disabilities. Peers can then volunteer after the announcement or at some other time. Given the number of peers that volunteer, fixed or rotating support groups are then typically arranged. Results for this approach suggest that it is effective for both recruiting and retaining peers for up to one school year (Hunt, Staub, et al., 1994; Kennedy, Cushing, et al., 1997; Kennedy & Itkonen, 1994).

Identifying Curricular Adaptations

A third component of peer support programs is the identification of curricular adaptations for the student with severe disabilities. Once these activities are identified, one must consider what modifications in activities may be needed. The typical approach to curricular adaptation has been for teachers to develop the general strategies to be used and then either modify the materials directly themselves (e.g., Dugan et al., 1995) or teach peers how to modify class materials (e.g., Cushing & Kennedy, 1997). Both approaches have been used by researchers but not directly compared. Because the activities and their modifications provide the context for student and peer interactions, assessment of the potential effects of these different approaches is warranted. For example, directly engaging a peer without disabilities in the initial efforts of modifying curricular materials may allow for incorporation of peer interests into the process. This action has the potential to enhance interest in the activities by the various people involved in the interactions.

Structuring and Monitoring Support

Perhaps the most critical issue affecting the quality of social interactions within peer support programs is the structuring and monitoring of the groups. An important aspect of the structure of support groups is who is involved and to what extent. A related issue is the role teachers serve in influencing social interactions. The triadic conceptualization of social interactions presented in Figure 10.1 indicates that socially relevant events occur among various individuals, not just between student–peer dyads. Research suggests that the roles of students with disabilities and each peer without disabilities need to be individualized based on the social dynamics within a peer support group. A review of recent studies highlights the pertinent issues for each constituency.

Variables that influence the participation of students with severe disabilities within peer support groups are diverse. Student preferences are clearly a critical component (Dattilo & Rusch, 1985; Haring & Lovinger, 1989). Among the possible preferences that might be assessed, choices regarding activities and peers seem the most germane. For example, decreases in engagement or increases in problem behavior can result if a particular peer or teacher who is a preferred interactant does not participate at some level. In addition, activities should reflect a student's interests to maximize his or her engagement (Logan, Bakeman, & Keefe, 1997).

Providing systematic instruction to the student with disabilities also has the potential to improve interactions with peers. The reasons for general education participation are twofold. The first reason is to facilitate the development of social relationships; the second reason is to develop new skills and competence. There does not appear to be any conflict between increasing a student's social participation and increasing his or her personal competence (Hunt, Farron-Davis, et al., 1994; Kamps et al., 1992; Shukla, Kennedy, & Cushing, 1998, 1999). Indeed, the two goals appear to be complementary (Haring, 1991).

Social skills training is particularly well-suited to peer support contexts. Social skills interventions serve the dual role of improving social competence and increasing inclusion (Guralnick, 1990; Haring, 1991; Strain, 1990). This is particularly the case for peer-mediated interactions that form the basis of peer supports (Haring, 1991; Odom et al., 1992). As long as training of skills occurs within typical contexts, the outcomes associated with this type of process appear desirable and appropriate (Gaylord-Ross et al., 1984).

Similar issues are apparent for peers without disabilities. An emerging issue in the peer support literature is the role of peer preferences and interests in the structuring of peer supports. Studies assessing this aspect of peer support groups provide some evidence that peer preferences can be involved both in the quality of social interactions and the continued participation of peers in the support program (Cushing & Kennedy, 1997; Shukla et al., 1998, 1999).

Although it has often been taken at face value that the primary reason a peer is involved in a peer support program is an interest in the student with disabilities, other social interests may exist. For example, a peer also may be interested in interactions with adults that being a peer support provides. Another reason is that the presence of another peer within the support program may provide some influence on a particular individual's participation and quality of interaction. Current data suggest that formally or informally assessing peer social interests may provide important information regarding peer support membership (Cushing & Kennedy, 1997; Cushing, Kennedy, Shukla, Davis, & Meyer, 1997; Shukla et al., 1998, 1999).

An often encountered concern with peer support programs and with general education participation for students with severe disabilities is that the quality of instruction may be reduced for peers without disabilities (Kauffman & Hallahan, 1995). Although intuitively appealing, the data for systematic inclusion efforts do not support this concern. Research has indicated that including peer supports groups in general education classrooms does not have a negative impact on overall class performance (Cushing et al., 1997; Dugan et al., 1985) or the performance of peer supports (Cushing & Kennedy, 1997; Shukla et al., 1998, 1999). In fact, data summarized from the Cushing and colleagues (1997) and Shukla and colleagues (1998, 1999) studies suggest a pattern of academic improvement resulting from being a peer support (Figure 10.4). The figure shows the relative change in grades received by peers prior to beginning as a peer support and during their time as a peer support, as a function of their baseline performances. The data suggest no adverse effects of being a peer support and some potentially positive outcomes for some peers.

Although the importance of peer interests and preferences is only beginning to be appreciated by researchers focusing on adolescent social development, from the studies that have been conducted, it appears as if the role of peer preferences may be very influential. Those influences may include the peers who participate in support groups, their respective roles, and the activities in which they engage. A better understanding of peer interests may not only affect the frequency and quality of social interactions within peer support groups but may play a pivotal role in the long-term maintenance of social interactions (a topic covered in the following section).

Supporting Durable Relationships

Social interactions function at many levels—they provide social support, shape social competence, and form the foundation for friendships. If adolescent social interactions are successfully supported during their initial development, approximately 10% of the peers contacted go on to establish friendships lasting at least 1 year (Kennedy & Itkonen, 1994; Kennedy, Shukla, & Fryxell, 1997). Theoretically, there is no reason why that percentage could not be higher. Actually, little is known about the pattern of durable social relationships in adolescence or how to improve an individual's social outcomes.

Available information indicates that long-term interactions, such as those observed in Dan's graph, differ from more short-lived interactions. Whereas short-term interactions are characterized by an increase in the types of activities engaged in, it appears as if more durable interactions settle into a relatively stable pattern (Kennedy & Itkonen, 1994; Kennedy, Shukla, & Fryxell, 1997). That stability, in our research, has been observed in terms of the types of activities that form the context

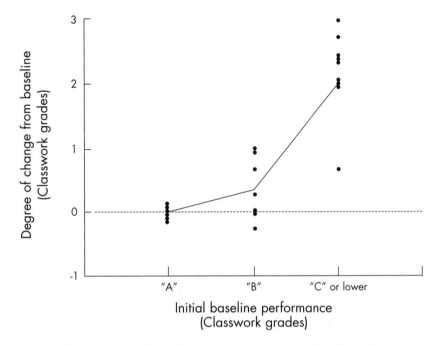

Figure 10.4. Summary of data from several studies assessing the effects of serving as a peer support on the academic performances of peers without disabilities. The horizontal axis shows peers' baseline grades prior to becoming a peer support. The vertical axis represents the change in peers' academic performances following their serving as a peer support. Data points represent individual students, and lines represent the mean for each set of data points.

for social interactions, as well as the days and times that those interactions occur. As long as the stability in interaction patterns remains, relationships appear to continue.

Interestingly, when this pattern of stability changes, it may signal a potential transition point in the relationship. For example, if a set of peers have been gathering for lunch at the same time each day throughout the first two quarters of the school year, a change in one or more peers' schedules may break this pattern. For a student with severe disabilities who has interacted regularly with a peer during those lunches, additional supports by adults may be necessary to overcome this disruption. If not, such subtle changes as an alteration in class schedule can have negative long-term consequences for adolescent social interactions (Coleman, 1961).

Adults' monitoring of durable social interactions provides one means of detecting when disruptions in stable contact patterns might occur. When such disruptions occur, one should assess potential causes of the disruption. A number of strategies may be effective in overcoming disruptions in stable patterns:

1. Have the individuals involved in durable relationships focus on multiple activities and/or engage in those activities in multiple environments. Such an arrangement might overcome disruptions that are localized (e.g., a change in part of a daily class schedule).
2. Facilitate interactions after school and on weekends to provide more contexts for interaction so that school-based interactions are only part of the social contact pattern.
3. If possible, have multiple peers involved in social interactions so that if one individual is unable to interact on a regular basis, others will still be available to maintain interactions.

Unfortunately, little research has focused on analyzing strategies for maintaining durable social relationships (Newton, Olson, & Horner, 1995). All that can be concluded at this point is that characteristic patterns of behavior emerge that identify relationships as becoming stable and durable, although those patterns differ among networks of interactants. Given both the complexity of analyzing durable social interactions and the important contribution these relationships make to a person's overall quality of life, it is a topic that deserves intensive study.

CONCLUSION

Enough is known about measuring and improving social interactions for adolescents with severe disabilities to be optimistic. It can be said with the assurance of empirical evidence that 1) social interactions develop within a predictable series of phases, 2) differing approaches to educational placement have a significant impact on social affiliation patterns, 3) peers without disabilities do form durable relationships with adolescents with severe disabilities, 4) more typical environments and activities occasion more frequent, and higher quality, social interactions, and 5) adolescents with severe disabilities are more socially competent when systematically supported in general education environments than in more traditional arrangements.

This review of the literature has identified a number of areas that have yet to be studied. Those areas include strategies for recruiting peers for social interactions, the costs and benefits of specific approaches to arranging peer supports within general education environments, and variables that contribute to the development and support of lasting social interactions. Also, the social interests and needs of peers without disabilities who participate in social interactions with adolescents with severe disabilities are clearly important but not well understood.

As each of these areas is further researched, undoubtedly, there will be important insights into the nature of social interactions. As basic knowledge of the development of social interactions progresses, it can be expected, and indeed demanded, that support technologies be improved and tested. This synergistic coupling of research and practice in the area of social interaction research has proven effective with younger learners with severe disabilities since the 1970s. It is anticipated that similar gains will be made for adolescents with severe disabilities.

REFERENCES

Argyle, M. (1969). *Social interaction.* Chicago: Aldine.

Argyle, M. (1993). *Experiments in social interaction.* Brookfield, VT: Dartmouth Publishing.

Barker, R.G. (1978). *Habitats, environments, and human behavior.* San Francisco: Jossey-Bass.

Bijou, S.W., Peterson, R.F., & Ault, M.H. (1968). A method to integrate descriptive and experimental field studies at the level of data and empirical concepts. *Journal of Applied Behavior Analysis, 1,* 175–191.

Bronfenbrenner, U. (1979). *The ecology of human development: Experiments by nature and design.* Cambridge, MA: Harvard University Press.

Buhrmester, D. (1990). Friendship, interpersonal competence, and adjustment in preadolescence and adolescence. *Child Development, 61,* 1101-1111.

Cartwright, D., & Harary, F. (1956). Structural balance: A generalization of Heider's theory. *Psychological Review, 63,* 277–293.

Cohen, L.B., DeLoache, J.S., & Strauss, M.S. (1979). Infant visual perception. In J.D. Osofsky (Ed.), *Handbook of infant development* (pp. 83–101). New York: John Wiley & Sons.

Coleman, J.S. (1961). *The adolescent society.* New York: Free Press.

Cook, K.S. (1987). *Social exchange theory.* Thousand Oaks, CA: Sage Publications.

Cushing, L.S., & Kennedy, C.H. (1997). Academic effects of providing peer support in general education classrooms on students without disabilities. *Journal of Applied Behavior Analysis, 30,* 139–152.

Cushing, L.S., Kennedy, C.H., Shukla, S., Davis, J., & Meyer, K.A. (1997). Disentangling the effects of curricular revision and social grouping in cooperative learning arrangements. *Focus on Autism and Other Developmental Disabilities, 12,* 231–240.

Darwin, C.R. (1989). *The descent of man, and selection in relation to sex.* New York: New York University Press. (Original work published 1871)

Dattilo, J., & Rusch, F.R. (1985). Effects of choice on leisure participation for persons with severe handicaps. *Journal of The Association for Persons with Severe Handicaps, 10,* 194–199.

Downing, J.E. (1996). *Including students with severe and multiple disabilities in typical classrooms.* Baltimore: Paul H. Brookes Publishing Co.

Dugan, E., Kamps, D., Leonard, B., Watkins, N., Rheinberger, A., & Stackhaus, J. (1995). Effects of cooperative learning groups during social studies for students with autism and fourth-grade peers. *Journal of Applied Behavior Analysis, 28,* 175–188.

Falvey, M.A. (1995). *Inclusive and heterogeneous schooling: Assessment, curriculum, and instruction.* Baltimore: Paul H. Brookes Publishing Co.

Fryxell, D., & Kennedy, C.H. (1995). Placement along the continuum of services and its impact on students' social relationships. *Journal of The Association for Persons with Severe Handicaps, 20,* 259–269.

Gaylord-Ross, R.J., Haring, T.G., Breen, C., & Pitts-Conway, V. (1984). The training and generalization of social interaction skills with autistic youth. *Journal of Applied Behavior Analysis, 17,* 229–248.

Gaylord-Ross, R.J., & Pitts-Conway, V. (1984). Social behavior development in integrated secondary autistic programs. In N. Certo, N. Haring, & R. York (Eds.), *Public school integration of severely handicapped students: Rational issues and progressive alternatives* (pp. 197–219). Baltimore: Paul H. Brookes Publishing Co.

Gewirtz, J.L., & Petrovich, S.B. (1983). Early social attachment learning in the framework of organic and cultural evolution. In T.M. Field, A. Huston, H.C. Quay, L. Troll, & G.E. Finley (Eds.), *Review of human development* (pp. 3–19). New York: John Wiley & Sons.

Goldstein, H., Kaczmarek, L., Pennington, R., & Shafer, K. (1992). Peer-mediated intervention: Attending to, commenting on, and acknowledging the behavior of preschoolers with autism. *Journal of Applied Behavior Analysis, 25,* 289–306.

Gottlieb, B.H. (1997). *Coping with chronic stress.* New York: Kluwer Academic/Plenum Publishers.

Guerin, B. (1994). *Analyzing social behavior: Behavior analysis and the social sciences.* Reno, NV: Context Press.

Guralnick, M.J. (1990). Social competence and early intervention. *Journal of Early Intervention, 14,* 3–14.

Guralnick, M.J., Connor, R.T., Hammond, M., Gottman, J.M., & Kinnish, K. (1995). Immediate effects of mainstreamed settings on the social interactions and social integration of preschool children. *American Journal on Mental Retardation, 100,* 359–377.

Hallinan, M.T. (1978/1979). The process of friendship formation. *Social Networks, 1,* 193–210.

Hamblin, R.L., & Kunkel, J.H. (1977). *Behavior theory in sociology: Essays in honor of George C. Homans.* Piscataway, NJ: Transaction Publishers.

Haring, T.G. (1991). Social relationships. In L.H. Meyer, C.A. Peck, & L. Brown (Eds.), *Critical issues in the lives of people with severe disabilities* (pp. 195–217). Baltimore: Paul H. Brookes Publishing Co.

Haring, T.G., & Breen, C.G. (1992). A peer-mediated social network intervention to enhance the social integration of persons with moderate and severe disabilities. *Journal of Applied Behavior Analysis, 25,* 319–334.

Haring, T.G., & Lovinger, L. (1989). Promoting social interaction through teaching generalized play initiation responses to preschool children with autism. *Journal of The Association for Persons with Severe Handicaps, 14,* 58–67.

Haring, T.G., Roger, B., Lee, M., Breen, C., & Gaylord-Ross, R. (1986). Teaching social language to moderately handicapped students. *Journal of Applied Behavior Analysis, 19,* 159–172.

Hoffman, H.S. (1997, May). *A search for the causes of social attachment.* Invited address presented at the annual meeting of the Association for Behavior Analysis, Chicago.

Holland, P.W., & Leinhardt, S. (1971). Transitivity in structural models of small groups. *Comparative Group Studies, 2,* 107–124.

Homans, G.C. (1974). *Social behavior: Its elementary forms.* Orlando, FL: Harcourt Brace & Co.

Hughes, C., Harmer, M.L., Killian, K.J., & Niarhos, F. (1995). The effects of multiple-exemplar self-instructional training on high school students' generalized conversational interactions. *Journal of Applied Behavior Analysis, 28,* 201–218.

Hughes, C., Lorden, S.W., & Scott, S.V. (1997, May). Social validation of critical social interaction skills for high school students. In C.H. Kennedy (Chair), *Peer-mediated interventions in general education settings.* Symposium presented at the annual meeting of the Association for Behavior Analysis, Chicago.

Hunt, P., Farron-Davis, F., Beckstead, S., Curtis, D., & Goetz, L. (1994). Evaluating the effects of placement of students with severe disabilities in general education versus special classes. *Journal of The Association for Persons with Severe Handicaps, 19,* 200–214.

Hunt, P., Staub, D., Alwell, M., & Goetz, L. (1994). Achievement by all students within the context of cooperative learning groups. *Journal of The Association for Persons with Severe Handicaps, 19,* 290–301.

Jackson, S., & Rodriguez-Tomé, H. (1993). *Adolescence and its social worlds.* Mahwah, NJ: Lawrence Erlbaum Associates.

Jansson, I. (1997). Clique structure in school classroom data. *Social Networks, 19,* 285–301.

Johnson, E.C. (1985). Network macrostructure models for the Davis-Leinhardt set of empirical sociomatrices. *Social Networks, 7,* 203–224.

Kagan, J. (1970). Attention and psychological change in the young child. *Science, 170,* 826–832.

Kamps, D.M., Leonard, B.R., Vernon, S., Dugan, E.P., Delquadri, J.C., Gershon, B., Wade, L., & Folk, L. (1992). Teaching social skills to students with autism to increase peer interactions in an integrated first-grade classroom. *Journal of Applied Behavior Analysis, 25,* 281–288.

Kauffman, J.M., & Hallahan, D.P. (1995). *The illusion of full inclusion: A comprehensive critique of a current special education bandwagon.* Austin, TX: PRO-ED.

Keller, F.S., & Schoenfeld, N.W. (1950). *Principles of psychology.* New York: Appleton-Century-Crofts.

Kennedy, C.H., Cushing, L., & Itkonen, T. (1997). General education participation increases the social contacts and friendship networks of students with severe disabilities. *Journal of Behavioral Education, 7,* 167–189.

Kennedy, C.H., & Fisher, D. (2001). *Inclusive middle schools.* Baltimore: Paul H. Brookes Publishing Co.

Kennedy, C.H., Horner, R.H., & Newton, J.S. (1989). Social contacts of adults with severe disabilities living in the community: A descriptive analysis of relationship patterns. *Journal of The Association for Persons with Severe Handicaps, 14,* 190–196.

Kennedy, C.H., & Itkonen, T. (1994). Some effects of regular class participation on the social contacts and social networks of high school students with severe disabilities. *Journal of The Association for Persons with Severe Handicaps, 19,* 1–10.

Kennedy, C.H., & Shukla, S. (1995). Social interaction research for people with autism as a set of past, current, and emerging propositions. *Behavioral Disorders, 21,* 21–36.

Kennedy, C.H., Shukla, S., & Fryxell, D. (1997). Comparing the effects of educational placement on the social relationships of intermediate school students with severe disabilities. *Exceptional Children, 64,* 31–47.

Kirke, D.M. (1996). Collecting peer data and delineating peer networks in a complete network. *Social Networks, 18,* 333–346.

Logan, K.R., Bakeman, R., & Keefe, E.B. (1997). Effects of instructional variables on engaged behavior of students with severe disabilities in general education classrooms. *Exceptional Children, 63,* 481–497.

Logan, K.R., & Keefe, E.B. (1997). A comparison of instructional context, teacher behavior, and engaged behavior for students with severe disabilities in general education and self-contained classrooms. *Journal of The Association for Persons with Severe Handicaps, 22,* 12–19.

McConnell, S.R. (1987). Entrapment effects and the generalization and maintenance of social skills training for elementary school students with behavior disorders. *Behavior Disorders, 12,* 252–263.

Meehl, P.E. (1986). Trait language and behaviorese. In T. Thompson & M.D. Zeiler (Eds.), *Analysis and integration of behavioral units* (pp. 315–334). Mahwah, NJ: Lawrence Erlbaum Associates.

Moerk, E.L. (1992). *A first language taught and learned.* Baltimore: Paul H. Brookes Publishing Co.

Moreno, J.L. (1953). *Who shall survive?* Boston: Beacon Press.

Newton, J.S., & Horner, R.H. (1993). Using a social guide to improve social relationships of people with severe disabilities. *Journal of The Association for Persons with Severe Handicaps, 18,* 36–45.

Newton, J.S., Olson, D., & Horner, R.H. (1995). Factors contributing to the stability of social relationships between individuals with mental retardation and other community members. *Mental Retardation, 33,* 383–396.

Odom, S.L., McConnell, S.R., & McEvoy, M.A. (Eds.). (1992). *Social competence of young children with disabilities: Issues and strategies for intervention.* Baltimore: Paul H. Brookes Publishing Co.

Patterson, G.R., Reid, J.B., & Dishion, T.J. (1992). *Antisocial boys.* Eugene, OR: Castalia.

Piaget, J. (1971). *Biology and knowledge: An essay on the relations between organic regulations and cognitive processes.* Chicago: University of Chicago Press.

Pierce, G.R., Sarason, B.R., & Sarason, I.G. (1996). *Handbook of social support and the family.* New York: Kluwer Academic/Plenum Publishers.

Rainforth, B., & York-Barr, J. (1997). *Collaborative teams for students with severe disabilities: Integrating therapy and education services* (2nd ed.). Baltimore: Paul H. Brookes Publishing Co.

Samualson, M.A.K. (1997). Social networks of children in single-parent families. *Social Networks, 19,* 113–127.

Schnorr, R.F. (1997). From enrollment to membership: "Belonging" in middle and high school classes. *Journal of The Association for Persons with Severe Handicaps, 22,* 1–15.

Selman, R.L. (1980). *The growth of interpersonal understanding.* San Diego: Academic Press.

Shukla, S., Kennedy, C.H., & Cushing, L.S. (1998). Adult influence on the participation of peers without disabilities in peer support programs. *Journal of Behavioral Education, 8,* 397–413.

Shukla, S., Kennedy, C.H., & Cushing, L.S. (1999). Supporting intermediate school students with severe disabilities in general education classrooms: A comparison of two approaches. *Journal of Positive Behavior Intervention, 1,* 130–140.

Sidman, M. (1960). *Tactics of scientific research: Evaluating experimental data in psychology.* New York: Basic Books.

Skinner, B.F. (1953). *Science and human behavior.* New York: Free Press.

Skinner, B.F. (1957). *Verbal behavior.* New York: Appleton-Century-Crofts.

Storey, K. (1993). A proposal for assessing integration. *Education and Training in Mental Retardation and Developmental Disabilities, 28,* 279–287.

Strain, P.S. (1990). LRE for preschool children with handicaps: What we know, what we should be doing. *Journal of Early Intervention, 14,* 291–296.

Strain, P.S., Odom, S.L., & McConnell, W.C. (1984). Promoting social reciprocity of exceptional children: Identification, target behavior, selection and intervention. *Remedial and Special Education, 5,* 21–28.

Suitor, J., & Keeton, S. (1997). Once a friend, always a friend? *Social Networks, 19,* 51–62.

Thompson, T., & Lubinski, D. (1986). Units of analysis and kinetic structure of behavioral repertoires. *Journal of the Experimental Analysis of Behavior, 46,* 219–242.

11

Adolescents

Putting Research into Practice

Lisa Sharon Cushing and Craig H. Kennedy

Jamal is new to his middle school, as is his special education teacher, Mr. Washington. The school is composed of teams that cut across traditional academic and educational boundaries and are based on dividing each grade level into sections of 250 students and 12 teachers. Jamal and Mr. Washington are on the eighth-grade team called the Blue Crew. Jamal's individualized education program (IEP), which was developed for his previous self-contained classroom placement, focuses on his developing a few signs to communicate with others, increasing his independence, and following a picture schedule. Mr. Washington has the challenge of facilitating each of these IEP goals within the context of a new school, with new colleagues and students with and without disabilities. How can Mr. Washington facilitate communication, inclusion, and independence? How can Jamal's IEP goals, which were developed for a special education environment, be applied to general education classrooms in his new middle school, and how can Mr. Washington support Jamal and six other students with severe disabilities who are dispersed throughout various classrooms and grades?

Chapter 10 surveys the foundations of research and theory as they apply to quantifying and improving the social interactions of adolescents with severe disabilities. This chapter provides real-world illustrations of how to accomplish those outcomes. The examples are derived from actual experiences, such as those of Jamal, and answer many of the questions facing Mr. Washington as a special educator working in a general education environment. Several challenges emerged in the 1990s to which special educators and related services personnel had to adapt. Foremost among those changes was the evolution toward greater general education participation. As research demonstrated the social benefits of increased general education participation and illustrated the models that could achieve those goals, the direction that special education took for students with severe disabilities was clear (Hunt, Farron-Davis, Beckstead, Curtis, & Goetz, 1994; Kennedy, Shukla, & Fryxell, 1997; Logan & Keefe, 1997; Salisbury, Wilson, & Palombaro, 1994; Schnorr, 1997; Staub, Spaulding, Peck, Gallucci, & Schwartz, 1996). Support that once was provided only by special education teachers in special education environments was now provided in more typical environments with the help of general education teachers and peers without disabilities.

Changes in professional responsibilities necessarily entail changes in professional behavior. The following examples illustrate the importance of considering scheduling and curricular adaptation, as well as deciding who will provide direct support and how the adults will coordinate their educational activities and goals. Although these changes are implicit in Chapter 10, this chapter addresses these issues more explicitly.

It is instructive to remember that social relationships in school environments involve a number of different individuals. For example, how a general and special education teacher communicate and interact with each other can have substantial effects on the interactions between peers with and without disabilities (Downing, 1996; Jorgensen, 1998; Kennedy & Fisher, 2001; Rainforth & York-Barr, 1997). For instance, Mr. Washington may want to suggest that a social studies teacher, Ms. Finnefrock, try to teach her class using cooperative learning groups; however, in the absence of a collaborative relationship between the special and general education teacher, such suggestions may be threatening or insulting to Ms. Finnefrock. Thus, the general education teacher may feel hurt despite evidence that cooperative learning groups may be a better teaching approach to use (Cushing, Kennedy, Shukla, Davis, & Meyer, 1997; Dugan et al., 1995; Slavin, Madden, & Leavey, 1984).

Similarly, how special and general education personnel interact with students with severe disabilities and peers without disabilities affects student–peer interactions. Very different social interactions occur between students with severe disabilities and peers without disabilities depending on how teachers define their support roles (Shukla, Kennedy, & Cushing, 1998, 1999). If an adult provides direct assistance to Jamal, his interactions with peers without disabilities may be as sparse as if he were in a self-contained special education classroom (Giangreco, Edelman, Luiselli, & MacFarland, 1997; Shukla et al., 1999); however, if Mr. Washington and Ms. Finnefrock use peer-mediated instruction to support Jamal, social interactions and academic progress for Jamal will be the most likely outcomes.

The remainder of this chapter illustrates various procedures for improving the social interactions of adolescents with and without severe disabilities within general education environments. The following sections focus on different phases of relationship development discussed in Chapter 10: 1) encouraging initial social encounters, 2) facilitating additional social interactions, and 3) supporting durable social relationships. In each section, critical concepts are highlighted followed by a real-life example to illustrate how these ideas can be put into practice.

INITIAL SOCIAL ENCOUNTERS

As noted in the previous chapter, more initial social encounters occur when adolescents with severe disabilities are systematically included in general education contexts. Those contexts can encompass science, art, history, math, English, physical education, vocational sites, and other typical areas around campus or in the community. Research indicates that participating in typical activities in ordinary environments is an effective way to establish initial social encounters (Logan, Bakeman, & Keefe, 1997).

Teachers need to use active planning in general education environments to facilitate social interactions (Shukla et al., 1999). For example, it would not be enough for Mr. Washington and Ms. Finnefrock to agree that Jamal should attend Ms. Finnefrock's social studies class. Mr. Washington also will need to identify the activities that Jamal will participate in, potential peers without disabilities he will interact with, and a monitoring system that will keep track of his progress. The following example illustrates the process designed to establish social interactions within general education contexts.

Missy

Missy was an eighth-grade student with severe disabilities attending a middle school in an economically, culturally, and ethnically diverse suburb of a metropolitan city. Her earlier educational experience was in a self-contained classroom in an elementary school. Missy had Rett syndrome and was a quiet student who would shake or cry when upset. If she was interested in an object or person, she would look at the individual or object and smile. Her time at the middle school was focused on basic skills and communication within general education environments.

Prior to the school year, the special education teacher met with Missy's family and discussed general education class options. The biggest issue for her family was the absence of same-age friends in her life as well as experiences typical of a 13-year-old girl. Input during this family-centered meeting helped the special education teacher identify general education courses that would provide both academic and social inclusion opportunities.

Inclusion was a new concept for all the teachers at the middle school, and the special education teacher and administrators felt it was important to collaborate with general education teachers who expressed a willingness to include students with severe disabilities. The special education teacher met with the general education teachers who volunteered. She described Missy's abilities and why it was important that she be included in general education classes. The teachers discussed their teaching approaches and what they expected to gain from Missy's participation in their classes. The special education teacher then shared examples of goals and objectives that Missy could work on while in the general education class. Following this meeting, the special educator conducted ecological assessments of the general education classrooms to identify specific instructional objectives for Missy (see Rainforth & York-Barr, 1997). This process entailed identifying key routines that peers engaged in and opportunities for embedding IEP goals into those routines. In addition, it was decided that the special educator would meet weekly with the general education teacher to brainstorm about curricular adaptations and to keep abreast of the classroom social dynamics.

Missy was initially included in six classes: English, computers, home economics, physical education, social studies, and art. She attended classes with her peers beginning the first day of school. In each classroom, the general education teacher made a brief announcement asking if any peers without disabilities would like to help Missy in the class. Several peers showed an interest in working with Missy. In computer class, for example, a peer named Annie approached the teacher on the first day and asked if she could help Missy. A few days later, Tawny, another peer, approached a special education assistant and asked about ways that she could help Missy feel more comfortable in class. Similar events occurred in other classes, sometimes initiated by peers, sometimes by adults.

Concurrent with the classroom announcements, a peer support program was created. A notice was posted in the school bulletin during the first few weeks of school asking for peers without disabilities to help students with disabilities. The peer support announcement was extremely successful in recruiting peers. Those peers who were in classes with students with disabilities were asked to assist the students in class. Peers who shared no classes with a student with disabilities were asked to assist a student in another school context (e.g., transitions between the bus to class, during lunch).

Through discussions with teachers and through personal experience, peer supports learned how Missy communicated, interacted, and learned. Adult support was systematically faded. Eventually, adults took a consultative role for Missy and her peer supports. Such an arrangement allowed adults to engage in various other activities while monitoring Missy and her peer supports. A checklist was created consisting of goals and objectives from Missy's IEP. This checklist was easy to follow and allowed the peers to check off the objectives they worked on in class. During most classes, a special educator was available to assist the peers and to address their concerns. The peer support programs increased social interactions among Missy and her peers and helped to alleviate the fears of some general education teachers who then began to consider Missy just another student in the school.

Summary

Missy's example highlights a number of themes outlined in Chapter 10. Two basic strategies are especially important for establishing initial interactions between students with severe disabilities and their peers in general education environments. First, active communication and collaboration among special and general educators is essential. Special educators need to be liaisons and facilitators of general education participation for students with disabilities. Without active recruitment of general education teachers and classrooms, social participation for students with severe disabilities is unlikely.

Second, special educators must establish peer support networks. This responsibility entails recruiting peers without disabilities, encouraging initial encounters between students and peers, and routinely monitoring those interactions. Unless special educators take an active role in developing peer support programs, these interactions rarely materialize by themselves. These two messages suggest a significant departure from the traditional roles of special educators; however, as the environments in which educational goals are targeted for instruction evolve, special educators' roles change accordingly.

FACILITATING CONTINUED SOCIAL INTERACTIONS

Facilitating regular social interactions presents a further challenge. Because social interactions occur within the context of larger networks of social relationships, facilitating continued interactions necessitates a broader perspective than may be necessary when attempting to initiate social contact. For example, teachers may need to tailor how frequently they interact with a particular peer support group based on the social interests of the student with severe disabilities and, just as importantly, the peer(s) without disabilities (Shukla et al., 1998). In addition, issues such as what activities the peer support groups will focus on, how many peers without disabilities should be involved, how curricular adaptations are made (and by whom), and the type of instruction students with disabilities receive appear to be related to the ongoing success of peer support programs (see Chapter 10).

The ongoing support of peer support programs within general education environments is analogous to juggling. Getting things started requires one set of skills; keeping things going and in functioning order requires different skills. Jamal's teachers, for example, will need to be aware of feedback from Jamal and his peers about what is working and what is not. In addition, Mr. Washington will need to maintain open communication with Ms. Finnefrock so that her feedback is incorporated into the fine-tuning that occurs in peer support programs (Jorgensen, Fisher, Sax, & Skoglund, 1998).

Dave

The following illustration helps elucidate the various parameters of peer support groups that teachers need to consider to help facilitate adolescent social interactions. Dave was an eleventh grader with moderate-to-severe disabilities who needed assistance in various academic activities and required adaptations for reading, writing, and speech clarity. Dave was included in a variety of academic and nonacademic courses throughout the school day. This particular example focuses on an English class he attended.

Dave's IEP objectives focused on reading, writing, and speaking. His social goals involved interacting appropriately with adults and peers without disabilities. Dave was working on initiating, continuing and ending conversations, and learning classroom social behaviors (e.g., when to raise his hand, how to pass around handouts, saying "here" during roll call). His objectives also related to personal responsibility and self-determination, including remembering to bring papers and books to class and to and from school, getting to classes by himself or with a peer, and requesting help when needed.

Dave had several friends who served as peer supports in English class. Typically, Dave was allowed to choose a peer he wanted to work with that day, and, if the peer agreed, the two would work together.

During the semester, five peers became regular supports, with one peer in particular working with Dave 2 or 3 days per week. Initially, the special education assistant worked with Dave and his peer, but eventually she faded her assistance to occasional monitoring (e.g., every 10 minutes) and answering of questions. This fading process allowed Dave and his peers to interact but still complete their work assignments under adult supervision.

One strategy that helped Dave and his peers interact on a regular basis was the establishment of daily routines for them. For example, every day the English teacher checked all of the peers' assignment notebooks to see if they had completed their homework assignments and brought them to class. If a peer had completed and brought his or her homework assignment to class, the assignment notebook was stamped. Dave was responsible for stamping peers' notebooks. At the beginning of the semester, a peer walked alongside Dave to assist him. Eventually, Dave learned to do the task independently. This activity gave Dave the opportunity not only to be involved in daily class activities but also to interact with each of his peers in class on a regular basis.

Another activity that helped facilitate regular interactions with peers involved journal writing. During each class, the English teacher would require peers to write in their journals for approximately 10 minutes on an assigned topic. One of Dave's peers developed the idea of asking Dave the question and letting him respond verbally while the peer wrote down his answer. The English teacher or special education assistant would then read the response and select a few sentences for Dave to copy in his notebook. The role of the special educator was to make sure Dave and a peer worked together, to monitor and praise the work of both students, and to assist the English teacher in other classroom roles.

Dave and his peers often needed help to adapt curricular activities. Initially, the special educator would work with Dave and his peers to explain class assignments and problem-solve ways to adapt them. To the maximum extent possible, the adaptations were similar to what other peers in the class were working on, only adjusted to Dave's needs. Some adaptations were quite creative, and peers seemed to enjoy developing novel curricular adaptations. For example, one assignment involved writing a short story. The English teacher introduced essential elements and discussed how to construct a short story. Dave's peer supports decided that Dave would dictate his story while one of the peers typed it into a computer; other peers helped Dave keep a linear structure to his emerging short story. Once the story was completed, the peers and Dave took turns reading the work and making changes. The story was a success with Dave, his peer supports, and others in the class.

Through a combination of structured activities, curricular adaptations, and regular monitoring by adults, the peer support program was maintained throughout the school year. The peer support groups went through a continual process of evaluation and evolution to establish a successful and enjoyable learning environment for Dave and his peers.

Summary

Repeated social interactions among adolescents are dynamic events. Successful development and monitoring of peer support groups requires that adults, particularly special educators, be aware of interpersonal connections and how those relationships may change over time. In Dave's case, those ongoing changes were manifested in adult support roles during activities performed by Dave with his peers. Initially, adults were heavily involved in structuring the interactions of Dave and his peers. As Dave and his peers got to know each other, however, the role of adults became more peripheral. The special educator, for instance, changed her role from developing curricular adaptations, to assisting peers in making adaptations, to providing them with constructive feedback on a regular basis. In a sense, the initial role of adults was to make sure that interactions were appropriate and educationally relevant. Later, the adults sought to ensure that the peer support programs were successful in meeting the needs of all students.

One basic strategy Dave's special and general education teachers used was to involve Dave and his peer supports in ongoing decision making. The teachers tried to avoid imposing predetermined adaptations when introducing new assignments. Instead, they sought input from Dave and his peers and incorporated their suggestions into future activities. This practice also provided opportunities for peers to offer additional suggestions. For example, a peer might suggest a new type of curricular adaptation and also suggest that the special educator does not need to check in so frequently.

Successful social relationships often emerge when interactions extend beyond a particular classroom (Epstein & Karweit, 1983). In fact, an underlying goal of peer support programs is to develop friendships that are exhibited beyond the interactions structured by adults. Once social interactions are initially established, regular in-class contacts may be an important vehicle for facilitating out-of-class contacts. Peer-mediated supports may be necessary to begin establishing continued social interactions. Getting those interactions to extend to other parts of school life may require additional adult support to occasion their occurrence. The final section of this chapter discusses promoting durable social relationships.

SUPPORTING DURABLE SOCIAL RELATIONSHIPS

An important goal of social interaction strategies is to facilitate durable social relationships or friendships. Obviously, maintaining a relationship with another person is difficult without regular contact. How regular contact is maintained can vary widely. Maintaining durable relationships requires creative problem solving to identify effective strategies (see Chapter 10). For some individuals, opportunities to interact outside of class may not have been identified. Even if times have been identified, appropriate adult supports may be needed to make interactions possible. In the first instance, it may be a matter of helping a student and peer coordinate their schedules to identify potential interaction times. The second instance may be a matter of how to coordinate the students' and peers' schedules with the adults' schedules. For example, there may be a reciprocal interest between Jamal and Tami (a peer without disabilities) in having lunch together a few days a week. They may have identified times and activities, but they may need additional assistance from Mr. Washington or his assistant to make sure Jamal can be at the right place at the right time.

Many of the barriers to facilitating long-term relationships at school appear to be structural. General education participation often allows for the development of social interactions between adolescents with severe disabilities and some peers without disabilities within those classrooms (e.g., Kennedy, Shukla, & Fryxell, 1997); however, there does not appear to be spillover from those specific classroom interactions unless deliberate attempts are made to promote generalization of those interactions. Logistical events such as student, peer, and adult schedules, class blocking, and staggered lunch times can have profound influences on opportunities for sustaining durable social interactions. Although Jamal and Tami may be interested in interacting with each other outside of social studies, if opportunities are not identified, then afterschool activities may not be possible. Such planning, however, is typically beyond the scope of most school-based supports (see Skrtic & Sailor, 1996).

Structural barriers place a substantial responsibility on the adults who support student and peer social interactions. Unfortunately, little research is available to elucidate strategies for overcoming barriers to out-of-school social interactions for adolescents. As interest grows in extending social interactions beyond general education environments to community environments, the barriers to generalized interaction should become increasingly apparent. Creative problem solving on a barrier-by-barrier basis appears to be the focus of best practices at this time.

Jamal

A discussion of Jamal and his social network offers an illustration of strategies for expanding social interactions beyond classroom environments. By the end of the semester, Jamal had developed several friends in Ms. Finnefrock's class, two of whom (Alex and Tami) wanted to continue their interactions with Jamal next semester and in other places. Jamal indicated that he felt the same way. Interestingly, Jamal's parents noticed an important change in his behavior—Jamal was more cooperative getting up in the morning and getting to school. By the end of fall semester, Jamal looked forward to going to school and complained when he had to stay home on the weekends.

Prior to the school year, Jamal's parents had expressed their concerns to Mr. Washington about the absence of friends in Jamal's life. They thought social relationships were essential and wished that Jamal could experience the benefits of friendship. A daily logbook and telephone conversations were maintained between Jamal's parents and the special education staff. They worked together to develop ways of supporting potential friendships. Given Alex, Jamal, and Tami's interest in continuing their interactions, the spring semester seemed an important time to coordinate additional supports for their social contacts.

At school, Mr. Washington talked with the school registrar about possible classes that Jamal could take with Alex and Tami. Three possible classes were identified, one class with Alex, one with Tami, and one with both of them. Because of Jamal's scheduling needs, there were conflicts with two of those classes. This predicament left only the class with Tami. Subsequently, Jamal was enrolled in an algebra class with Tami, who was his peer support; however, there were no scheduled activities between Alex and Jamal.

Mr. Washington and Jamal's team decided to target out-of-class activities for Alex and Jamal (and Tami, if she was interested). It was suggested to Alex that he and Jamal identify a couple of times during the school day or school week when they could interact. After some discussion, Alex and Jamal identified two possibilities: meeting when they arrived at school and eating lunch together. Based on these ideas, a schedule was worked out between Alex, Jamal, and Mr. Washington that could be flexible over the semester but allowed several times each week when Alex and Jamal could interact. Although Alex and Jamal were the ones interested in interacting, an important responsibility fell to Mr. Washington to support the interactions as unobtrusively as possible.

Along with these school-based efforts, Jamal's parents began actively inviting Jamal's friends to participate in family activities, such as coming over for dinner or going to the movies. Alex was interested in several of these activities and participated approximately once a week. Tami also showed an interested in community-based social interactions and participated once or twice per month—sometimes with Jamal, sometimes with Jamal and Alex. Interestingly, Tami began inviting several of her other friends to outings with Jamal, which led to peer group outings of four or five adolescents. Over the course of the spring semester, school-based contacts coordinated by Mr. Washington and community-based interactions coordinated by Jamal's parents settled into a routine of frequent social interactions that the various individuals appeared to enjoy. Jamal's parents and Mr. Washington maintained contact via a home–school journal so that they could each keep informed about developments in Jamal's growing social life.

Summary

The long-term benefits of sustained social relationships are undeniable. Supporting long-term social interactions, in particular, requires participation beyond the general education classroom to include additional environments, activities, and individuals. Once social interactions seem to stabilize and fall into a routine, support strategies tend to focus on maintaining the status quo. When changes in schedules or routines occur, it is important that multiple people—including the student with disabilities, peers without disabilities, various teachers, administrators, and family members—be involved in resolving the problems.

CONCLUSION

For special educators interested in developing procedures for various policy initiatives such as inclusive education, outcomes-based education, national standards, and school reform, it is a time of promise and a time of challenge. When the Education for All Handicapped Children

Act, PL 94-142, was enacted in 1975, the roles and responsibilities of every professional in special education were changed. Clearly, the changes resulting from PL 94-142 have benefited people with severe disabilities immensely. Nonetheless, one must acknowledge that there is a long way to go to make the educational opportunities and outcomes for students with severe disabilities equal to their peers without disabilities.

In this chapter, we have endeavored to provide concrete examples of how to improve the social development of adolescents with severe disabilities. Although this is only one aspect of the larger picture of educational change, it is a component that has not been studied enough for youth with disabilities. Viable and effective educational strategies for teaching daily living and job skills to these individuals are available. Indeed, effective instructional strategies, such as task analysis, general case programming, and time delay, have been adopted by many educators, families, and others interested in improving the lives of people with other types of intellectual disabilities; however, it was only in the 1990s that national and state policy initiatives began to include the social outcomes of education as valued goals.

There are many parallels between the changes initiated in the 1990s regarding improving social outcomes and the changes that occurred in the 1970s regarding improving functional living skills. The shift in the 1970s from making adolescents with severe disabilities piece together children's puzzles to encouraging them to bus tables at fast-food restaurants was dramatic for those who were required to change what they did as educators. In the 1990s, a similar process required teachers to move from their special education classrooms into the classrooms of general educators. In effect, special educators are becoming consultants rather than classroom teachers.

Nevertheless, a strong empirical literature is emergent to support the multiple social benefits that are accruing for adolescents with severe disabilities as a result of such changes in professionals' behavior. Chapter 10 documents what is known about improving the social interactions of adolescents with severe disabilities. This chapter provides everyday illustrations of the processes and outcomes discussed in the previous chapter. The field's knowledge of social development for this group of students is only beginning to emerge. One thing, however, is perfectly clear at this juncture—there are concrete and practical strategies for improving the social interactions of adolescents with severe disabilities. We hope that this chapter has provided the readers with some new ideas, or empirical support for their own ideas, about how to improve the social lives of this group of students.

REFERENCES

Cushing, L.S., Kennedy, C.H., Shukla, S., Davis, J., & Meyer, K.A. (1997). Disentangling the effects of curricular revision and social grouping in cooperative learning arrangements. *Focus on Autism and Other Developmental Disabilities, 12,* 231–240.

Downing, J.E. (1996). *Including students with severe and multiple disabilities in typical classrooms.* Baltimore: Paul H. Brookes Publishing Co.

Dugan, E., Kamps, D., Leonard, B., Watkins, N., Rheinberger, A., & Stackhaus, J. (1995). Effects of cooperative learning groups during social studies for students with autism and fourth-grade peers. *Journal of Applied Behavior Analysis, 28,* 175–188.

Education for All Handicapped Children Act of 1975, PL 94-142, 20 U.S.C. §§ 1400 *et seq.*

Epstein, J.L., & Karweit, N. (1983). *Friends in school: Patterns of selection and influence in secondary schools.* San Diego: Academic Press.

Giangreco, M.F., Edelman, S., Luiselli, T.E., & MacFarland, S.Z. (1997). Helping or hovering?: Effects of instructional assistant proximity on students with disabilities. *Exceptional Children, 64,* 7–18.

Hunt, P., Farron-Davis, F., Beckstead, S., Curtis, D., & Goetz, L. (1994). Evaluating the effects of placement of students with severe disabilities in general education versus special classes. *Journal of The Association for Persons with Severe Handicaps, 19,* 200–214.

Jorgensen, C.M. (1998). *Restructuring high schools for all students: Taking inclusion to the next level.* Baltimore: Paul H. Brookes Publishing Co.

Jorgensen, C.M., Fisher, D., Sax, C., & Skoglund, K.L. (1998). Innovative scheduling, new roles for teachers, and heterogeneous grouping: The organizational factors related to student success in inclusive, restructured schools. In C.M. Jorgensen, *Restructuring high schools for all students: Taking inclusion to the next level* (pp. 49–70). Baltimore: Paul H. Brookes Publishing Co.

Kennedy, C.H., & Fisher, D. (2001). *Inclusive middle schools.* Baltimore: Paul H. Brookes Publishing Co.

Kennedy, C.H., Shukla, S., & Fryxell, D. (1997). Comparing the effects of educational placement on the social relationships of intermediate school students with severe disabilities. *Exceptional Children, 64,* 31–47.

Logan, K.R., Bakeman, R., & Keefe, E.B. (1997). Effects of instructional variables on engaged behavior of students with severe disabilities in general education classrooms. *Exceptional Children, 63,* 481–497.

Logan, K.R., & Keefe, E.B. (1997). A comparison of instructional context, teacher behavior, and engaged behavior for students with severe disabilities in general education and self-contained classrooms. *Journal of The Association for Persons with Severe Handicaps, 22,* 13–20.

Rainforth, B., & York-Barr, J. (1997). *Collaborative teams for students with severe disabilities: Integrating therapy and educational services* (2nd ed.). Baltimore: Paul H. Brookes Publishing Co.

Salisbury, C.L., Wilson, L., & Palombaro, M.M. (1994, December). *Collaborative innovations project: Practitioners as partners in research and reform.* Session presented at the annual meeting of The Association for Persons with Severe Handicaps, Atlanta, GA.

Schnorr, R.F. (1997). From enrollment to membership: "Belonging" in middle and high school classes. *Journal of The Association for Persons with Severe Handicaps, 22,* 1–15.

Shukla, S., Kennedy, C.H., & Cushing, L.S. (1998). Adult influence on the participation of peers without disabilities in peer support programs. *Journal of Behavioral Education, 8,* 397–413.

Shukla, S., Kennedy, C.H., & Cushing, L.S. (1999). Supporting intermediate school students with severe disabilities in general education classrooms: A comparison of two approaches. *Journal of Positive Behavior Interventions, 1,* 130–140.

Skrtic, T.M., & Sailor, W. (1996). School-linked services integration: Crisis and opportunity in the transition to postmodern society. *Remedial and Special Education, 17,* 271–283.

Slavin, R.E., Madden, N.A., & Leavey, M.B. (1984). Effects of cooperative learning and individualized instruction on mainstreamed students. *Exceptional Children, 50,* 434–443.

Staub, D., Spaulding, M., Peck, C.A., Gallucci, C., & Schwartz, I.S. (1996). Using nondisabled peers to support the inclusion of students with disabilities at the junior high school level. *Journal of The Association for Persons with Severe Handicaps, 21,* 194–205.

12

Relationships Between Social-Communicative Skills and Life Achievements

Charles R. Greenwood, Dale Walker, and Cheryl A. Utley

Social communication and social competence are keystones from which other forms of competence emerge and remain linked (see Chapters 1–2). Without social competence, other important forms of competence (e.g., emotional, cognitive, economic) are impossible to achieve. Thus, in order for a child to grow into a responsible and contributing adult, it is important that he or she develop good social-communicative skills during early childhood (Bates, O'Connell, & Shore, 1987; Kaiser, 1993). Young children need communication skills to gather information and experience, to achieve cognitive competencies, and to interact appropriately with others in their environments (Crais & Roberts, 1996; Walker, Greenwood, Hart, & Carta, 1994).

Delay in developing communication skills leads to additional developmental problems (see Chapter 2). Evidence exists that the social-communicative skills of young children at school entry affect both what they are taught and how fast they learn additional keystone skills such as reading and literacy. Thus, social-communicative skills affect growth and competence in academic skills and future opportunities for secondary and postsecondary education and employment. For example, children with delays in communication often experience delays in early literacy, school achievement, emotional and behavioral development, and establishing relationships with friends and family (McCathren, Warren, & Yoder, 1996; Schuele, 1999). Unfortunately, delays in social communication are not readily identified until the preschool years with the onset of delays in the use of spoken language (Wetherby & Prizant, 1992). Earlier efforts to identify and intervene remain highly desirable (see Chapter 4); research indicates that children who receive intervention services for communication develop improved language (Yoder &

Warren, 1999), which may also reduce their risk for early school failure (e.g., learning to read) and other future problems (Cole, Dale, &
Mills, 1991).

The purpose of this chapter is to reflect on what is known as well
as what still needs to be learned about the relationship between social-
communicative skills and the attainment of life achievements. Because
a primary educational goal is to intervene to accelerate the competence
of children with developmental disabilities, a life span rather than a
cross-sectional age perspective is applied. Suggestions of how such interventions, and policies linked to their provision, can be systematically
improved and sustained over time are offered. The following questions
are addressed:

1. What is the role and importance of social communication and so-
    cial competence in the lives of children and youth?
2. Are the identified social skills likely to relate to life achievements,
    and what should be important to families, educators, and society?
3. What are the clinical applicability and generality of the proposed
    assessments and interventions?
4. What knowledge is still needed to prepare all students for the de-
    mands of the educational system or to prepare the education sys-
    tem to accommodate the needs of students with developmental
    disabilities?

RELATIONSHIP BETWEEN IDENTIFIED
SOCIAL SKILLS AND VALUED LIFE ACHIEVEMENTS

Life-Related Skills

Communication problems are one of the most prevalent reasons for
referring young children for special education services (Marcovitch,
Chiasson, Ushycky, Goldberg, & MacGregor, 1996). At least 70% of
preschool children with disabilities have communication impairments
(Wetherby & Prizant, 1993), and 12% of all services provided to infants
and toddlers in 1995 were for speech and language problems (U.S. Department of Education, 1998). Children with communication delays
also are at risk for development of later problems (Fey, Catts, & Lar-
rivee, 1995). These include behavior problems that result from frustra-
tion at the difficulty they have communicating needs, wants, and ideas
to others (Conroy & Brown, 1997) and reading and other academic difficulties in school (Scarborough & Dobrich, 1994; Wetherby & Prizant,
1993).

Childhood development must equip a child to meet the demands of schooling (Collins, 1988). Hence, childhood is characterized by expanding capacities for social relationships, by emotional behavior that is influenced by socialization, and by increasingly complex cognitive behavior. The transmission of social-communicative and cognitive competence is considered to be a function of the combination of biological and sociocultural factors (Collins & Gunnar, 1990; Horowitz & O'Brien, 1989; Sameroff & Fiese, 1990). These sociocultural factors include the cumulative set of interactions and transactions children have with their parents, siblings, teachers, and peers as well as the influence of broader societal factors. Individual differences in children's abilities interact with the early learning and social opportunities provided to children by their parents or caregivers to establish a foundation for future learning (Garcia Coll, 1990; Heath, 1989). The social and learning opportunities provided to children through their interactions with teachers and peers in school act on and contribute to acquired skills and provide the context for learning and for establishing social relationships (Greenwood, 1991b; Greenwood, Delquadri, & Hall, 1989; Hops & Greenwood, 1988).

The 10-year longitudinal research of Hart and Risley (1995) and Walker and colleagues (1994) demonstrated that social communication in early childhood is linked to later achievement in elementary school. The emergence of spoken language was observed in a representative sample of children whose first language was English. Results of the school assessments up to 7 years later indicated that language (assessed using the Peabody Picture Vocabulary Test–Revised [Dunn & Dunn, 1981]) and other cognitive abilities such as reading achievement (assessed using standardized achievement tests) were well predicted by the 36-month home data (Walker et al., 1994). Children with lower expressive language skills at 36 months of age also had significantly lower scores in indices of language and academic achievement in first through fourth grades.

Young children who fail to learn to read by third grade are on an early trajectory for school failure (e.g., Greenwood et al., 1989; Greenwood, Hart, Walker, & Risley, 1994; McKinney, Osborne, & Schulte, 1993; Reid & Patterson, 1991). The majority of children referred for special education services are linked to slow reading progress (Snow, Burns, & Griffin, 1998), and most qualify for special education services in reading (Council for Exceptional Children, 1994). The extent of this national problem is monumental; 40% of American children read below the basic level on national reading assessments (Wasik, 1997). Children who are particularly likely to have difficulty with learning to read in the primary grades are those who begin school with less prior knowledge and skill in relevant domains, most notably general verbal abilities, the ability to attend to the sounds of language as distinct from meaning, familiarity with the basic purposes and mechanisms of reading, and letter knowledge.

It is widely recognized that failed efforts to remediate basic reading skills in the primary grades further deprive students of opportunities to learn advanced subjects such as science (U.S. Department of Education, 1997). Consequently, children with developmental disabilities may not realize their potential to learn subject content needed for success and maximal life achievement (Blackorby & Wagner, 1996). Early failure to learn is compounded, limiting individuals' access to education, employment, and independent living opportunities as well as their contributions to society (Heal, Khoju, & Rusch, 1997; Wagner, D'Amico, Marder, Newman, & Blackorby, 1992). Preventing early and life-long trajectories of low academic achievement of children with developmental disabilities is necessary and increasingly possible. As noted by Snow and colleagues (1998), each child presents the teacher with a unique history of earlier language and literacy experiences and beginning reading skills.

Classwide Peer Tutoring

The longitudinal findings supporting the classwide peer tutoring program (CWPT, Greenwood et al., 1989) show how early reading failure can be prevented through early intervention. CWPT is a form of intraclass, same-age, reciprocal peer tutoring. In CWPT, all students assigned to a general education teacher for instruction participate in peer tutoring sessions over specific content materials at the same time. Special materials, peer correction, and teacher supervision of tutors reduce the need for older or upper-grade level students from serving as peer tutors. CWPT sessions are reciprocal because each student serves as both the tutor and the tutee during each daily session. The potential benefits of CWPT are reported to be academic (Greenwood et al., 1989), behavioral (Greenwood, 1991a), and prosocial. The social benefits include increases in peer interaction skills such as talking, teaching, helping, and group participation (Kamps & Tankersley, 1996; Kohler & Greenwood, 1990; Kohler, Richardson, Mina, & Greenwood, 1985).

The first phase of CWPT research sought to demonstrate that students' engagement with academic subject matter and their mastery of content could be accelerated compared with traditional forms of instruction (Delquadri, Greenwood, Stretton, & Hall, 1983; Greenwood, 1991a, 1991b; Greenwood et al., 1989; Maheady, Harper, & Mallette, 1991). These and other experiments demonstrated clearly that students are able to learn more in less time in the presence of teaching strategies based on CWPT (Greenwood, Maheady, & Delquadri, in press).

In one 12-year study, students who experienced CWPT in reading, spelling, and arithmetic during first through fourth grade were significantly higher achievers on standardized achievement tests in both elementary and middle school (Greenwood et al., 1989; Greenwood, Terry, Utley, Montagna, & Walker, 1993). Follow-up results demonstrated that students using CWPT continued higher growth in achievement into middle school and received fewer special education services [e.g., learning disabilities, educable mentally retarded, behavior disorders, conduct disorders, attention-deficit/hyperactivity disorder] after sixth and seventh grades (Greenwood et al., 1993); and fewer students dropped out of school prior to graduation (Greenwood & Delquadri, 1995). Other longitudinal intervention studies provide equally interesting and important information on the life-long benefits of early intervention (e.g., Learning Experiences: An Alternative Program for Preschoolers and Parents; Strain & Hoyson, 2000).

Socially Important Skills

In addition to these important empirical relationships between social communication and life-related skills, one might also question the social validity of social-communicative skills. Do parents and early childhood practitioners value them? Priest and his colleagues (in press) conducted a survey to assess the social validity of 15 general outcome statements developed for the purpose of guiding the development of progress monitoring measures deemed socially important. The survey was sent to a nationally representative sample of 1,099 parents of children with and without disabilities in kindergarten through third grade and 1,275 professionals (i.e., early childhood and elementary level general and special educators and school psychologists). The completed return rate was 351 (32%) for parents and 672 (53%) for professionals.

Using a three-level rating differential of importance (e.g., critically, very, somewhat), they evaluated general outcome statements. Three of these were designed to reflect competency in social communication. Evaluated outcome statements were

- The child uses gestures, sounds, words, or sentences to convey wants and needs or to express meaning to others.
- The child responds to other's communication with appropriate gestures, sounds, words, or word combinations.
- The child uses gestures, sounds, words, or sentences to initiate, respond to, or maintain reciprocal interactions with others.

Results indicated that all three were nearly always rated as either *very important* (range = 8%–23% across items and stakeholders) or *critically important* (range = 72%–92%) for children this age (see Figure 12.1). With respect to the first two outcomes, professionals rated them more critically important than did parents, 92% versus 85% for Outcome 1 and 83% versus 78% for Outcome 2. Professionals and parents rated Outcome 3 nearly the same at 75% versus 77%.

These data provide converging evidence of the perceived importance of social-communicative skills. First, based on available developmental, correlational, and experimental studies, it is clear that social-communicative skills and competencies are associated with and predictive of later life outcomes. Second, longitudinal, developmental studies demonstrate that growth in social competence in early childhood is linked to social, emotional, and cognitive competence in children during their school years. Finally, it also is clear that parents and practitioners recognize and value the importance of social communication and language acquisition in children's development.

KNOWLEDGE NEEDED TO PREPARE STUDENTS FOR SCHOOL AND FOR SCHOOLS TO ACCOMMODATE STUDENTS WITH DISABILITIES

Social-Communicative Behavior within the School

In middle childhood and continuing through adolescence and early adulthood, the most significant opportunities for social and cognitive growth take place in the context of interactions with peers in school rather than within the home (Parker & Asher, 1987; Stevenson & Baker, 1987). It has been argued that peer relationships are an absolute necessity for social and cognitive development and socialization. Peer social relationships appear to have a great influence on the development of social-communicative and cognitive competence in children. They may function as a protective factor for ensuring competence under adverse circumstances (e.g., Collins & Gunnar, 1990). If peers contribute substantially to the teaching of social-communicative competence, it follows that children who do not communicate, are not accepted, or who are antisocial might be more vulnerable to later problems due to limited opportunities for positive peer interactions (Parker & Asher, 1987). This appears to be the case, in that uncommunicative, unaccepted, or antisocial children are more likely to exhibit negative behavior (i.e., anger, aggression) toward their peers. This negative behavior also leads to pervasive peer rejection, association with other antisocial peers, poor

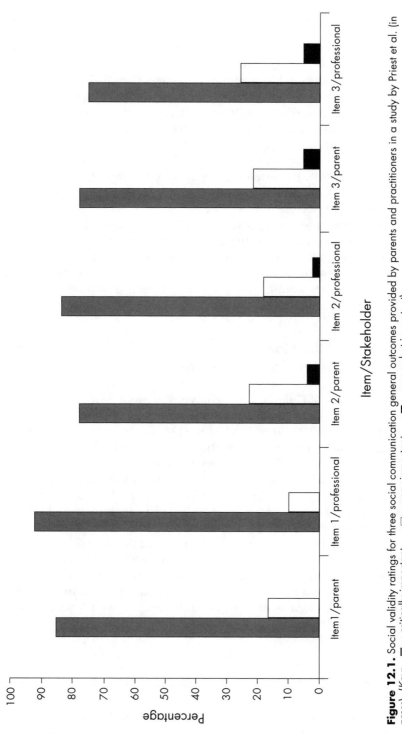

Figure 12.1. Social validity ratings for three social communication general outcomes provided by parents and practitioners in a study by Priest et al. (in press). (Key: ■ = critically important □ = very important ■ = somewhat important)

academic adjustment, and school dropout (Dishion, Patterson, Stool-miller, & Skinner, 1991; Dunlap & Kern, 1997; Parker & Asher, 1987).

In this regard, children with developmental disabilities are at high risk, and the procedures described by Kamps and others in this volume are critically important. Students who experience limited and poor peer relationships may not only miss out on prosocial interactions (e.g., camaraderie allows for collaboration on schoolwork), they may also be denied important opportunities to learn academic material (e.g., Collins & Gunnar, 1990). Because of lower social competence, children with developmental disabilities are at risk for social isolation and rejection by typical peers. Assessment of the transactions between children and their peers in school, the characteristics of their social relationships over time, and the longitudinal development of behavior patterns within the context of those relationships is critically important to determining the most salient aspects of social-communicative competence, effects for children with developmental disabilities, and how these transactions modulate later social and emotional aptitude.

Influence of the Home
Environment on Cognitive Behavior

Characteristics of children's home environments are closely associated with cognitive development and subsequent school performance (e.g., Bradley, Caldwell, & Rock, 1988; Walker et al., 1994). Parenting factors related to early cognitive development and language learning include active participation in reciprocal social interactions, frequency of verbal interactions, and encouragement of intellectual skills (e.g., Bradley et al., 1988; Hart & Risley, 1992; Slaughter & Epps, 1987). Similarly, the extent to which parents are involved with their children's school-related activities and the degree of mutual respect and cooperation between families and schools have been associated with the school-specific cognitive skills, social aptitude, and later performance of children (Slaughter-Defoe, Nakagawa, Takanishi, & Johnson, 1990; Stevenson & Baker, 1987). Parents' monitoring and involvement in their children's homework, at least as early as the fourth grade, has been found to be a powerful determinant of subsequent academic achievement (Reid & Patterson, 1991).

Influences of the School on Cognitive Behavior

Middle childhood and adolescence are characterized by normative, transitional periods during which children spend increasingly less time in the direct care of their parents. During these periods when there are considerably more new demands and changing intellectual and social expectations, students spend more time under the supervision of teachers and in the company of peers (Collins & Russell, 1991; Dunn, 1988). The unique experiences that children have in school during this period contribute to their social-communicative and cognitive development, academic performance, and eventually to school success or failure (Greenwood, 1991a; Maughan, 1988; Reynolds, 1991). Comparatively few studies have identified the specific school processes such as variation in exposure to academic subject matter, behavioral factors, and school practice factors that affect school success or failure of students (Jordan, 1990; Wachs, 1992).

Interrelations Between Social-Communicative and Cognitive Factors

The school environment may further constrain cognitive competence by failing to provide optimal instructional practices and opportunities. The unfortunate result is maintenance of lower cognitive trajectories (Eccles, Lord, & Midgley, 1991; Greenwood, 1991a; Greenwood et al., 1994; Walker et al. 1994). Poor achievement in early elementary school not only places children at an increased risk for learning and accelerating antisocial behaviors, attitudes, and values in early adolescence (Cairns, Cairns, & Neckerman, 1989) but also acts as an important predictor of later delinquency (e.g., Farrington, 1987). Thus, the interrelations between social-communicative and cognitive experiences of children, and the differential effects of the varied contexts in which children interact, support the contention that home and schooling factors either advance or limit developmental outcomes in childhood, adolescence, and throughout the life span. For children with developmental disabilities, these processes operate in similar ways putting them at continued levels of elevated risk depending on how their opportunities for social interaction with the myriad environments and people that constitute their social environments are affected.

THE APPLICABILITY AND GENERALITY OF PROPOSED ASSESSMENTS AND INTERVENTIONS

Conroy and Brown in Chapter 7 discuss the issue of applicability and translation of research-validated techniques and models into practice. The applicability of research-validated procedures is a broader national concern with respect to research, practice, and policy (e.g., Carnine,

1997; Malouf & Schiller, 1995). Conroy and Brown note with concern that too much of this work has yet to undergo translation into common practice. They also write that too few researchers have sought to evaluate techniques used in actual preschool environments with parents and teachers implementing treatment and completing the needed assessments. Instead, the majority of what is known has involved researchers and research assistants responsible for implementation. Thus, whereas strong evidence indicates that these procedures work, it is not yet known if they can be used effectively and sustained by practitioners in natural environments (Gersten, Carnine, & Woodward, 1987; Gersten, Vaughn, Deshler, & Schiller, 1997).

The clinical applicability and potential scale of use of the intervention technology can be considered a function of at least two constructs in future research and development efforts: How effective are the interventions, and how sustainable are they when they are used as intended by practitioners? Issues that influence the effectiveness of an intervention include intervention design and method, context management, behavior management, and instructionally relevant assessment. Each contributes an important dimension to the potential acceleration of outcomes beyond baseline levels.

Effectiveness Principles

Researchers know that students with developmental disabilities learn more when intervention designs are based on explicit, rather then implicit, strategies. In explicit strategies, the learner is guided, rather than left to mediate learning of new skills alone (Cazden, 1992). Alternately, in implicit instruction, learners are left to their own guidance. Implicit instruction is typically used in general education environments. Some examples of explicit intervention strategies include

- Establishing routines and embedding milieu teaching strategies (Chapter 4)
- Arranging the physical environment and reinforcement contingencies for social-communicative behaviors (Chapter 6)
- Using scripts for structuring social interactions or for guiding the teaching of peer tutors, enabling them to present specific prompts and learning trials, check tutees for responses, and provide differential forms of correction and help depending on the accuracy of the response (Chapter 8)
- Setting up support networks using precision assessments to capture peer availability across microenvironments within the school (Chapter 10)

Additional examples of explicit strategies used to better teach reading to students with developmental disabilities in general education environments include requiring students to retell stories they have read and asking students to predict events based on current information and to check the accuracy of their predictions (Brown & Palincsar, 1989; Mathes, Fuchs, Fuchs, Henley, & Sanders, 1994; Rosenshine & Meister, 1994). Strategies designed around *well-connected* knowledge structures that guide learning using *big ideas* to promote generalization and the hierarchical teaching of skills are explicit strategies that can be used to teach challenging subject matter (Rosenshine, 1997; Rosenshine & Stevens, 1986).

Students with developmental disabilities learn better when treatments are applied across multiple contexts, thereby supporting generalization and increasing time in treatment. Examples include using incidental or responsive teaching procedures across multiple hours and embedding them within caregiving routines in the home and child care center (see Chapter 4). Similarly, extending procedures across time and environments in the school (see Chapter 10) can increase the opportunities for social interactions and the development of peer relationships and friendships. Also, more continuous use of procedures across home, child care, and preschool environments further strengthens the impact of the use of specific interventions on social-communicative development.

Students with developmental disabilities learn better when behavioral principles are used. The use of behavioral principles optimizes the number of interactions with higher probabilities of promoting competent behavior. An example would be arranging social contingencies so that children's social initiations are immediately reinforced and expanded, as in incidental teaching or in peer-mediated strategies (see Chapters 4, 6, 8, and 9). These procedures increase the probability of children responding again at a future time. The use of natural reinforcers helps children to learn about the temporal rhythm of natural social contexts and to discriminate between specific social situations and how one must draw on one's social behavioral repertoire.

Another condition in which students with developmental disabilities learn more is when instructionally relevant assessments are used to monitor their progress toward socially desired outcomes and when these assessments serve as a basis for decision making (Deno, 1997; see Chapter 3). Part C of the Individuals with Disabilities Education Act (IDEA) Amendments of 1997 (PL 105-17) requires that an evaluation be conducted to determine a child's progress toward the goals contained in the individual family service plan (IFSP) or the individualized education program (IEP). A variety of assessments are available (see Chapter 3), but most can only be administered intermittently and few can be administered by practitioners or interventionists. These assessments indicate the presence of a delay (standardized norm-referenced tests), the child's level of skill mastery (criterion-referenced tests), a change in developmental age scores, or the number of IEP objectives mastered following intervention (Carta, 1999; McLean, 1996).

None of these intermittent approaches tells practitioners whether the child is making progress toward a meaningful outcome (Deno, 1997). Practitioners are more likely to employ measures that reflect progress if they are repeatable and can be quickly administered. The advantage of repeated measurement is that practitioners and interventionists can monitor the rate of progress in terms of days, weeks, and months needed in deciding when to change treatment, implement a new treatment, or continue using an effective treatment. One example of the use of repeated measurement is the behavioral observations employed by Leew, Warren, and Yoder (Chapter 5). In this form of behavioral measurement, individual target behaviors are defined and observed repeatedly to reveal change over time. Mastery monitoring is another form of repeated measurement useful for tracking growth in learning academic or preacademic skills (Deno, 1997; Fuchs & Fuchs, 1999). In mastery monitoring, a skills hierarchy is monitored repeatedly including separate assessments for each subskill in the hierarchy.

General outcome measurement (GOM) is a third form of repeatable measurement suitable for progress monitoring (Deno, 1997; McConnell, 2000). GOMs are designed to reflect progress toward an identified general outcome, such as a child's ability to express his or her wants and needs using social communication. GOMs have been constructed to monitor development of expressive communication (Greenwood, Luze, & Carta, in press; Luze et al., in press) and emerging literacy skills (Kaminski & Good, 1996). Central to GOMs are repeated measurement of a few key skill elements that serve as indicators of progress toward the GOM. Thus, increasing proficiency is indicated by improved performance on the same key skill elements measured repeatedly.

GOMs used in pediatric medicine, such as height and weight charts, provide information about how well a child is growing and whether a need exists for additional evaluation or a change in care. Curriculum-based measurement (CBM) is the best-known educational GOM. It is used most often to measure the individual progress of children learning basic reading, math, and writing skills (Fuchs & Fuchs, 1986; Fuchs, Fuchs, Hamlett, & Bentz, 1994; Marston, 1989). CBM provides quick, reliable, and accurate measurement of growth toward long-term IEP goals (e.g., Fuchs & Deno, 1991). The critically important feature of all these measures, like height and weight charts and CBM, is the ability to detect when a child is falling below growth expectation, when intervention is needed, whether the intervention is moving the child toward the desired outcome, or when a change is needed to accelerate growth (Deno, 1997).

Taken together, issues of intervention design and method, context management, behavior management, and instructionally relevant assessment provide foundations for improving intervention effectiveness. They are the key ideas guiding intervention research and development; however, whether effective interventions can be used to obtain maximal benefits in the home and school is another question.

Sustainability Principles

For parents, caregivers, and teachers to sustain effective intervention practices, the practices must be accessible and useable (Carnine, 1997). Products and tools designed for practitioners must be available to support training, implementation, and professional development. Effective practices described only in journal articles will not readily be applied because parents and teachers are infrequent consumers of research literature (Abbott, Walton, Tapia, & Greenwood, 1999; Greenwood & Abbott, in press). Classroom teachers, for example, have a difficult time gaining access to research findings and often find the results to have little relevance to classroom practice. Researchers find teachers to be uninformed about research methods and findings and often unwilling or unable to follow through with procedures designed by researchers. Teacher educators rarely assign research-based articles for teachers in training, nor do they teach intervention research methods with implications for improving classroom practice. In addition, teachers in training are often unaware that a gap between research and application exists. As a result, training and support of teachers' use of effective practices is a critically important part of sustainability.

In contrast to traditional forms of in-service teacher training, more effective efforts have sought to involve teachers actively in the research process by establishing and sustaining interactions between researchers and practitioners around issues of classroom practice. These efforts required researchers to spend more time in local schools and classroom teachers to collaborate with researchers in the use of research-based practices and the conduct of new research on instructional interventions (Baker & Smith, in press; Boudah & Knight, 1999; Fuchs & Fuchs, 1998; Logan et al., 1999).

Some of the effective strategies included establishing: 1) formal partnerships between researchers and local school faculty; 2) professional development organized around research on issues of interest to teachers; and 3) involving teachers in stages of research addressing initial discovery, replication and refinement, and going to scale. The technique of collaboration with teachers very often was designed to respond to and incorporate teachers' interests and concerns into research (Baker & Smith, in press; Boudah & Knight, 1999; Fuchs & Fuchs, 1998; Logan et al., 1999). Collaboration also involved consulting and directly working with teachers to help them establish and sustain measurement and intervention activities. Consequently, these researchers made measurable progress improving practice, child outcomes, and teachers' views of the contribution of research to what teachers actually did in the classroom (Abbott et al., 1999; Fuchs & Fuchs, 1998). Descriptions and details of such models and their results are available at the web site for the Juniper Gardens Children's Project: http://www.lsi.ukans.edu/jg/blueprnt.htm.

In summary, researchers know that more is needed than just information on the effectiveness of a technique. Knowledge of its usability and accessibility is needed. This requires additional forms of research, development, demonstration, and dissemination designed to translate effective techniques into procedural manuals, forms of training, assessment for practitioners, implementation and adoption models, and computer software supporting access and use.

CONCLUSION

This chapter has examined the relationships between social-communicative skills and life achievements by considering the advances in the research and pointing out gaps in our knowledge. Because a primary goal in research on developmental disabilities is to enhance the social-communicative competence of children with developmental disabilities, a life span rather than a cross-sectional age perspective was used to examine how intervention strategies and policies might be improved. Despite the obvious value of changing specific social-communicative behaviors and developing specific intervention technology, it is vitally important that we also address the question of how to implement this technology in order to change a life trajectory. We still lack longitudinal intervention studies employing interventions and measurement models that integrate social, emotional, and cognitive measures with measures of social interaction taken in the contexts of the home, the school, and the peer group. Thus, we conclude with the following points:

- Prior research has focused rather exclusively on either home or on school contexts and not both as causal processes in developmental outcomes. Although this narrow focus is necessary for intervention component building and effectiveness research, it may overemphasize the contributions of either home or school to the development of social-communicative competence. We know little about how they combine and operate together to affect growth in social-communicative competence (Greenwood et al., 1992). For example, Spencer (1995) argued that research has looked too narrowly at the relationships between environmental conditions and developmental outcomes. Research that integrates home and school sources of influence with interventions is needed.
- Research should address the transactional or reciprocal quality of interactions experienced by children. Much of the current research is short-term in duration and unidirectional in nature. As a result, many current findings contradict one another. For example, McLloyd and Wilson (1991) reported that some parents might unintentionally promote antisocial behavior in their children through harsh and inconsistent discipline principles. Yet, Vuchinich, Bank, and Patterson (1992) reported that a difficult child might induce ineffective parenting. Thus, research designed to examine bidirectionality in causal relationship across specific periods of development with and without the use of social-communicative interventions is needed.
- The current literature is only beginning to incorporate data on the effects of home and school transitions into analyses of social interaction and developmental trajectories. Data on adolescence and transition to secondary schooling (e.g., Seidman, Allen, Aber, Mitchell, & Feinman, 1994) are especially sparse. Research is needed to examine the type, onset, and impact of normative and nonnormative transitions in home and school contexts experienced by children with disabilities as they make the transition from home to child care, preschool, elementary school, secondary school, and beyond.
- Explanatory models that consider how risk, protection (intervention), and transition contexts affect developmental trajectories and especially social-communicative development are relatively new. Research is needed to determine whether models based on typical developmental experiences are common or unique to differences in gender and disability.
- Longitudinal early intervention studies for children with developmental delays are vitally important with respect to the previous concerns but also with respect to our growing ability to prevent and ameliorate the life course effects of developmental disabilities.

PROMOTING SOCIAL COMMUNICATION: CLOSING REMARKS

This book details the development of social-communicative skills from birth through young adulthood for children with developmental disabilities. Beginning with infants and toddlers and progressing across preschool, school-age, and adolescence, the authors review the conceptual and empirical foundations of social communication and how social communication is promoted across environments (e.g., home, preschool, elementary and secondary schools). Compared with what was known even as recently as the 1970s, these reviews represent an impressive advance in knowledge, particularly in what is needed to enhance the lives of children with developmental disabilities. Some of these advances include

1. The linking of reciprocal social behavior and language conceptually as social communication in empirical research and intervention when both have traditionally been considered apart
2. The understanding that, after movement, social communication is the skill class most used by humans to regulate their physical, social, and cognitive needs and to pursue quality in life
3. The knowledge that in conjunction with the physical environment and architecture, social communication used in interactions with others defines the human ecology. Social communication surrounds and affects individual social interactions in ways that signal culturally appropriate opportunities to respond and that differentially reinforce responding and reciprocally influence the social communication of others in ways that transact.
4. The understanding that social communication represents the effects of socialization, teaching, and the promotion of increasingly more desired, adaptive, functional, and proficient behavior

The first three chapters in this book provide the broader context for the subsequent chapters focused on interventions for children of different ages. Goldstein and Morgan (Chapter 1) set forth the theoretical perspectives that underlie social-communicative development with implications for intervention. Most important for children with developmental disabilities, they pinpoint commonalities among these perspectives that suggest approaches to intervention. Converging outcomes include the importance of proximity, common goals, and linking of social skills to friendship through cumulative histories of mutually reinforcing interactions. In order to engineer these outcomes in the lives of specific children, they argue convincingly for the necessity of targeting both children with developmental disabilities and their typically developing peers in interventions in order to move from occasional interaction to real friendship between these groups of children.

Abbeduto and Short-Meyerson (Chapter 2) focus directly on the use of language in social interaction. They contribute to our understanding of how linguistic skills affect social communication among typically developing children and how these skills may reflect changes or barriers for children with developmental disabilities. They also identify the effects that shared knowledge and recurring, scripted contexts of language have on the social communications of children of specific ages in the environments in which they live. According to Abbeduto and Short-Meyerson, interventions for children with developmental disabilities must be designed to be sensitive to and build on shared knowledge of the participants.

Interventions for these children also must be informed and guided by measurement. In Chapter 3, Kaczmarek organizes the measurement of social and communicative competence into an interdisciplinary framework based on the interrelatedness of two common themes: social competence (three levels) and a dimension reflecting appropriateness and effectiveness (also three levels). Represented in the cells of this matrix are measurements of the functions and forms of social communication. Three targets of these measures are discussed with respect to intervention problem solving including the child, aspects of social situations, and the specifics of social-communicative tasks. Measurement of the child reveals social-communicative skill level and growth in skills over time and intervention, whereas measurement of social situations reveals aspects of the social ecology and contexts that set the occasion for social-communicative responding and reinforcement of this responding. Measurement of social-communicative tasks reveals features of tasks that are more or less likely to promote social-communicative behavior in children of differing ages and skills.

The context, methods, and informants of measurement also are described. Specific situational contexts are used that are designed to assess social communication in natural, analogue, and role-play situations and in recall reports by multiple informants (e.g., parents, teachers) familiar with the child. Within these situational contexts, measurement methods include direct observation, language sampling, play-based assessment, functional analyses of challenging behaviors, adult and peer ratings, behavioral checklists, and tests. The majority of these measures can be seen in the work reported in subsequent chapters used to identify skills and behaviors in need of intervention, to identify and select

social situations for use in interventions, to monitor change and progress over time, and to reveal levels of peer acceptance, friendship, and
rejection.

The remaining chapters in this volume teach us that social-
communicative development and intervention in early childhood are
strongly influenced by caregiving and parenting in the home. In middle childhood and adolescence, social communication increasingly is
influenced by the amount of time spent in school, the quality of instruction and schooling experiences received, and a growing number of
peer interactions and relationships. Competence at any single point of
time during this period from birth to adulthood is thought to result
from the interplay of multiple influences caught in a process of change
over time that includes parents', teachers', and peers' responses to a
child during social interaction. Conversely, parents', teachers', and
peers' responses are thought to be moderated by differences in specific
features of the home and school environment and fluctuations in the
child's competence.

For example, Warren and his colleagues in Chapters 4 and 5 discuss specific methods of arranging the environment of infants and toddlers to evoke young children's prelinguistic communication skills and
later use of spoken language. They describe how to arrange the interactions between adults and young children in ways that follow the
child's lead, so that the child's communicative behavior is reinforced by
adult responses, and ultimately to ensure that children learn that communication is a functional tool for addressing their needs, wants, and
interests.

Brown and Conroy in Chapters 6 and 7 extend this knowledge to
older children who have transitioned to preschool by training teachers
to program similar contingencies using teacher- and peer-mediated interventions. In their work, they are concerned with the challenges of
learning how to program the generalization and maintenance of social
behavior for all children. They also are concerned with developing a
technology for implementing more comprehensive intervention strategies for promoting both short- and long-term peer relations and friendships among children with and without delays.

Kamps and her colleagues (Chapters 8 and 9) are engaged in work
extending similar issues and interventions to school-age children with
developmental delays. In their work, there are extensions to augmentative and alternative communication systems, such as signing, picture
pointing, and the Picture Exchange Communication System (Bondy &
Frost, 1994). They also are actively engaged in designing effective and
sustainable teacher- and peer-mediated environmental arrangements

capable of promoting social interactions (e.g., through peer tutoring and peer networks) but also peer support and friendship.

Kennedy and Cushing in Chapters 10 and 11 further extend the analysis of interaction from dyadic to triadic units involving adolescents and their teachers and adult caregivers. Their work enables research on issues of how teacher support affects peer interactions of youth with and without developmental disabilities.

A common principle in all this work is arranging the behavioral ecology of youth through specific changes in what parents, teachers, peers, and caregivers do and where, when, and how long they do it. Not to be ignored is the important goal of determining precisely how special and general education teachers can collaborate effectively to take advantage of the general education classroom's rich social ecology to promote the child's social and academic competence. Nevertheless, there are unique dimensions of these age-related transitions and environments. The interaction partners and the increasing sophistication of social-communicative skills present different expectations and challenges in these distinctly different environments within the social ecology (Capaldi & Patterson, 1991).

Central to these authors' work is the general principle that growth in competence is acquired one interaction at a time, which accumulates into one's evolving history of prosocial and negative social interactions (Bijou & Baer, 1978). The unique contexts that exist in childhood and adolescence (including those of the home, the school, and the peer group) regulate these interactions. This social interactionist perspective suggests that these unique contexts mediate the developmental paths between individual differences in initial ability and outcome trajectories (e.g., Ramey & Ramey, 1998); however, questions still remain: How are social interactions with multiple agents regulated by the unique contextual factors of childhood? How do social interactions affect trajectories of social, emotional, and cognitive competence? How do subsequently changed trajectories affect contexts and interactions in home and school? The chapters in this volume provide us some new insights based on experimental interventions and case studies.

The metaphor of a vortex with a narrowing funnel aptly describes how interaction regulates growth in competence (Patterson, 1982; 1986). In the vortex, interaction and social-communicative acts are the individual and reciprocal units wherein an individual's behavior contacts and potentially affects that of another. The funnel narrowing from top to bottom suggests competence that has become concentrated while strengthened by a history of opportunities to respond and consequences for social responding. This mechanism is lifelong and dynamic; social communication is shaped by everyday life experiences. For children with developmental disabilities, early interventions defined in IFSPs or in the IEPs of school-age youth supplement children's normative life experiences. These supports provide specially designed services and instruction intended to assist and to accelerate development with these children and their families.

The importance of examining human development within a social context of multiple, interrelated relationships has increasingly been acknowledged (Bronfenbrenner, 1979; Collins & Gunnar, 1990; Dunn, 1988). The patterns of action and reciprocal influences between parents and their children provide a foundation for examining the significance of these relationships for later development between teachers and students in the school and between children and their peer groups (e.g., Collins & Russell, 1991). The papers in this volume and elsewhere (e.g., Collins, 1988) suggest that later optimal outcomes are associated with environments that offer many and varied opportunities to interact with caregivers and others who are responsive (Hart & Risley, 1995, 1999). The specific child-rearing practices and interventions that promote or accelerate these later optimal social-communicative outcomes await further research (e.g., Baumrind, 1993; Sameroff & Fiese, 1990).

REFERENCES

Abbott, M., Walton, C., Tapia, Y., & Greenwood, C.R. (1999). Research to practice: A "blueprint" for closing the gap in local schools. *Exceptional Children, 65*(3), 339–352.

Baker, S., & Smith, S. (in press). Linking school assessments to research-based practices in beginning reading: Improving programs and outcomes for students with and without disabilities. *Teacher Education and Special Education.*

Bates, E., O'Connell, B., & Shore, C. (1987). Language and communication in infancy. In J.D. Osofsky (Ed.), *Handbook of infant development* (2nd ed., pp. 149–203). New York: John Wiley & Sons.

Baumrind, D. (1993). The average expectable environment is not good enough: A response to Scarr. *Child Development, 64,* 1299–1317.

Bijou, S.W., & Baer, D.M. (1978). *Behavior analysis of child development.* Upper Saddle River, NJ: Prentice-Hall.

Blackorby, J., & Wagner, M. (1996). Longitudinal postschool outcomes of youth with disabilities: Findings from the national longitudinal transition study. *Exceptional Children, 62*(5), 399–413.

Bondy, A., & Frost, L. (1994). The picture exchange communication system. *Focus on Autistic Behavior, 9,* 1–19.

Boudah, D.J., & Knight, S.L. (1999). Creating learning communities of research & practice: Participatory research and development. In D. Byrd & J. McIntyre (Eds.), *Teacher education yearbook* (Vol. 7, pp. 97–114). Thousand Oaks, CA: Corwin Press.

Bradley, R.H., Caldwell, B.M., & Rock, S.L. (1988). Home environments and school performance: A ten-year follow-up and examination of three models of environmental action. *Child Development, 59*, 852–867.

Bronfenbrenner, U. (1979). Contexts of child rearing: Problems and prospects. *American Psychologist, 34*, 844–850.

Brown, A.L., & Palincsar, A.S. (1989). Guided, cooperative learning and individual knowledge acquisition. In L.B. Resnick (Ed.), *Knowing, learning, and instruction: Essays in honor of Robert Glaser* (pp. 393–451). Mahwah, NJ: Lawrence Erlbaum Associates.

Cairns, R.B., Cairns, B.D., & Neckerman, H.J. (1989). Early school dropout: Configurations and determinants. *Child Development, 60*, 1437–1452.

Capaldi, D.M., & Patterson, G.R. (1991). Relation of parental transitions to boys' adjustment problems: I. A linear hypothesis. II. Mothers at risk for transition and unskilled parenting. *Developmental Psychology, 27*, 489–504.

Carnine, D. (1997). Bridging the research-to-practice gap. *Exceptional Children, 63*(4), 513–521.

Carta, J. (1999, December). Implications of general outcome measurement for young children. In D. Walker (Chair), *Measuring growth and development of infants and toddlers for the 21st century.* Symposium presented at the Fifteenth Annual Meeting of the Division for Early Childhood, Council for Exceptional Children, Washington, DC.

Cazden, C.B. (1992). *Whole language plus: Essays on literacy in the United States and New Zealand.* New York: Teachers College Press.

Cole, K.N., Dale, P.S., & Mills, P.E. (1991). Individual differences in language delayed children's responses to direct and interactive preschool instruction. *Topics in Early Childhood Special Education, 11*, 99–124.

Collins, W.A. (1988). Research on the transition to adolescence: Continuity in the study of developmental processes. In M.R. Gunnar & W.A. Collins (Eds.), *Minnesota Symposia on Child Psychology, 21*, 1–15. Mahwah, NJ: Lawrence Erlbaum Associates.

Collins, W.A., & Gunnar, M.R. (1990). Social and personality development. *Annual Review of Psychology, 41*, 387–416.

Collins, W.A., & Russell, G. (1991). Mother–child and father–child relationships in middle childhood and adolescence: A developmental analysis. *Developmental Review, 11*, 99–136.

Conroy, M.A., & Brown, W.H. (1997). Promoting language for children with developmental delays in inclusive settings: Effective strategies for early childhood educators. In W.H. Brown & M.A. Conroy (Eds.), *Including and supporting preschool children with developmental delays in early childhood programs* (pp. 65–78). Little Rock, AR: Southern Early Childhood Association.

Council for Exceptional Children. (1994). Statistics profile of special education in the United States, 1994. *Teaching Exceptional Children, 26* (Supplement).

Crais, E.R., & Roberts, J.E. (1996). Assessing communication skills. In M. McLean, D.B. Bailey, & M. Wolery (Eds.), *Assessing infants and preschoolers with special needs* (pp. 334–397). New York: Merrill.

Delquadri, J., Greenwood, C.R., Stretton, K., & Hall, R.V. (1983). The peer tutoring spelling game: A classroom procedure for increasing opportunity to respond and spelling performance. *Education and Treatment of Children, 6*, 225–239.

Deno, S.L. (1997). Whether thou goest . . . Perspectives on progress monitoring. In J.W. Lloyd, E.J. Kameenui, & D. Chard (Eds.), *Issues in educating students with disabilities* (pp. 77–99). Mahwah, NJ: Lawrence Erlbaum Associates.

Dishion, T.J., Patterson, G.R., Stoolmiller, M., & Skinner, M.L. (1991). Family, school, and behavioral antecedents to early adolescent involvement with antisocial peers. *Developmental Psychology, 27,* 172–180.

Dunlap, G., & Kern, L. (1997). Modifying instructional activities to promote desirable behavior: A conceptual and practical framework. *School Psychology Quarterly, 11*(4), 297–312.

Dunn, J. (1988). Normative life events as risk factors in childhood. In M. Rutter (Ed.), *Studies of psychosocial risk: The power of longitudinal data* (pp. 227–244). New York: Cambridge University Press.

Dunn, L.M., & Dunn, L.M. (1981). *Peabody Picture Vocabulary Test–Revised.* Circle Pines, MN: American Guidance Service.

Eccles, J.S., Lord, S., & Midgley, C. (1991). What are we doing to early adolescents? The impact of educational contexts on early adolescents. *American Journal of Education, 99,* 521–542.

Farrington, D.P. (1987). Early precursors of frequent offending. In J.Q. Wilson & G.C. Loury (Eds.), *From children to citizens: Vol. 3. Family, schools, and delinquency prevention* (pp. 27–50). New York: Springer-Verlag.

Fey, M.E., Catts, H.W., & Larivee, L.S. (1995). Preparing preschoolers for the academic and social challenges of school. In S.F. Warren & J. Reichle (Series Eds.) & M.E. Fey, J. Windsor, & S.F. Warren (Vol. Eds.), *Communication and language intervention series: Vol. 5. Language intervention: Preschool through the elementary years* (pp. 3–37). Baltimore: Paul H. Brookes Publishing Co.

Fuchs, D., & Fuchs, L. (1998). Researchers and teachers working together to adapt instruction for diverse learners. *Learning Disabilities Research and Practice, 13*(3), 162–170.

Fuchs, L.S., & Deno, S.L. (1991). Paradigmatic distinctions between instructionally relevant measurement models. *Exceptional Children, 57,* 488–500.

Fuchs, L.S., & Fuchs, D. (1986). Linking assessment to instructional intervention: An overview. *School Psychology Review, 15,* 318–323.

Fuchs, L.S., & Fuchs, D. (1999). Monitoring student progress toward the development of reading competence: A review of three forms of classroom-based assessment. *School Psychology Review, 28,* 659–671.

Fuchs, L.S., Fuchs, D., Hamlett, C.L., & Bentz, J. (1994). Classwide curriculum-based measurement: Helping general educators meet the challenge of student diversity. *Exceptional Children, 60,* 518–537.

Garcia Coll, C.T. (1990). Developmental outcome of minority infants: A process-oriented look into our beginnings. *Child Development, 61,* 270–279.

Gersten, R., Carnine, D., & Woodward, J. (1987). Direct instruction research: The third decade. *Remedial and Special Education, 8*(6), 48–56.

Gersten, R., Vaughn, S., Deshler, D., & Schiller, E. (1997). What we know about using research findings: Implications for improving special education practice. *Journal of Learning Disabilities, 30*(5), 466–476.

Greenwood, C.R. (1991a). Classwide peer tutoring: Longitudinal effects on the reading, language, and mathematics achievement of at-risk students. *Reading, Writing, and Learning Disabilities International, 7,* 105–124.

Greenwood, C.R. (1991b). A longitudinal analysis of time, engagement, and academic achievement in at-risk vs. non-risk students. *Exceptional Children, 57,* 521–535.

Greenwood, C.R., & Abbott, M. (in press). Bridging the gap between research and practice. *Teacher Education and Special Education.*

Greenwood, C.R., Carta, J.J., Hart, B., Kamps, D., Terry, B., Arreaga-Mayer, C., Atwater, J., Walker, D., Risley, T., & Delquadri, J.C. (1992). Out of the laboratory and into the community: 26 years of applied behavior analysis at the Juniper Gardens Children's Project. *American Psychologist, 47,* 1464–1474.

Greenwood, C.R., & Delquadri, J. (1995). Classwide peer tutoring and the prevention of school failure. *Preventing School Failure, 39*(4), 21–25.

Greenwood, C.R., Delquadri, J.C., & Hall, R.V. (1989). Longitudinal effects of classwide peer tutoring. *Journal of Educational Psychology, 81,* 371–383.

Greenwood, C.R., Hart, B., Walker, D., & Risley, T.R. (1994). The opportunity to respond revisited: A behavioral theory of developmental retardation and its prevention. In R. Gardner, III, D.M. Sainato, J.O. Cooper, T.E. Heron, W.L. Heward, & J.W. Eshleman (Eds.), *Behavior analysis in education: Focus on measurably superior instruction* (pp. 213–239). Pacific Grove, CA: Brooks/Cole Thomson Learning.

Greenwood, C.R., Luze, G.J., & Carta, J.J. (in press). Assessment of intervention results with infants and toddlers. In A. Thomas & J. Grimes (Eds.), *Best practices in school psychology (IV).* Washington, DC: National Association for School Psychologists.

Greenwood, C.R., Maheady, L., & Delquadri, J. (in press). Classwide peer tutoring. In G. Stoner, M.R. Shinn, & H.M. Walker (Eds.), *Interventions for achievement and behavior problems* (2nd ed.). Washington, DC: National Association for School Psychologists.

Greenwood, C.R., Terry, B., Utley, C.A., Montagna, D., & Walker (1993). Achievement, placement, and services: Middle school benefits of classwide peer tutoring used at the elementary school. *School Psychology Review, 22,* 497–516.

Hart, B., & Risley, T.R. (1992). American parenting of language-learning children: Persisting differences in family–child interaction observed in natural home environments. *Developmental Psychology, 28,* 1096–1105.

Hart, B., & Risley, T.R. (1995). *Meaningful differences in the everyday experience of young American children.* Baltimore: Paul H. Brookes Publishing Co.

Hart, B., & Risley, T.R. (1999). *The social world of children learning to talk.* Baltimore: Paul H. Brookes Publishing Co.

Heal, L.W., Khoju, M., & Rusch, F.R. (1997). Predicting quality of life of youth after they leave special education high school programs. *Journal of Special Education, 31*(3), 279–299.

Heath, S.B. (1989). Oral and literate traditions among Black Americans living in poverty. *American Psychologist, 44,* 441–445.

Hops, H., & Greenwood, C.R. (1988). Social skill deficits. In E.J. Mash & L.G. Terdal (Eds.), *Behavioral assessment of childhood disorders* (2nd ed., pp. 263–314). New York: Guilford Press.

Horowitz, F.D., & O'Brien, M. (1989). In the interest of the nation: A reflective essay on the state of our knowledge and the challenges before us. *American Psychologist, 44,* 441–445.

Individuals with Disabilities Education Act (IDEA) Amendments of 1997, PL 105-17, 20 U.S.C. §§ 1400 *et seq.*

Jordan, J.I. (1990). *Black students and school failure: Policies, practices, and prescriptions.* Westport, CT: Greenwood Publishing Group.

Kaiser, A.P. (1993). Introduction: Enhancing children's social communication. In S.F. Warren & J. Reichle (Series Eds.) & A.P. Kaiser & D.B. Gray (Vol. Eds.), *Communication and language intervention series: Vol. 2. Enhancing children's communication: Research foundations for intervention* (pp. 3–9). Baltimore: Paul H. Brookes Publishing Co.

Kaminski, R.A., & Good, R.H. (1996). Toward a technology for assessing basic early literacy skills. *School Psychology Review, 25,* 215–227.

Kamps, D.M., & Tankersley, M. (1996). Prevention of behavioral and conduct disorders: Trends and research issues. *Behavioral Disorders, 22*(1), 41–48.

Kohler, F.W., & Greenwood, C.R. (1990). Effects of collateral peer supportive behaviors within the classwide peer tutoring program. *Journal of Applied Behavior Analysis, 23*(3), 307–322.

Kohler, F.W., Richardson, T., Mina, C., & Greenwood, C.R. (1985). Establishing cooperative peer relations in the classroom. *Pointer, 25*(4), 12–16.

Logan, K.R., Stein, S.S., Nieminen, P., Wright, H., Major, P., & Hansen, C. (1999). *The research lead teacher model: A local school model for bridging the gap from research to practice.* Kennesaw, GA: Kennesaw State University.

Luze, G.J., Linebarger, D., Greenwood, C.R., Carta, J.J., Walker, D., Leitschuh, C., & Atwater, J.B. (in press). Developing a general outcome measure of growth in the expressive communication of infants and toddlers. *School Psychology Review.*

Maheady, L., Harper, G.F., & Mallette, B. (1991). Peer-mediated instruction: A review of potential applications for special education. *Journal of Reading, Writing, & Learning Disabilities, 7,* 75–104.

Malouf, D.B., & Schiller, E.P. (1995). Practice and research in special education. *Exceptional Children, 61,* 414–424.

Marcovitch, S., Chiasson, L., Ushycky, I., Goldberg, S., & MacGregor, D. (1996). Maternal communication style with developmentally delayed preschoolers. *Journal of Children's Communication Development, 17,* 23–30.

Marston, D.B. (1989). A curriculum-based measurement approach to assessing academic performance: What it is and why do it. In M.R. Shinn (Ed.), *Curriculum-based measurement: Assessing special children* (pp. 18–78). New York: Guilford Press.

Mathes, P., Fuchs, D., Fuchs, L.S., Henley, A.M., & Sanders, A. (1994). Increasing strategic reading practice with Peabody classwide peer tutoring. *Learning Disabilities Research and Practice, 8*(4), 233–243.

Maughan, B. (1988). School experiences as risk/protective factors. In M. Rutter (Ed.), *Studies of psychosocial risk: The power of longitudinal data* (pp. 200–220). New York: Cambridge University Press.

McCathren, R.B., Warren, S.F., & Yoder, P.J. (1996). Prelinguistic predictors of later language development. In S.F. Warren & J. Reichle (Series Eds.) & K.N. Cole, P.S. Dale, & D.J. Thal (Vol. Eds.), *Communication and language intervention series: Vol. 6. Assessment of communication and language* (pp. 57–74). Baltimore: Paul H. Brookes Publishing Co.

McConnell, S.R. (2000). Assessment in early intervention and early childhood special education: Building on the past to project into the future. *Topics in Early Childhood Special Education, 20,* 43–48.

McKinney, J.D., Osborne, S.S., & Schulte, A.C. (1993). Academic consequences of learning disability: Longitudinal prediction of results at 11 years of age. *Learning Disabilities Research and Practice, 8*(1), 19–27.

McLean, M. (1996). Assessment and its importance in early intervention/early childhood special education. In M. McLean, D.B. Bailey, & M. Wolery (Eds.), *Assessing infants and preschoolers with special needs* (pp. 1–22). Columbus, OH: Charles E. Merrill.

McLloyd, V.C., & Wilson, L. (1991). The strain of living poor: Parenting, social support, and child mental health. In A.C. Huston (Ed.), *Children in poverty:*

Child development and public policy (pp. 105–133). New York: Cambridge University Press.

Parker, J.G., & Asher, S.R. (1987). Peer relations and later personal adjustment: Are low-accepted children at risk? *Psychological Bulletin, 102,* 357–389.

Patterson, G.R. (1982). *Coercive family process.* Eugene, OR: Castalia.

Patterson, G.R. (1986). Performance models for antisocial boys. *American Psychologist, 41,* 432–444.

Priest, J.S., McConnell, S.R., Walker, D., Carta, J.J., Kaminski, R.A., McEvoy, M.A., Good, R.H., Greenwood, C.R., & Shinn, M.R. (in press). General growth outcomes for children between birth and age eight: Where do you want young children to go today and tomorrow? *Journal of Early Intervention.*

Ramey, C.T., & Ramey, S.L. (1998). Early intervention and early experience. *American Psychologist, 53*(2), 109–120.

Reid, J.B., & Patterson, G.R. (1991). Early prevention and intervention with conduct problems: A social interactional model for the integration of research and practice. In G. Stoner, M.R. Shinn, & H.M. Walker (Eds.), *Interventions for achievement and behavior problems* (pp. 715–739). Silver Spring, MD: National Association of School Psychologists.

Reynolds, A.J. (1991). Early schooling of children at risk. *American Educational Research Journal, 28,* 392–442.

Rosenshine, B. (1997). Advances in research on instruction In J.W. Lloyd, E.J. Kameenui, & D. Chard (Eds.), *Issues in educating students with disabilities* (pp. 197–220). Mahwah, NJ: Lawrence Erlbaum Associates.

Rosenshine, B., & Meister, C. (1994). Reciprocal teaching: A review of research. *Review of Educational Research, 64*(4), 479–530.

Rosenshine, B., & Stevens, R. (1986). Teaching functions. In M.C. Wittrock (Ed.), *Handbook of research on teaching* (pp. 745–799). New York: Macmillan.

Sameroff, A.J., & Fiese, B.H. (1990). Transactional regulation and early intervention. In S.J. Meisels, & J.P. Shonkoff (Eds.), *Handbook of early childhood intervention* (pp. 119–149). New York: Cambridge University Press.

Scarborough, H.S., & Dobrich, W. (1994). On the efficacy of reading to preschoolers. *Developmental Review, 14,* 245–302.

Schuele, C.M. (1999, December). *Phonological awareness training: A 12-week incentive program for kindergartners and first graders.* Presentation at the Fifteenth Annual Meeting of the Division for Early Childhood, Council for Exceptional Children, Washington, DC.

Seidman, E., Allen, L., Aber, J.L., Mitchell, C., & Feinman, J. (1994). The impact of school transitions in early adolescence on the self-system and perceived social context of poor urban youth. *Development Psychology, 65,* 507–522.

Slaughter, D., & Epps, E. (1987). Home environment and academic achievement of black American children and youth. *Journal of Negro Education, 56,* 3–20.

Slaughter-Defoe, D.T., Nakagawa, K., Takanishi, R., & Johnson, D.J. (1990). Toward cultural/ecological perspectives on schooling and achievement in African- and Asian-American children. *Child Development, 61,* 363–383.

Snow, C.E., Burns, M.S., & Griffin, P. (Eds.). (1998). *Preventing reading difficulties in young children.* Committee on the Prevention of Reading Difficulties in Young Children, Commission on Behavioral and Social Sciences and Education, National Research Council. Washington, DC: National Academy Press.

Spencer, M.B. (1995). Old issues and new theorizing about African-American youth: A phenomenological variant of ecological systems theory. In R.L. Taylor (Ed.), *African-American youth: Their social and economic status in the United States* (pp. 37–69). New York: Praeger.

Stevenson, D.L., & Baker, D.P. (1987). The family-school relation and the child's school performance. *Child Development, 58,* 1348–1357.

Strain, P.S., & Hoyson, M. (2000). The need for longitudinal, intensive social skill intervention: LEAP outcomes for children with autism. *Topics in Early Childhood Special Education, 20*(2), 116–122.

U.S. Department of Education. (1997). *Nineteenth Annual Report to Congress on the Implementation of the Individuals with Disabilities Act.* Washington, DC: Office of Special Education Programs, Department of Education.

U.S. Department of Education. (1998). *Twentieth Annual Report to Congress on the Implementation of the Individuals with Disabilities Act.* Washington, DC: Office of Special Education Programs, Department of Education.

Vuchinich, S., Bank, L., & Patterson, G. (1992). Parenting, peers, and the stability of antisocial behavior in preadolescent boys. *Developmental Psychology, 28,* 510–521.

Wachs, T.D. (1992). *The nature of nurture.* Thousand Oaks, CA: Sage Publications.

Wagner, M., D'Amico, R., Marder, C., Newman, L., & Blackorby, J. (1992). *What happens next? Trends in postschool outcomes of youth with disabilities.* Menlo Park, CA: SRI International.

Walker, D., Greenwood, C.R., Hart, B., & Carta, J.J. (1994). Improving the prediction of early school academic outcomes using socioeconomic status and early language production. *Child Development, 65,* 606–662.

Wasik, B. (1997). Volunteer tutoring programs: Do we know what works? *Phi Delta Kappan, 79,* 282–287.

Wetherby, A.M., & Prizant, B.M. (1992). Profiling young children's communicative competence. In S.F. Warren & J. Reichle (Series & Vol. Eds.), *Communication and language intervention series: Vol. 1. Causes and effects in communication and language intervention* (pp. 217–253). Baltimore: Paul H. Brookes Publishing Co.

Wetherby, A.M., & Prizant, B.M. (1993). Profiling communication and symbolic abilities in young children. *Journal of Childhood Communication Disorders, 15,* 23–32.

Yoder, P.J., & Warren, S.F. (1999). Facilitating self-initiated proto-declaratives and proto-imperatives in prelinguistic children with developmental disabilities. *Journal of Early Intervention, 22,* 337–354.

Author Index

Page references followed by *f* or *t* indicate figures or tables, respectively.

Subject Index

Page references followed by *f* or *t* indicate figures or tables, respectively.